Jean Carper is one of America's best-known authorities on health and nutrition. She is the author of sixteen books, including *The Food Pharmacy* and *The Food Pharmacy Guide to Good Eating*.

ALSO BY JEAN CARPER
The Food Pharmacy
The Food Pharmacy Guide to Good Eating
Health Care USA
Jean Carper's Total Nutrition Guide

FOOD –

YOUR MIRACLE

MEDICINE

HOW FOOD
CAN PREVENT AND TREAT OVER
100 SYMPTOMS AND PROBLEMS

JEAN CARPER

SIMON & SCHUSTER

LONDON · SYDNEY · NEW YORK · TOKYO · SINGAPORE · TORONTO

First published in Great Britain by Simon & Schuster Ltd, 1994
A Paramount Communications Company
This paperback edition first published 1995.
Copyright © Jean Carper, 1994

The right of Jean Carper to be identified as author of this work has been asserted in accordance with sections 77 and 78 of the Copyright, Designs and Patents Act 1988.

Simon & Schuster Ltd
West Garden Place
Kendal Street
London W2 2AQ

Simon & Schuster of Australia Pty Ltd

A CIP catalogue record for this book is available from the
British Library.

ISBN 0-671-71336-1

Printed and bound in Great Britain by Butler & Tanner Ltd,
Frome and London

In memory of Lola

CONTENTS

ACKNOWLEDGMENTS

My ultimate appreciation must go to the pioneering scientists who use their talents, imagination and energy to study the age-old secrets of food's medicinal powers and how to apply them to today's critical health problems. This book is a distillation of their many years of work, creativity and discovery. I have read thousands of their research papers and communicated with hundreds of them in personal interviews, on the telephone, by fax and at conferences. They have given me countless hours of their time.

I cannot thank them all in this limited space, but I would like to express my gratitude to the following scientists and physicians, whom I have consulted and interviewed, some several times: James W. Anderson, University of Kentucky; Stephen Barnes, University of Alabama; Gary Beecher, U.S. Department of Agriculture; George L. Blackburn, Harvard Medical School; Elliott Blass, Cornell University; Mark Blumenthal, American Botanical Council; Arun Bordia, Tagore Medical College, India; David Buchholz, Johns Hopkins University; Michael L. Burr, MRC Epidemiology Unit, Cardiff, Wales; Tim Byers, Centers for Disease Control and Prevention; Donald Castell, University of Pennsylvania School of Medicine; Donald Castelli, Framingham (Mass.) Heart Study; Leonard Cohen, American Health Foundation; Leroy Creasy, Cornell University; Stephen L. DeFelice, The Foundation for Innovation in Medicine; Ara H. DerMarderosian, Philadelphia College of Pharmacy and Science; James Duke, U.S. Department of Agriculture; Martin A. Eastwood, Western General Hospital, Edinburgh, Scotland; John Erdman, Jr., University of Illinois at Urbana; Norman Farnsworth, University of Illinois at Chicago; Gary Fraser, Loma Linda University; Balz Frei, Harvard School of Public Health; Harinder S. Garewal, Tucson V.A. Medical Center and University of Arizona; Cedric Garland, University of California at San Diego; Judith Gavaler, University of Pittsburgh; Stanley Goldfarb, University of Pennsylvania School of Medicine; Sherwood Gorbach, Tufts University; William B. Greenough III, Johns Hopkins University; Peter Greenwald, National Cancer Institute; Richard Griffith, Indiana University; Roland Griffiths, Johns Hopkins University; Victor Gurewich, Harvard Medical School; Georges Halpern, University of California at Davis; Yukihiko Hara,

Food Research Laboratories, Mitsui Norin Co. Ltd., Shizuoka, Japan; Robert Heaney, Creighton University; Douglas C. Heimburger, University of Alabama at Birmingham; Paul F. Jacques, USDA Human Nutrition Research Center on Aging, Tufts University; Mahendra K. Jain, University of Delaware; David J. A. Jenkins, University of Toronto; Ishwarial Jialal, University of Texas Southwestern Medical Center; Dean Jones, Emory University; Frederick Khachik, U.S. Department of Agriculture; David M. Klurfeld, Wistar Institute; Joel M. Kremer, Albany (New York) Medical College; David Kritchevsky, The Wistar Institute; William E. M. Lands, National Institutes of Health; Benjamin H. S. Lau, Loma Linda University School of Medicine; Alexander Leaf, Harvard Medical School; Terrance Leighton, University of California at Berkeley; Robert I. Lin, Nutrition International Company; Donald Lisk, Cornell University; Armar N. Makheja, George Washington University Medical Center; Frank L. Meyskens Jr., University of California at Irvine; Jon Michnovicz, Institute of Hormone Research, New York; Forrest Nielsen, U.S. Department of Agriculture; Paul J. Nestel, CSIRO Division of Human Nutrition, Australia; Talal Nsouli, Georgetown University Medical School; Richard Panush, Saint Barnabas Medical Center, New Jersey; Michael Pariza, University of Wisconsin; James Penland, U.S. Department of Agriculture; Herbert F. Pierson, consultant, formerly National Cancer Institute; John D. Potter, University of Minnesota School of Public Health; Nicholas Read, University of Sheffield, England; David Rose, American Health Foundation; Norman Rosenthal, National Institute of Mental Health; Harold Sandstead, University of Texas at Galveston; Joel Saper, Michigan State University; Marvin Schuster, Johns Hopkins University; Joel Schwartz, Environmental Protection Agency; Kenneth D. R. Setchell, Children's Hospital Medical Center, Cincinnati, Ohio; Helmut Sies, University of Dusseldorf Medical School, Germany; Artemis Simopoulos, The Center for Genetics, Nutrition and Health; Peter Singer, Institute of Clinical Chemistry, Berlin, Germany; Gene A. Spiller, The Health Research & Studies Center Inc., Los Altos, California; Krishna C. Srivastava, Odense University, Denmark; Roy Swank, Oregon Health Sciences University; Michael Thun, Amercian Cancer Society; Varro Tyler, Purdue University; Thomas Uhde, National Institute of Mental Health; A. R. P. Walker, the South African Institute of Medical Research, Johannesburg; Andrew Weil, University of Arizona College of Medicine; John Weisburger, American Health Foundation; Jay Whelan, Cornell University; Joseph L. Witztum, University of California at San Diego; Judith Wurtman, Massachusetts Institute of Technology; Irwin Ziment, UCLA School of Medicine.

Others who were a vital part of the creation of this book are my publisher, Gladys Justin Carr, and my agent, Raphael Sagalyn, both of whom buoyed me with their spirited support. My endless gratitude also goes to my friend Thea Flaum, who read every word of the manuscript in all three of its incarnations and gave me priceless and lovingly dispensed advice for revisions.

For the origin of my curiosity that inspired me to write this book, I must credit my maternal grandmother, Lola, who kept me enthralled as a child by her joyful enthusiasm for home remedies and medical books. One that passed to me after her death is titled *The Favorite Medical Receipt Book and Home Doctor, Comprising the Favorite Remedies of Over One Hundred of the World's Best Physicians and Nurses. Compiled and edited by Josephus Goodenough, M.D.* (F. B. Dickerson Co., 1907). Although it is a treasured part of my library, it was not a reference for this book.

INTRODUCTION

"Whatsoever was the father of a disease, an ill diet was the mother."
–Chinese proverb

To know the right food to eat – or not to eat – depending on your health circumstances, is to have an unprecedented wealth of knowledge with which to treat and prevent health problems, ranging from colds to cancer. That's the purpose of *Food – Your Miracle Medicine*.

My earlier book *The Food Pharmacy*, published in Britain in 1989, examined the then-existing scientific evidence on the pharmacology of common foods. That book, like Columbus's first voyage, revealed exciting, largely unexplored new worlds. At the time, the idea that food had legitimate and scientifically validated medicinal properties was little recognized. Now the idea is being passionately pursued. Prestigious governmental and scientific bodies around the world agree that diet does broadly influence health and disease. Research on the subject has exploded. Dozens of international conferences, some devoted entirely to a single topic – such as garlic, tea, fish oils, antioxidants, fibre or monounsaturated fats – have unveiled astonishing new scientific findings on the healing and preventive powers of foods. Scientists have uncovered totally new disease-fighting agents in foods like broccoli and cabbage.

At the same time, new evidence and theories illuminating precisely how food affects cellular behaviour, leading to health or disease, have emerged or been refined. For example, scientists now believe they have uncovered the real secrets of what makes blood cholesterol so dangerous to arteries, and how you can eat to combat the hazard in totally new ways. Researchers now know that if you have any type of inflammatory disease, such as arthritis or asthma, eating fish oil is likely to soothe it and corn oil to exacerbate it. There's also mounting evidence that certain foods have disastrous health consequences for a surprising number of people with unsuspected food intolerances or "allergies".

Mainly, it is becoming much clearer which foods are most likely to influence a wide array of health problems. Thus, this book not only documents the expanding knowledge of food's healing and preventive powers, but also suggests specific foods that may help promote or alleviate everything from minor troubles to life-threatening diseases. The Food Pharmacy proved there was a new world. Food – Your Miracle Medicine explores that new world and what it means to you personally. It offers practical scientific "maps" you can use to master your health concerns, ward off disease and treat existing troubles.

For me the book has been an exciting adventure of tracking down new and astonishing scientific findings on the connection between diet and health. In that pursuit, I interviewed hundreds of scientists, studied thousands of pages of references and abstracts from computer searches, attended a dozen or so international scientific conferences and read countless medical and scientific papers. A major source of information was the huge database of scientific and medical articles known as MEDLARS at the National Library of Medicine in Bethesda, Maryland. I also consulted the large database on pharmacological properties of foods and plants, called Natural Products Alert, or NAPRALERT, at the University of Illinois at Chicago. As a conservative estimate, the book is based on more than 10,000 studies which I have consulted in abstract or total text or learned about directly through individual researchers.

It's important to note that the scientific information in this book comes from prominent researchers, affiliated with leading scientific centres around the world, whose findings have been published in prestigious scientific journals. These are men and women on the cutting edge, who nevertheless represent the scientific standards of mainstream medicine. They are also, perhaps without realizing it, participants in an unstoppable and benevolent trend – the mainstreaming of alternative medicine. Surveys report that at least one-third of Americans use some form of alternative medicine. Diet is undoubtedly our best, safest and cheapest form of alternative medicine. That it is being legitimized by mainstream medicine can only spare us much needless suffering, as well as give us some relief from astronomical medical costs and the monopoly of the pharmaceutical industry. One economic analysis, reported in the Journal of the American Medical Association in 1988, found that substituting oat bran for a specific cholesterol-lowering drug could slash an individual's drug bills by 80 per cent. Of course, oat bran also does not have the drug's potentially serious side effects.

Food – Your Miracle Medicine is witness to a new frontier – not just of discoveries, but of personal solutions. It explores the magnificent powers of food to direct biochemical events at the cellular level, which is where all health matters begin and end. Despite our man-made wonder drugs, Mother Nature is truly the world's oldest and greatest pharmacist, the source of major and minor health miracles. Listening to science's new revelations about this ageless wisdom gives you unprecedented control over your health.

––––––––

"Diet has the distinction of being the only major determinant of health that is completely under your control. You have the final say over what does and does not go into your mouth and stomach. You cannot always control the other determinants of health, such as the quality of the air you breathe, the noise you are subjected to, or the emotional climate of your surroundings, but you can control what you eat. It is a shame to squander such a good opportunity to influence your health." – Andrew Weil, M.D., Natural Health, Natural Medicine

––––––––

Important: Diet is but one factor in the genesis of disease. Critical also are genetic susceptibility and environmental exposure to pathogens and pollutants. Thus, you should not rely on diet alone to treat or prevent disease, nor should you substitute foods for medications without consulting your physician. Further, no single food, or foods of one type, should be eaten to the exclusion of others for the purpose of preventing or treating a specific disease or maintaining health, except on the advice of your own physician. Various types of foods provide known and unknown substances vital to health; varying your diet is an essential part of achieving and maintaining better health. The information in this book is not medical advice and is not given as medical advice. For individual medical advice, you should consult your own physician. Further, unless specifically noted, the information and research reported in this book applies to adults, not children.

THE MIRACLE OF FOOD

To most of us, miracle drugs are the brainstorms of pharmaceutical geniuses – magic bullets concocted in a laboratory to use in the fight against all our ailments, large and small. Many scientists are increasingly engaged in a search for a far different treasure of drugs that were created on this planet millions of years ago. These drugs come from other living creatures and plants. They are the stuff we put in our mouths, often unconsciously, every day.

These substances, too, are miraculous – awesome in their ability to affect our well-being. In the larger scheme of things, the miracles these food essences continually perform inside our cells, outside our awareness, are very tiny, but they are major miracles in the lives of cells. They are changing forever their destiny – and consequently our destiny, with their cumulative effects.

Who can say that these are not minor miracles? Garlic can kill cancer cells. Substances in spinach can imprison and paralyze the virus that otherwise would cause cervical cancer. An obscure compound in asparagus and avocados in test-tube experiments stopped the proliferation of the virus responsible for the greatest infectious tragedy of our day – AIDS. Cabbage compounds can help detoxify our bodies of twentieth-century air pollutants – a job never anticipated at the time of the plant's creation. Compounds, spun out by plants to fight off their own destruction, become angels of mercy inside our bodies to prevent blood clots fomented by a fatty diet out of control. Particles freed by digestion from the fibrous structure of plants can tell our liver to cool down its cholesterol output. Chemicals from the plant kingdom can enter our brains and affect the transmission of messages among neurons, influencing our mood, our memories, our alertness – everything we cherish as distinguishing our humanness.

Make no mistake about it, eating is not a trivial event for the billions upon billions of cells that constitute your being. As scientists, for the first time in human history, have begun to investigate the act of eating vigorously and appreciate it is of great consequence; a communion with nature that promotes life or death. The choice is increasingly ours, as new scientific discoveries uncover the enormous impact of our everyday diets on our prospects for health and longevity.

New research shows that food can bestow health and vigour, freeing us of minor discomforts and protecting us from devastating diseases or it can make us ill and miserable.

Food can quicken the brain and lift our mood. It can infuse our brains with spurts of electrical energy that make us think faster and perform better. It can quiet our distress as surely as a prescription tranquillizer can, or it can make us drowsy and play havoc with our concentration. It can pull us out of depression or reduce us to panic. Food can set in progress silent attacks that erode our joints and clog our arteries – and it can help reverse the damage. The type of food we eat as children or young adults may subtly alter our brain chemistry, leaving us in middle age the victims of muscle-destroying multiple sclerosis or in old age with the tremors of Parkinson's disease.

Food can promote aberrant activity within cells that years later end up as cancerous growths. Conversely, food can release agents that literally vaporize cancer-causing chemicals or extinguish chain reactions of molecules that roar through the body, ripping apart the membranes of healthy cells, corrupting their genetic good intentions or leaving them to die. Even after abnormal cell growths have emerged on their way to becoming cancer, food can cause them to shrink or disappear. When the wandering cells from a breast cancer are scouting for new places to attach and grow, food's emissaries can create a hostile surface that cannot be colonized by cancer cells.

Foods can also

- keep the lens of the eye from becoming opaque with cataracts in old age
- dilate air passages, easing breathing
- rejuvenate cilia, the tiny beating hair-wings in the lungs that help wave off emphysema and chronic bronchitis
- create substances that cause flare-ups of rheumatoid arthritis or mute the arthritic's pain and swelling
- trigger headaches and asthma attacks as well as prevent them
- increase the stomach's resistance to ulcers
- reverse the redness, itching and pain of psoriasis
- stimulate the body to make more natural killer cells and interferon to ward off infections
- attack bacteria and viruses with a vigour equal to that of laboratory-made drugs
- cure diarrhoea in infants and constipation in the elderly
- alter immunity, chasing away common colds and hay fever

In heart disease, food is a prime player. Food can set in motion destructive processes that leave arteries narrow and stiff, just right for the formation of blood clots that cause heart muscle to suffocate and die. Conversely, food can supply a chemical armada that circulates in the blood, disarming the artery's enemies and even scrubbing away some of their dangerous handiwork from artery walls. Food can create blood-clot solvents, blood thinners and cholesterol reducers. Food can stimulate insulin release and control blood sugar surges. Food can send hormones to relax artery walls, reducing blood pressure.

Food can interfere with the so-called natural processes of ageing. Food can deter the body's deterioration.

There is hardly a health problem or natural bodily process that is not influenced in some fashion by the substances you put in your mouth. Food is being redefined as powerful medicine – medicine you can use in preventing and curtailing diseases of all kinds and in boosting mental and physical energy, vigour and well being.

Food is the breakthrough drug of the twenty-first century.

"Food folktales are not just fairy tales." – David Kritchevsky, Ph.D., Wistar Institute, Philadelphia

---

FROM ANCIENT MYTH TO MODERN MEDICINE

Until recently, modern medicine neglected the medicine in everyday foods, viewing it as folklore, lacking proven scientific validity. Now mainstream scientists are increasingly reaching back to the truths of ancient food folk medicine and dietary practices for clues to remedies and antidotes for our modern diseases. Research on nature's medicine is fast-paced.

Why is all this attention to the medicinal aspects of food accelerating now? Why are prestigious research institutions like Johns Hopkins and Harvard telling us with great fanfare that broccoli is full of powerful anticancer agents and that eating more carrots seems dramatically to prevent strokes and heart disease?

The reason is that for the first time in history, science is vigorously validating that what we eat is of urgent importance in determining events at the basic cellular level. That is where the real mystery and drama take place – where battles are continuously won or lost, affirming health and longevity or dooming us to illness and death. That is where life begins and ends – in those seas of cellular fluids and genetic and structural material, where destiny may hang on the presence of a particular enzyme or a fatty acid metabolized from a molecule of food.

If you know what is going on in your cells, you know what is happening to your health. About 60 trillion cells make up your body. Each cell is a complex and awe-inspiring miniature universe that experiences billions of chemical reactions every minute of your life. And what dictates the chemical reactions within these cells? Their sole source of energy is the food you give them. For the first time science can now probe how food promotes health or disease at the cell level, documenting the long-held human wisdom that food does have medicinal powers.

Unquestionably, early physicians used food as the mainstay prescription against disease. In a recent medical journal, Dr. John Potter, of the University of Minnesota, recounted some of the early medicinal uses of food: "In ancient Egypt, Pliny declared that consumption of cabbage would cure as many as 87 diseases and that consumption of onions would cure 28. Garlic was considered a holy plant. Cruciferous vegetables (cabbage and broccoli) were cultivated primarily for medicinal purposes and were used therapeutically against headache, deafness, diarrhoea, gout, and stomach disorders . . . The ancient Romans believed that lentils were a cure for diarrhoea and conducive to an even temper. Raisins and grapes had many medicinal uses and were incorporated into oral preparations, enemas, inhalations, and topical applications."

Since the dawn of civilization, we have relied on the forests, fields and gardens for our medicines. About 75 per cent of the world's population still does. Such a body of human wisdom should not be discounted, says James Duke, Ph.D., a botanist and specialist in medicinal plants at the U.S. Department of Agriculture. In his view, if a food has a wide folk-lore reputation as a remedy for specific diseases, this constitutes some proof of its potential validity. After all, he points out, such folk usage has often led scientists to discover strong medicines in plants. At least 25 per cent of our prescription drugs are derived from plants, including a powerful new anticancer medicine, taxol.

Ancient physicians and healers who used natural medicines to treat diseases were guided by their own experience and that of their ancestors and kinspeople. They, of course, knew nothing of germs they could not see, or of hormones or cholesterol and how painkillers and anticoagulants actually work, let alone how to test foods for such pharmacological properties.

NEW PROOF OF FOOD POWER

Today scientists with new technology can detect, isolate and test minute quantities of bioactive plant compounds. Using sophisticated laboratory tests, they can ferret out the biological activities of whole foods and their constituents and their impact on disease processes.

Scientists also scrutinize the diets of populations with low rates of disease – for example, Mediterranean peoples and the Japanese – to determine how they eat differently from people with high disease rates. In "case-control" studies, nearly identical groups of individuals are studied, except one group has a particular disease and the other does not, then their diets are compared. A lot of clues come from such so-called epidemiological or population studies.

The best are *intervention studies*, in which researchers actually put people with a certain malady, such as heart disease or precancerous lumps, on very specific but different diets. They then keep track of who gets worse or better in the next two or three years. In this way a food is tested much like a drug to judge the potency of the therapy. Such intervention studies are rare, but the advice derived from them is golden.

Tests using such precise scientific methods convince many leading scientists of food's extraordinary effects on bodily functions and leave no doubt that foods induce druglike reactions. Countless tests confirm that foods can act as anticoagulants, antidepressants, antiulcerants, anti-thrombotics, analgesics, tranquillizers, sedatives, cholesterol reducers, cancer fighters and cancer chemopreventives, hormones, fertility agents, laxatives, antidiarrhoeal agents, immune stimulators, biological response modifiers, antihypertensives, diuretics, decongestants, anti-inflammatory agents, antibiotics, antiviral agents, antinausea agents, cough suppressants, blood-vessel dilators, bronchial dilators, and so on. A mammoth computer data base called NAPRALERT, at the University of Illinois at Chicago, contains more than 102,000 entries on the pharmacological attributes of plants worldwide, many of them edible.

The food pharmacy is as viable as the pill pharmacy, and more complex. Nobody has yet invented a "broccoli pill" that can match eating the real thing, for example, and probably never will. A single food contains hundreds or thousands of chemicals, most unidentified, that make up each bite's varied pharmacological activity.

At the same time, some strong theories are emerging to account for food's pharmacological powers. Better medical understanding of the biochemical changes underlying the progression of chronic disease, from events in single cells to disease symptoms, gives scientists reasons to believe in food's enormous potential for influencing disease. These recent scientific happenings have catapulted the study of food-power out of the realm of folklore into mainstream medicine.

"*Already two millennia ago, the Greeks were eating a delicious diet as healthful as any we now know in the world. Instead of playing sorcerer's apprentice, we have to look at Mother Nature and see what people have been doing for thousands of years.*" — Serge Renaud, a biologist and epidemiologist at INSERM, the French government's main research institution

---

THREE THEORIES OF
FOOD'S HEALING POWERS

There are dozens of scientifically plausible ways food can affect health. However, three umbrella theories fuel and shape much new research into food's healing and preventive powers. These three theories focus on:

- disease-fighting **antioxidants** in foods
- the unappreciated pharmacological powers of **fat**
- new kinds of food "allergies", intolerances or **sensitivities**

If you understand these theories, you can better appreciate how food can counteract or promote disease and how you can best protect yourself.

ANTIOXIDANTS

Many of our health misfortunes are due to the perversity of oxygen. Yes, the very stuff that gives life can also help take it away. It's a remarkable proposition – that our cells are perpetually besieged by toxic forms of oxygen, our existence wiped out, a molecule at a time, by the element's fierce destructive powers. Attacks by continual bursts from oxygen reactions help clog our arteries, turn our cells cancerous, make our joints give out and our nervous systems malfunction. In fact, this new theory about oxygen has revolutionized the way scientists look at the genesis of disease and its prevention. It is the single most significant line of inquiry behind science's strong new belief in the power of food to thwart bodily deterioration. So far, scientists have linked destructive oxygen reactions to at least 60 different chronic diseases, as well as to ageing itself.

"The older we are, the more oxidized we get," observes Helmut Sies, M.D., chairman of the department of physiological chemistry at the University of Dusseldorf Medical School in Germany, and a leading scholar on the subject. In less gentle terms, we are all somewhat like a piece of meat that has lain around too long. We are going rancid, some of us at a faster rate than others. These are the crucial questions. Why do certain people go bad more quickly, or conversely, why do some better resist oxygen-induced deterioration? Why do some folks age less rapidly and seem less prone to disease? How can we slow down the destructive process?

As Dr. Sies explains, the oxygen theory of disease is not very subtle. Two formidable forces are in combat in our bodies: renegade oxygen molecules called *oxidants*, and the body's police force, known as antioxidants. Although some oxidants can be beneficial and are routinely spawned by normal metabolic processes, many are malevolent foreign invaders. You can envisage destructive oxidants as wanton molecular gangs that roam your body, mugging cells, ripping their membranes, corrupting their genetic material, turning fat rancid and leaving cells to die. Of course, the process is so gradual and internally painless, occurring over years in incessant microsecond bursts of destruction, that you don't notice it until the cumulative damage gives rise to what we call symptoms of disease, including inflammation, deteriorating vision, chest pain, poor concentration and cancer.

On the other hand, various antioxidants, put into your body mostly by foods, strive to protect cells by fending off the destructive oxygen molecules. Essentially, when the bad-guy oxidants consistently outnumber and outwit the good-guy antioxidants, your body enters the "oxidative stress" zone and you are in high-disease-risk territory.

BEWARE THE FREE RADICALS

Oxidants come in various forms and guises. The most notorious and best-studied are so-called oxygen free radicals. These molecules are charged up and looking for trouble. They have lost one of the electrons that keep them chemically stable. In their frenetic search for another one, they will try to grab it from anywhere, destroying healthy cells in their path and creating still more gangs of free radicals in split-second reactions that become out-of-control chain reactions. One of the laws of nature is that "radicals beget radicals that beget more radicals," explains Dr. Sies.

Oxygen free radicals can attack DNA, the genetic material of cells, causing them to mutate, which is a first step on the path to cancer. Perhaps even more awesome – free radicals attack the fatty parts of cell membranes. Left defenceless without enough antioxidants, these fatty molecules become *peroxidized*, another word for rancid. This can completely disrupt the cell membrane's architecture. Worse, each peroxidized fat molecule is now like a torch, capable of peroxidizing any new fat molecule it contacts, fomenting a chain reaction that can continue until it is interrupted or exhausted, and ends up sullying millions of other fat molecules.

Where do oxidants come from? Some are simply the waste products of ordinary metabolic processes, such as breathing and immune reactions. Thus, some oxidant activity eludes control and is beneficial but many oxidants come from the environment and are destructive, such as ionizing radiation, air pollutants, toxic industrial chemicals, pesticides, cigarette smoke and drugs. Obviously, you can influence your fate mightily by not doing hazardous things like smoking cigarettes and exposing yourself to dangerous chemicals. You can also try to outwit the oxidants to varying degrees by mounting a better antioxidant defence against their assaults.

ENTER THE FOOD WARRIORS

One of the great revelations of the last few years, according to a massive and growing body of evidence, is that you may be able to eat your way out of this dilemma, in so far as the boundaries of human life span and genetics allow. You can supply your cells with antioxidant food compounds that strike down, intercept and extinguish rampaging oxygen molecules and even repair some of their damage. Foods, notably plant food – fruits and vegetables – are packed with a variety of ferocious antioxidants. When you eat these antioxidants, they are infused into your tissue and fluids where they can help resist the oxidant invasions. Scientists, now that they understand the awesome potential powers of antioxidants, are busy analysing foods for their presence. The search has already turned up a bundle of potent plant antioxidants with exotic names like *quercetin*, *lycopene*, *lutein* and *glutathione*, as well as familiar nutrients, namely vitamins C and E, beta carotene and the trace mineral selenium.

So persuasive is the new antioxidant research that William A. Pryor, Ph.D., head of biomedical research at Louisiana State University, has called for the development and widespread use of a blood test to reveal your "antioxidant status," just as tests now measure blood cholesterol. Such a test would measure the level of damaging oxidative activity in your body

---

WHAT OXIDANTS CAN DO THAT DIETARY ANTIOXIDANTS MAY PREVENT

- Turn LDL cholesterol into a form that can clog arteries
- Attack cells' genetic material, causing mutations that can lead to cancer
- Destroy cells of the eyes, leading to cataracts and macular degeneration
- Interfere with normal processes, raising blood pressure
- Destroy nerve cells, leading to neurological deterioration, such as Parkinson's disease and Lou Gehrig's disease
- Promote inflammation, as in arthritis and asthma
- Damage sperm, leading to infertility and birth defects

---

and also whether you are eating enough neutralizing antioxidants. If you had high oxidative activity and low antioxidant intake, you would be judged a high risk for disease and be advised to increase your intake of antioxidants. Nothing you can do for your health and survival is more important than consistently eating foods packed with disease-fighting antioxidants. (For antioxidants in foods, see below and pages 428–32.

HOW TO GET THE MOST DISEASE-FIGHTING ANTIOXIDANTS

When you choose fruits and vegetables, look for those with colour; usually the deeper the colour, the more antioxidants. Also, fresh and frozen fruits and vegetables have more antioxidants than those that are canned, processed or heated.

Generally you get more antioxidants if you eat
- Red grapes rather than green or white grapes
- Red and yellow onions instead of white onions
- Cabbage, cauliflower and broccoli raw or lightly cooked
- Garlic raw and crushed
- Fresh and frozen vegetables rather than canned ones
- Microwaved vegetables instead of boiled and steamed ones
- Extra virgin cold-processed olive oil
- The deepest, darkest green leafy vegetables
- Pink grapefruit instead of white grapefruit
- Whole fruits rather than juices
- Fresh and frozen juices instead of canned ones
- The deepest orange carrots. sweet potatoes and pumpkins

FAT

The fat in food wields surprising power over your cells. A cell's biological activity – thus its propensity to promote or discourage disease processes – often hangs on a fragile balance of food-derived fatty acids within the cell. *That means the type of fat you eat is of enormous consequence to your overall health.*

New research shows that eating any type of fat sets off biochemical fireworks of exquisite complexity in cells. The result may be the dispatching of hormone-like messengers to stimulate inflammation, immune responses, blood clotting, headaches, constriction of blood vessels, pain and growth of malignant tumours. In contrast, certain fats incite cells to make chemicals that break up undesirable blood clots, fight off joint pain and frustrate cancer cells. Although fat pharmacology is a very complex process, involving enzymes, many metabolic steps and a delicate balance of fats in cells, it has thrilling possibilities for deterring and ameliorating disease.

The knowledge of how fat reigns over certain critical cellular functions hinges on two recent major discoveries. First came the discovery that numerous bodily processes, such as blood clotting and inflammation, are largely controlled by very potent hormone-like substances – *prostaglandins, thromboxanes* and *leukotrienes* – collectively called *eicosanoids*. Then, even more momentous, researchers learned that the raw material from which these mighty eicosanoid messengers are made is fat from food. In other words, the diet serves up raw material of fatty acids for the cellular factories that turn out these all-important eicosanoids. Not surprisingly, the type and quantities of specific fatty acids that go in determine the type and amounts of eicosanoids that come out. They can be biologically friendly or dangerous. In any event, the profound message is that, through the type of fat you eat, you can manipulate the levels and biological activity of eicosanoids circulating in your body.

YOU ARE THE FAT YOU EAT

Very quickly after you eat fat, it shows up in the membranes of your cells where its metabolic fate is determined. Although fatty acids come in many subtle variations of molecular arrangement, two major categories are most important in making eicosanoids: *omega-3 fatty acids,* concentrated in marine life as well as a few land plants, and *omega-6 fatty acids,* concentrated in land-based vegetable oils such as corn oil, safflower and sunflower oil, as well as in animal foods raised on land-based feeds.

When you consume land-based omega-6 fatty acids from a piece of meat or corn oil, they are likely to be changed into a substance called *arachidonic acid*, which in turn spawns substances that are highly inflammatory or promote blood stickiness and blood vessel constriction. Fat from seafood is radically different and more benign. Its omega-3 fatty acids are apt to be converted into substances that counteract blood platelet clumping, dilate blood vessels and reduce inflammation and cell damage.

Since food is made of mixtures of omega-3s and omega-6s, obviously these two fatty acids are continuously giving contradictory instructions to cells. Which prevails – those for health or those for disease – depends on the ratio of the two fatty acids in your diet and hence your cells says William E. M. Lands, Ph.D., a pioneering researcher on fish oils and formerly a professor of biochemistry at the University of Illinois at Chicago. If your cells are flooded with omega-6 fatty acids, the resulting oversupply of overactive prostaglandins is apt to run amok, generating disease. If you have sufficient omega-3 fatty acids, they can check or cool down the arachidonic engine that is spewing out the disease-producing eicosanoids.

THE BATTLES BETWEEN FISH AND CORN OILS

At the cellular level the stakes are high. In short, as Dr. Lands explains, your cells are a battleground where omega-3 and omega-6 fatty acids compete for supremacy. Which one wins day after day helps determine the state of your health. The truth is that for most people of Western countries, it is continual defeat. We get far too much omega-6 and too little omega-3 in our diet. Dr. Lands says Americans eat at least 10–15 times more terrestrial omega-6s than marine omega-3s – a "horrible proportion". By contrast, Eskimos, who are known for their very low rates of chronic diseases, eat three times more omega-3s than omega-6s, primarily because they eat so much seafood. Proof of the problem is found in the tissues of Americans. In recent studies Phyllis Bowen, associate professor in the Department of Nutrition and Medical Dietetics at the University of Illinois at Chicago, found that omega-6s comprised 80 per cent of the unsaturated fatty acids circulating in Americans' cell membranes. In comparison, omega-6 levels were closer to 65 per cent in the French, 50 per cent in the Japanese and only 22 per cent in Greenland Eskimos.

Omega-6 excesses worry experts, such as Professor Emeritus Alexander Leaf of the Harvard University Medical School. When our bodies evolved eons ago they were nourished by lots of omega-3s and virtually no omega-6s, he notes. Now, with the invention of processed vegetable oils, the ratio is upside-down in many cultures. Today's fish-deficient diets leave our cells starved of marine oil and overburdened by modern processed oils and meat fats – Big Macs and Mazola oil – foreign to our cells. He believes our relatively new fatty-acid imbalance throws cells into major malfunction, precipitating our current epidemic of chronic illnesses, such as heart disease, cancer, diabetes and arthritis. Dr. Leaf suggests human bodies require a minimum dose of fish oil and that not getting it brings revenge by way of multiple diseases.

"Our epidemic of heart disease and cancer may be the result of a human fish oil deficiency state so enormous we fail to recognize it." – Ewan Cameron, M.D., Linus Pauling Institute of Science and Medicine in California

---

New research underscores the enormous lifesaving power of fat in fish. Eating fatty fish can directly intervene to save people from death and disability from heart attacks. Studies have found that atherosclerosis – diseased and clogged arteries – worsens, the less marine oil a person eats. Dr. Lands has developed a formula that he says can precisely predict an individual's odds of heart attack; a simple finger-prick test measures a person's blood ratio of omega-3 and omega-6 fatty acids. The higher the proportion of marine omega-3s to omega-6s, the lower the risk of heart attack. Similarly, studies reveal that a high ratio of omega-3 fatty acids to omega-6 fatty acids in the blood cuts your chances of cancer.

Although it's largely unappreciated, our overconsumption of omega-6 oils, prevalent in margarines, salad oils, cooking oils and processed foods, is helping create a health disaster, says Artemis Simopoulos, M.D., president of the Center for Genetics, Nutrition and Health in Washington, D.C. True, heart authorities first encouraged the widespread use of such vegetable oils to lower blood cholesterol, not suspecting the oils could have detrimental effects on other aspects of health, such as fostering inflammatory diseases, lowering immunity and promoting cancer. Such omega-6 oils are well-documented villains in augmenting cancer incidence, cancer spread and deaths in laboratory animals.

The only way to correct this abnormal and alarming fat imbalance in cells is to cut back drastically on foods rich in omega-6s and increase the intake of marine omega-3s, say experts. The impact is almost immediate. Within 72 hours, you can see a beneficial biochemical impact in tissue by eating 3½ oz (100g) of fish a day, studies indicate.

It is smart to eat fish, especially fatty fish such as salmon, sardines, mackerel, herring and tuna, at least two or three times a week. However, adding any amount of seafood to a seafood-poor diet can readjust our fatty acid balance somewhat, helping curtail not only heart disease, but the many modern disorders linked to a "seafood fat deficiency". Research shows that eating just 1oz (30g) of fish a day may help restore our cells to healthy functioning, saving countless people from disability and premature death inflicted by the unimagined consequences of fat's pharmacological powers. (For the best sources of omega-3 fatty acids, see page 463.)

DISORDERS THAT FISH OIL MAY ALLEVIATE OR PREVENT

- **Rheumatoid arthritis:** Reduces joint pain, soreness, stiffness, fatigue.
- **Heart attacks:** Cuts the odds of subsequent heart attacks by one-third.
- **Clogged arteries:** Keeps arteries open and clear. (Eaters of fatty fish have less atherosclerosis.) Reduces risk of reclosure of arteries after angioplasty surgery by 40–50 per cent.
- **High blood pressure:** Eliminates or reduces the need for pharmaceutical pressure-lowering medications.
- **Ulcerative colitis** (inflammatory bowel disease): In one test, eating 4.5g of fish oil a day – equal to that in 7oz (200g) of mackerel – for eight months depressed disease activity by 56 per cent. Another test reduced need for prednisone, a steroid, by one-third.
- **Psoriasis:** Reduces itching, redness, pain in some patients, and cuts the amount of medication needed.
- **Multiple sclerosis:** Helps reduce symptoms in some patients.
- **Asthma:** Curtails attacks in some individuals.
- **Migraine headaches:** Lessens severity and frequency in some sufferers.

WHERE TO GET THE MOST DISEASE-FIGHTING OMEGA-3S

You usually find the most omega-3 fat in the fattiest fish from the coldest deep seas. Richest sources are mackerel, anchovies, herring, salmon, sardines, lake trout, Atlantic sturgeon and tuna. Moderate amounts are found in turbot, bluefish, striped bass, shark, rainbow smelt, swordfish and rainbow trout. Shellfish – crab, lobster, shrimp, mussels, oysters, clams and squid – contain lesser amounts of omega 3s. (For a complete list, see the Appendix.)

To get the most omega-3 benefits, bake or poach fish. Frying or otherwise adding fat, especially vegetable oils high in omega-6s, decreases the omega-3 potency in the fish.

Choose tuna packed in water and sardines canned without oil, unless it is sardine oil, noted on the label as sild. Added oils, such as soya bean oil, can diminish the omega-3s. Also, draining oil from canned tuna washes away from 15–25 per cent of the omega-3s, whereas draining water off washes away only 3 per cent.

You also get some omega-3s in certain plant foods. The highest concentrations are in walnuts, flaxseed and rapeseed and purslane, a green leafy vegetable that is commonly eaten in Europe and the Middle East. However, plant omega-3s appear to be only one-fifth as potent as marine omega-3s in fostering beneficial reactions in cells.

THE BEST OF FISH, THE WORST OF FISH

Unfortunately, fish, such an ancient natural benefactor, is sometimes contaminated with modern poisons, such as pesticides and other industrial chemicals. Here are ways to get the most health benefits from fish with the least hazards:

- Choose saltwater ocean fish over freshwater fish from streams, rivers and lakes, which are more likely to be polluted.
- Avoid sport fish caught by recreational fishermen in lakes and streams. They are most likely to be contaminated.
- Choose smaller fish over larger fish. Small fish, like sardines, have had fewer years of exposure to pollutants.
- Eat a variety of fish instead of just one type. This reduces the risk of overdosing on one contaminated source.
- Don't eat fish skin, which is a prime depository of toxic chemicals.
- For a safer bet, you can choose farm-raised fish, such as catfish and salmon, not likely to be contaminated; however, they usually

have less omega-3 type oil than wild fish.

- Don't overdo it. Although some populations, such as Japanese fishermen and Eskimos, with low disease rates eat fish every day, sometimes as much as 1lb (450g), it's not necessary to eat so much to reap the benefits of fish. Most studies suggest that regularly eating fish two or three times a week can make a tremendous dent in heart disease, cancer and other chronic diseases.

- A special caution for pregnant women whose foetuses could be damaged by toxic chemicals: Forgo fish from inland waters, and restrict swordfish, shark and fresh tuna to once a month. Some experts also advise pregnant women not to eat more than 7oz (200g) of canned tuna a week.

FOOD SENSITIVITIES

Do you have headaches? Hives? Asthma? Eczema? Irritable bowel syndrome? Ulcerative colitis? Rheumatoid arthritis? Chronic fatigue syndrome? Are you depressed, moody, sluggish? Does your baby have colic? Rashes? Diarrhoea? Do your kids have wheezing? Ear infections? Migraines? Epileptic seizures? There is growing scientific recognition that such maladies can be triggered or aggravated by the body's innate objection to certain foods. These are not ordinary allergies; they are a strange sort of food torture, unique to certain individuals, and nobody understands exactly why they occur. One thing is certain; they are real, and recognizing them has solved many a health mystery. Overlooking the possibility of such adverse food reactions, as often happens, dooms many to needless years of ill health and suffering.

The recognition of such weird food "allergies" is revolutionary. Some leading experts believe hidden intolerances to food are widely incriminated in a variety of diseases. Such reactions, although popularly called allergies, do not meet the classic definition of a food allergy. Consequently, authorities often refer to such reactions as "intolerances," "sensitivities," "metabolic reactions" or just plain "adverse reactions".

Here's the difference between the old and new food allergy theories. In the classical clear-cut food allergy that doctors have long recognized, if you eat the merest morsel of a food to which you are allergic, you have an immediate, often dramatic reaction such as a sore mouth, an itchy red skin rash, an attack of asthma or anaphylactic shock. Blood and skin tests for the allergenic food are positive.

In a true classic case of food allergy, the immune system overreacts, and mistakenly identifies innocent compounds in, for example, cow's milk or nuts, as enemies like bacteria and viruses. This mistake throws the immune system into a chain reaction of alert. It produces antibodies called immunoglobulin E or IgE to launch an attack on the false threats (antigens), releasing histamines and other chemicals that provoke the symptoms of allergies. Traditionally, only reactions that involve IgE are considered true allergies.

THE FIVE MOST LIKELY ALLERGIC FOOD TRIGGERS OF CHRONIC DISORDERS

According to tests by British expert John O. Hunter, M.D., these foods most often provoke a variety of disease symptoms:

- Cereals based on wheat and corn
- Dairy products
- Caffeine
- Yeast
- Citrus fruits

DELAYED FOOD ALLERGIES

Now, a theory of food allergies, more accurately called intolerances or hypersensitivities, that is gaining medical attention suggests that when you eat an offending food, the reaction may be subtle and more difficult to detect. It may not set in for hours or a day or two, maybe even longer. It takes more food to trigger the reaction, and blood and skin tests for the food may turn up either positive or negative. There may be no typical involvement of the immune system. Such delayed food sensitivities, some believe, help bring on a range of maladies such as lethargy, headaches, mood problems and loss of concentration, as well as chronic conditions such as rheumatoid arthritis and irritable bowel syndrome.

Moreover, avoiding certain foods can bring remarkable reversals of so-called incurable, long-standing chronic conditions, including rheumatoid arthritis and digestive problems. According to pioneering British physician John O. Hunter, a gastroenterologist at Addenbrookes Hospital in Cambridge, "In controlled trials, exclusion (restricted) diets are effective in migraine, irritable bowel syndrome, Crohn's disease, eczema, hyperactivity and rheumatoid arthritis. Despite this huge variety of diseases, the foods concerned are strikingly similar – most commonly they are cereals, dairy products, caffeine, yeast and citrus fruits. Avoidance of some or all of these foods leads to relief of symptoms." In one study, Dr. Hunter found that wheat was the most troublesome all-around food, upsetting 60 per cent of subjects. Next came dairy products. Least offensive was honey, bothering only 2 per cent.

Oddly, with this type of food allergy, you may not always get a reaction if you infuse the specific offending food right into the bloodstream, says Dr. Hunter. This means the reaction is happening in the gut, he says, instead of in the blood and immune system. According to his theory, foods as they are broken down by bacteria in the intestinal tract release toxins and other chemicals that trigger reactions. The reaction comes and goes, depending on individual sensitivities and the delicate balance of various bacteria in the digestive tract.

Several other theories purport to explain these strange and debilitating food reactions. One possibility is that some people, because of chronic intestinal inflammation, have "leaky guts" that allow undigested food particles to pass through the colon wall into the bloodstream, where they are treated as foreign invaders by the immune system, creating an allergic uproar. Another explanation is that constituents in foods are direct instigators of symptoms. For example, coffee, fruit and particularly wine contain phenols, natural chemicals that are inactivated by enzymes during digestion. If a person has faulty enzymes and the phenols are not properly inactivated, they stir up trouble; phenols in wine are suspected of helping trigger migraine headaches. Further, some foods are straight-out carriers of potent allergic substances. Tests on milk have detected histamine, the prime substance in many allergic reactions, such as asthma. Milk and wheat contain natural opiates, morphine-like substances, that may affect brain cell activity, influencing mood and mental activity, and possibly inducing fatigue.

THE TWISTED-MIND SYNDROME

Can food reactions also trigger psychological ailments? "The mounting evidence is beginning to suggest that psychological symptoms such as depression and anxiety may be caused and/or exacerbated by food sensitivities in certain susceptible persons," concluded a recent review by Alan Gettis of the Columbia University College of Physicians and Surgeons. Dr. Talal Nsouli, an allergist on the faculty at Georgetown University Medical School, has found that chronic fatigue in a surprisingly high percentage of cases stems from delayed food allergies, especially to wheat, milk and corn.

Such newly discovered links between food intolerances and a long string of perplexing and seemingly incurable conditions at long last offer new hope for recovery to millions of people.

HOW TO DETECT A CHRONIC FOOD "ALLERGY"

If you suspect certain foods may disagree with you, bringing on or exacerbating chronic problems, such as arthritis, headaches, mood swings, abdominal pain, diarrhoea and other intestinal distress, you may be able to spot the causes by trial and error and eliminate them from your diet. Here are suggestions for doing so from Dr. Nsouli.

- For a week stop eating a suspect food. It makes sense to start with one of the most common culprits – milk and dairy products, wheat or corn products. Be careful to read food labels to detect the presence of the foods. For example, milk casein, wheat gluten and sweeteners made from corn (corn syrups) are very common in processed foods.

- During the week when you are avoiding the suspect food, keep close track of whether you feel better – whether, for example, your diarrhoea or headaches have diminished. If so, you must then try to confirm your suspicions.

- As proof that a specific food is troublesome, do a "challenge test". For a week, consume lots of the same food you have previously eliminated. If it is dairy products, eat low-fat milk, yoghurt and cottage cheese two or three times a day. If it is corn, eat lots of whole corn kernels, corn flakes, tortillas, corn bread and corn chips. If it is wheat, eat bread, wheat cereals and pasta. Notice whether you feel worse, whether your symptoms, such as pain, fatigue or abdominal distress have returned. If they have, the food may be partly at fault. Remember, the symptom may not appear until two or three days after you eat an offending food.

Warning: If you have ever had an acute reaction to a food, or believe you might be allergic to any foods, such as peanuts or shrimp, do not, *under any circumstances*, do a "food challenge test". Strictly avoid such foods; eating them could cause life-threatening reactions, including anaphylactic shock.

- Repeat the process, concentrating on different high-risk foods, including wheat, milk, corn, soya and eggs.
- Of course, you can also consult a physician who is a qualified specialist in food allergies. Typically, you will be given routine screening tests, including skin tests and/or a blood test called the RAST test, that detect immune reactions. These tests are helpful in detecting initial signs of food allergies, but they are not foolproof They may miss certain food intolerances and falsely report others. The only bottom-line test that really counts, insists Dr. Nsouli, is actually eliminating the food from your diet, then adding it back to see if it is the actual cause of trouble. That proof is the only real proof, even for allergists, he says.

If you do have an allergy or sensitivity to a particular food that is making your life miserable, avoiding it will bring an instant cure.

CARDIOVASCULAR
SYSTEM

HEART TROUBLE

Foods That Can Save Arteries and Prevent Heart Disease:
Seafood • Fruits • Vegetables • Nuts • Grains • Legumes •
Onions • Garlic • Olive Oil • Alcohol in Moderation • Foods
High in Vitamin C and E and Beta Carotene

Foods That Can Damage Arteries and the Heart: Meat and Dairy
Foods High in Saturated Fat • Excessive Alcohol

If you're afraid of heart disease – and who isn't in a land where it claims
some 179,000 lives every year? – one of the biggest clues to your survival is knowing what people eat who don't get heart disease or die of
it. Of course, genes and gender are partly at fault. So is lifestyle – smoking, exercise and stress. But even when scientists eliminate all those
things, diet still pops out as vital to whether your arteries clog or your
heart gives out. Curbing the progression of artery disease in the first
place – it invariably advances with age – is foremost in warding off heart
attacks and strokes. But remarkable new evidence shows that even if you
ate recklessly in earlier days, and even if you have already had heart
problems, including a heart attack, changing your diet now may prevent
future cardiac catastrophe and even halt or reverse arterial damage, helping restore arteries to health. It is not too early or too late.

HOW ARTERIES GET CLOGGED AND HOW FOOD CAN STOP IT

At birth, your arteries are clean, open and elastic. Early in life the process
of artery-clogging, known as atherosclerosis or coronary artery disease,
begins. Fatty streaks appear in and under the layer of cells that line artery
walls. Gradually the streaks are transformed into plaques – fatty scar
tissue that bulges into the artery opening, partly choking off blood
flow. If one of these plaques breaks down, the clotting mechanism may
be triggered. If the clot becomes large enough, it can block blood
flow, suffocating large patches of cardiac muscle, an event known as a

heart attack. Reduced blood flow can also trigger abnormal heart rhythms – tachycardia and fibrillation – sometimes causing sudden death. If a blood vessel to the brain closes off or ruptures, you suffer a stroke.

What you eat is a major determinant of how quickly and severely your arteries get clogged. The right diet can help keep vessels open, free of hazardous clots and flexible enough to serve as healthy conduits for blood flow. Food does this by combating the buildup of cholesterol and other blood fats, and most of all, by affecting blood-clotting factors. Here's what people eat who don't get heart disease, as confirmed by investigators around the world.

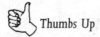 Thumbs Up

FISH: THE UNIVERSAL HEART MEDICINE

The best way to slash your chances of heart disease is, above all, eat fish, particularly fatty fish, overflowing with omega-3 fatty acids. The evidence of fish's preventive and therapeutic powers against cardiovascular disease is compelling. Seafood's probable main heart medicine is its unique marine fat.

Seafood eaters worldwide have less heart disease. Even eating tiny amounts of fish can have a monumental effect. A landmark Dutch study found that eating, on average, a mere 1oz (30g) of fish a day cut the chances of fatal heart disease in half. A study of 6,000 middle-aged American men revealed that those who ate the marine fat in a 1oz (30g) bite of mackerel or 3oz (85g) of bass a day were 36 per cent less likely to die of heart disease than men eating less fish. Another 25-year U.S. study of 17,000 men found that fatal heart attacks dropped the more fish they ate. Non-fish eaters had one-third more heart disease deaths than those who ate more than 1¼oz (35g) of seafood a day.

If you could look inside people's arteries, you would see that the healthiest ones belong to fish eaters and the most diseased ones to non-fish eaters. As an alternative, you could examine their arteries at autopsy. That's what Danish researchers did recently and came up with remarkable, unprecedented proof of the power of fish oil to prevent atherosclerosis.

The Danes obtained arteries and fat tissue from 40 consecutive autopsies at Frederiksberg Hospital in Denmark. They measured the fish oil in the fat tissue, which revealed how much fatty fish the individual had eaten while alive. Undeniably, the smoothest, cleanest arteries belonged to those with the most omega-3 fat in their tissue – who had eaten the most fish. The most seriously clogged arteries belonged to those with the least omega-3 fat in their tissue, indicating they had made the mistake of skimping on fatty fish.

Eating 1oz (30g) of fish a day, or a couple of servings a week, slashes your chances of heart attack by one-third to one-half, studies show.

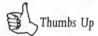 Thumbs Up

WHAT TO EAT TO SURVIVE A HEART ATTACK

If you have a heart attack, there's no question about what to do: make a preemptive strike. Get on a high-fish diet immediately. It can cut your chances of future deadly heart attacks by one third. In fact, eating fish boosts your odds of escaping subsequent heart attacks better than the traditional route of cutting down on foods high in saturated animal fat. So found a ground-breaking two-year study by Michael Burr, M.D., at the Medical Research Council in Cardiff. Dr. Burr studied 2,033 men who had all had at least one heart attack. He asked one group to eat a 5oz (140g) serving of oily fish, like salmon, mackerel or sardines, at least twice a week or take fish oil capsules. He instructed a second group to cut down on saturated fatty foods such as butter, cheese and cream and a third group to boost fibre intake by eating more bran cereal and whole wheat bread. For comparison, he gave no dietary advice at all to a fourth group.

After two years, there was no lifesaving effect from a low-fat or high-fibre diet but the impact from eating fish was startling. Deaths among the fish eaters dropped 29 per cent! "That's almost fantastic," says Harvard Medical School professor emeritus Alexander Leaf, an authority on fish oils.

• BOTTOM LINE • *If you suffer a heart attack, your odds of having another one go down more if you eat fish twice a week and lots of fruits and vegetables than if you simply follow the conventional advice of cutting down on fat in your diet.*

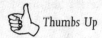 Thumbs Up

YOUR SECOND-CHANCE DIET AFTER HEART SURGERY

If you have a common surgical procedure called balloon angioplasty to open clogged arteries, eating fatty fish may help keep them unclogged. Such arteries tend to clog again in 40–50 per cent of cases. Yet, several studies show that fish oil may cut the chances of reclogging in half. Again, the fish oil may be superior to a low-fat diet. In one test by Mark R. Milner, a surgeon at the Washington, D.C., Hospital Center, only 19 per cent of 42 angioplasty patients who both ate a low-fat diet and took fish-oil capsules for six months after angioplasty had their arteries close up again. In contrast, an equal number of patients on a low-fat diet without fish oil had twice as much recurring blockage. The daily protective dose was the amount found in about 7oz (200g) of mackerel.

However, Dr. Milner says, people who ordinarily eat fish three times a week or more don't need the emergency catch-up provided by high doses of fish oil. That was documented in another study of angioplasty patients by Isabelle Bairati, M.D., professor of medicine at Laval University in Quebec City, Canada. She found that consistent fish eating alone before and after surgery kept arteries open just as well as taking fish-oil capsules. Those who ate more than 8oz (225g) of seafood a week were roughly half as likely to suffer reclogging as those who ate but 2oz (55g) a week. Not surprisingly, fatty fish, like salmon, mackerel and sardines, high in omega-3 fatty acids were more potent than other kinds.

TEN WAYS FISH OIL FIGHTS HEART DISEASE

- Blocks platelet aggregation (clotting)
- Reduces blood vessel constriction
- Increases blood flow
- Lowers fibrinogen (clotting factor)
- Revs up fibrinolytic (clot-dissolving) activity
- Blocks cell damage from oxygen free radicals
- Lowers triglycerides
- Raises good HDL cholesterol
- Makes cell membranes more flexible
- Lowers blood pressure

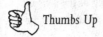 Thumbs Up

GARLIC TURNS BACK THE CLOCK ON CLOGGED ARTERIES

Eating garlic regularly can deter artery clogging, and, more remarkably, even reverse the damage, helping heal your arteries, says Arun Bordia, a cardiologist at Tagore Medical College in India. Dr. Bordia, a pioneering garlic researcher, discovered that feeding garlic to rabbits with 80 per cent arterial blockage reduced the degree of blockage, partially restoring the arteries to health.

He then tested garlic on a group of 432 heart-disease patients, most recovering from heart attacks. Half the group ate two or three fresh raw or cooked garlic cloves every day for three years. They squeezed the garlic into juice, put it in milk as a "morning tonic" or ate it boiled or minced. The other half ate no garlic. After the first year, there was no difference in the rate of heart attacks between the groups.

In the second year, however, *deaths among the garlic eaters dropped by 50 per cent and in the third year, they sank 66 per cent!* Nonfatal heart attacks also declined 30 per cent the second year and 60 per cent the third year. Further, blood pressure and blood cholesterol in the garlic eaters fell about 10 per cent. Garlic eaters also had fewer attacks of angina – chest pain. There were no significant cardiovascular changes in the non-garlic eaters.

Dr. Bordia suggests that, over time, steady infusions of garlic both wash away some of the arterial plaque and prevent future damage. Garlic's main weapon is probably a conglomeration of antioxidants. Garlic is said to possess at least 15 different antioxidants that may neutralize artery-destroying agents.

Note: Cooked garlic was as effective as raw garlic in warding off heart attacks and deaths, according to Dr. Bordia.

A Garlic Bonus. The garlic also produced unexpected health benefits. Dr. Bordia said the garlic eaters reported fewer joint pains, body aches and asthmatic tendencies; more vigour, energy and libido; and a better appetite. Particularly impressive was the diminished joint pain in those with osteoarthritis. Five per cent dropped out of the study, however, complaining of burning urine, bleeding piles, flatulence and irritability. Eating raw garlic elicited more complaints than eating it cooked.

Worldwide, eating garlic is linked to less heart disease. A 1981 study of the diets of 15 countries by researchers at the University of Western Ontario found that those nations with higher garlic consumption had lower rates of heart disease.

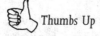 Thumbs Up

DISCOVER THE NUTTY HEART DRUGS

Eat a few nuts a day as an antidote to heart disease, suggests Gary Fraser, Ph.D., professor of medicine at Loma Linda (California) University. In a study of 31,208 Seventh-Day Adventists, Dr. Fraser found that nuts stood out as the number-one food among those who did not suffer heart attacks. Those who munched on nuts at least five times a week had roughly *half the chance of heart attack and coronary death* as those who ate nuts less than once a week. Even snacking on nuts once a week appeared to cut heart disease risk about 25 per cent. About 32 per cent of the nuts consumed were peanuts, 29 per cent almonds, 16 per cent walnuts and 23 per cent other nuts.

It's not as zany as it may seem. Nuts are rich in fibre and monounsaturated olive-oil type fats, known to counteract heart disease. Nuts are also packed with various antioxidants, including vitamin E, selenium (especially Brazil nuts) and ellagic acid (notably walnuts), that could guard arteries against the ravages of cholesterol. Since nuts are high in fat, although most is beneficial fat, you can't eat nuts with abandon if you are concerned about weight. In Dr. Fraser's study, however, enthusiastic nut-eaters were less obese than non-nut eaters. Dr. Fraser did not determine how many nuts people ate at one time. A sensible amount, depending on a person's weight, would be 1–2oz (30–55g) a day.

THE ITALIAN EXPERIMENT

What do Italian women eat who do and don't have heart attacks? To find out, Italian investigators at the Instituto di Ricerche Farmacologiche Mario Negri in Milan analysed the diets of 936 older women.

They found hat women who ate the most carrots and fresh fruit had a 60 per cent lower chance of heart attack; those who ate the most green vegetables and fish had a 40 per cent lower risk. Moderate alcohol consumption also reduced the risk 30 per cent, but heavy drinking increased it 20 per cent. Women with the highest risk ate more meat, specifically ham and salami, butter and total fat.

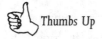 Thumbs Up

USE VEGETABLE POWER TO BLOCK HEART ATTACKS

Devouring fruits and vegetables can slash your chances of heart attacks and strokes, even if you have already suffered one. Unquestionably, dedicated fruit- and vegetable-eaters have better arteries. Vegetarians have the lowest rates of cardiovascular disease. Women who ate one additional large carrot or 4½oz (130g) of sweet potatoes (or other foods rich in beta carotene) every day slashed their risk of heart attack by 22 per cent and stroke by 40–70 per cent, according to recent Harvard studies.

Fruits and vegetables are also a good post-heart attack prescription. If you survive a heart attack, eating fruits and vegetables can save you from another cardiac event and death even better than just cutting back on high-fat meats and dairy foods, a recent year-long study of 400 heart attack patients in India found. Doctors put half the heart attack survivors on a standard low-fat diet, the other half on an "experimental" diet heavy on fruits, grains, nuts, legumes, fish and vegetables. Specifically, the diet called for about 14oz (400g) of fruits and vegetables a day. (This included guava, grapes, papaya, bananas, oranges, limes, apples, spinach, radishes, tomatoes, lotus root, mushrooms, onions, garlic, fenugreek seeds, peas and red beans.)

After a year, the fruit and vegetable eaters had had 40 per cent fewer cardiac events and 45 per cent fewer deaths from all causes than the low-fat eaters. The researchers concluded that if everyone immediately went on a high fruit-and-vegetable diet after a heart attack, countless lives could be saved. Important: For best results, a heart attack victim should get on the vegetarian-type diet as quickly as possible. In the Indian study, the diet was commenced within 72 hours of the attack.

Additionally, a recent Dutch study of heart patients found that switching to a vegetarian, low-saturated fat, low-cholesterol diet for two years both halted and reversed arterial damage.

The most likely explanation is that the vegetable carotenes and other antioxidants in fruits and vegetables help keep arteries unclogged and healthy, say researchers.

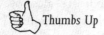 Thumbs Up

TRY THE JAPANESE HEART-SAVING DIET

Eat like the Japanese used to. For years, that country's low-fat, high-fish diet was a model for a heart-disease-free life, but with the invasion of westernized high-fat fast food, Japan's heart-disease rate is creeping upward. In 1957 Ancel Keys, then a professor at the University of Minnesota, began tracking heart-disease rates in seven countries: the United States, Finland, the Netherlands, Italy, Yugoslavia, Greece and Japan. He discovered that Western countries generally had five times more fatal heart disease than Japan, which had the lowest of all. For example, eastern Finland had the most heart disease, about eight times more than Japan. Striking was the fact that the Japanese ate only 9 per cent of calories in fat with only 3 per cent from animal fat, whereas the Finns' diet was 39 per cent fat with 22 per cent from animal fat.

Although the classic heart-saving Japanese diet is disappearing, University of Helsinki researchers recently interviewed Japanese villagers who said they still followed the traditional diet of their ancestors. This is what they ate on an average day: $1^{1}/_{2}$–2lbs (675-900g) of cooked rice, 5–8oz (140–225g) of fruit, about 9oz (255g) of vegetables, 2oz (55g) of beans, about 2oz (55g) of meat, 3–4oz (85–115g) of fish, 4fl oz (115ml) of milk, one egg or less, two teaspoons of sugar, one and one-half tablespoons of soya sauce. The men also drank 15fl oz (425ml) of beer, the women only a trace of beer.

Thus the classic Japanese diet is low in calories, fat and meat and high in fish, fruit, vegetables and rice. The one blot on the diet is excessive sodium, largely from soya sauce, which is partially blamed for their high rate of strokes. If you restrict the sodium, eating like the Japanese once did seems an excellent way to escape heart disease.

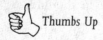 Thumbs Up

WHY MEDITERRANEAN PEOPLES HAVE BETTER HEARTS

Adopt the diet of people who live around the Mediterranean Sea, particularly in Greece, Italy, Spain and southern France. Such people are only half as likely to die of heart disease as Americans. Indeed, some researchers are convinced the Mediterranean diet is a more agreeable way to save hearts than is a lower-fat diet, generally advocated by health officials. No, the Mediterranean diet is not low-fat; in fact, Mediterraneans typically eat more fat than Americans do but there is a big difference. About three-quarters of all their fat calories come from monounsaturated fat, exemplified by olive oil; they also eat very little saturated animal fat. For example, residents of the island of Crete sometimes drink olive oil by the glass, running up their quota of calories from fat to over 40 per cent. Yet Dr. Keys found, in his landmark "Seven Countries Study," that Cretans rarely succumbed to heart disease. In a 15-year period only 38 out of 10,000 Cretans died of heart disease compared with 773 Americans, giving the United States 20 times as much deadly heart disease as Crete. Other Mediterranean populations also had low rates.

Here's the clincher: The most enthusiastic consumers of olive-oil-type fat among the Mediterranean peoples were least likely to die of cancer or anything else! Using "monos" as the major source of fat was the only dietary factor, according to Dr. Keys, that warded off death from all causes. No wonder olive oil is sometimes called the "longevity food".

FOODS HIGHEST IN ARTERY-PROTECTING FATS

	Percentage of fat as monounsaturated
Hazelnuts	81
Avocados	80
Olive oil	72
Almonds	71
Rapeseed oil	60

• BOTTOM LINE • *A relatively high-fat diet does not seem hazardous to the heart if it is very low in animal fat and high in olive-oil-type fat. A vocal group of Harvard physicians, in fact, favour a Mediterranean-style diet with 35–40 per cent of fat calories, mostly in monounsaturated fat, over the more restrictive 30-per-cent-of-calories-in-fat diet recommended as ideal by government heart officials.*

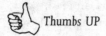 *Thumbs UP*

EAT OLIVE OIL: THE HEART-SAFE FAT

What makes monounsaturated fat, dominant in olive oil, better for the heart? Chemically, it is simply nicer to arteries. It lowers bad LDL cholesterol, but not good HDL cholesterol. Additionally, monoun–saturated fat has antioxidant activity that fends off artery damage from LDL cholesterol. In Italy, physicians have used olive oil as therapy after heart attacks. They find that such patients have better blood profiles, making them less vulnerable to future heart attacks. Further, Harvard's Dr. Walter Willett says, there are "centuries of epidemiological evidence about the benefits of olive oil".

Another reason olive oil is close to the hearts of health authorities is that nobody has found any danger in it. "It's the only really safe fat," insists Harry Demopoulos, M.D., a New York researcher on antioxidants. Monounsaturated fat is also concentrated in almond, hazelnut, rapeseed and avocado oils.

Note: Extra virgin, cold-pressed olive oil is best.

"In the [Mediterranean diet] olive oil is a major source of energy, fat averages 35–40 per cent of total calories, and rates of coronary disease are as low as in populations with very low-fat diets." – Frank Sacks, M.D., Harvard School of Public Health

---

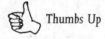 *Thumbs Up*

MORE HEART SECRETS OF THE MEDITERRANEAN DIET

Olive oil can't claim entire credit for healthy hearts among Mediterranean dwellers. Their diet also differs in other significant ways. To imitate the Mediterranean diet, here's what the typical American would have to do:

• double seafood intake
• increase vegetable consumption by 66 per cent and fruit by 10 per cent

- eat 20 per cent more whole grains and beans
- eat 45 per cent less red meat
- eat 16 per cent fewer eggs
- eat four times as much olive oil
- eat half as much of other vegetable oils
- eat 50 per cent less whole milk, cream and butterfat

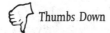 Thumbs Down

SURE WAY TO POISON ARTERIES

Shun animal fat. It is the real dietary demon in heart disease. It destroys arteries by raising blood cholesterol, encouraging blood stickiness and suppressing clot-dissolving mechanisms, leaving arteries clogged and constricted. Populations who eat a lot of animal fat have the highest rates of coronary heart disease in the world. As intake of animal fat goes up, so does heart disease. A 1990 World Health Organization report observes that populations eating from 3–10 per cent of their total calories in animal fat have little heart disease. Eating more saturated fat brings on "marked and progressive" fatal heart disease. In the United States and other Western countries, saturated fat often accounts for a deadly 15–20 per cent of calories.

Other good news is that you can reverse your mistakes and help unclog arteries by giving up animal fat. Several studies show that restricting fat, namely animal fat, can help block formation and growth of fatty deposits that clog arteries and may even help shrink such fatty buildup. David H. Blankenhorn, M.D., at the University of Southern California School of Medicine, who found such a low-fat diet (5 per cent of calories in saturated fat) successful in coronary bypass patients, said most people can save their arteries from animal-fat destruction by simply "substituting low-fat dairy products for high-fat dairy products."

"If I had to tell people just one thing to lower their risk of heart disease, it would be to reduce their intake of foods of animal origin, specifically animal fats, and to replace those fats with complex carbohydrates — grains, fruits and vegetables." – Ernst Schaefer, M.D., USDA Human Nutrition Research Center on Aging at Tufts University

---

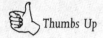Thumbs Up

A TOT A DAY KEEPS THE DOCTOR AWAY

Drink alcohol moderately, if you drink. A drink or two a day discourages heart disease, according to a couple of dozen studies. One study declared two-drink-a-day imbibers 40 per cent less likely than nondrinkers to be hospitalized for heart attacks. A major 1991 study by Eric Rimm at the Harvard University School of Public Health, showed that men who averaged one-half to one drink a day had 21 per cent less coronary artery disease than abstainers. One to one-and-a-half daily drinks shaved 32 per cent off their heart disease odds. Heavier drinking might depress heart disease odds even further, but the problem is more than two drinks a day puts you in high risk territory for other diseases.

"The maximum safe dose of alcohol is two drinks a day," says William Castelli, M.D., director of the Framingham Heart Study. Studies consistently find, he says, that the risk of heart disease falls slightly with one to two daily drinks, but that your chances of death from all causes, including cancer, rise with three drinks a day. One study showed that three to five alcoholic drinks a day increased death rates 50 per cent.

Some possible reasons for alcohol's heart benefits: alcohol boosts good type HDL cholesterol; wine, notably red wine, is an anticoagulant; alcohol relieves stress, and alcoholic beverages contain antioxidants.

"There is no other drug that is so efficient [at preventing heart attacks] as the moderate intake of alcohol." – Serge Renaud, M.D., a French researcher

---

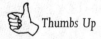Thumbs Up

STOUT-HEARTED FRENCHMEN – IS IT THE WINE?

Given the choice of an alcoholic beverage for the heart and health in general, it should probably be wine, a medicine dating back more than four thousand years. According to R. Curtis Ellison, M.D., chief of the Department of Preventive Medicine and Epidemiology at the Boston

University School of Medicine, research suggests wine reduces cardio-vascular disease better than distilled spirits or beer. The French are particularly keen on this idea.

Curiously, Frenchmen have one-third as many heart attacks as American men, even though the French indulge in fatty foods and have cholesterol and blood pressure as high as American men. This so-called "French paradox," some scientists suggest, is explained by the French habit of drinking wine, especially red wine, with meals. Dr. Alun Evans, of Queens University in Belfast, notes that Frenchmen have one-third fewer heart attacks than Irishmen. Both drink the same amount of alcohol, but there's one big difference, he says. The French mainly drink wine; the Irish drink more spirits.

It is true that some red wine, notably Bordeaux, acts as an anticoagulant. Thus, French health authorities suggest that wine consumed along with fatty meals *counteracts* the fat hazard. Fatty foods tend to make the blood more sluggish so it is likely to clot and plug up arteries. Wine may thwart that process. The scientists caution the wine drinking should be regular and "moderate – no more than two to three 4fl oz (115ml) glasses of wine a day".

However, white wine may also work in a different fashion to help ward off heart disease, according to research by Dr. Arthur Klatsky at Kaiser Permanente Medical Center in Oakland, California. In a major 10-year study of about 82,000 men and women, he concluded that all alcoholic beverages in moderation seem to discourage heart disease, and wine appeared better than beer and spirits in doing so. He did not find red wine more protective than white wine.

• BOTTOM LINE • *If you already drink and have no problems with alcohol, a drink or two a day on a regular basis may help protect your heart. More alcohol is dangerous, and binge-drinking is particularly harmful to your heart and general health. If you don't drink, do not take up drinking as a way to prevent cardiovascular disease. If you are a heavy drinker, cut down. Alcohol in heavy doses is definitely a heart poison, capable of inducing severe heart damage and sudden death.*

DOES COFFEE PROMOTE HEART DISEASE?

There's scant evidence that you need to give up coffee or caffeine to save your heart, although it may be wise for some people at high risk of heart disease to restrict their intake. A 1992 analysis of 11 major studies on the subject by Martin G. Myers, M.D., of the University of Toronto found no link between coffee consumption and heart disease whether subjects drank one cup or more than six cups a day.

On the other hand, a ten-year follow-up study of more than 100,000 individuals by Kaiser Permanente's Dr. Klatsky suggested that four or more cups of coffee a day boosted heart disease chances about 30 per cent in men and up to 60 per cent in women. There was no danger in tea, suggesting caffeine is not the culprit. Dr. Klatsky advises individuals at high risk of heart disease to limit coffee intake to less than four cups a day. Another recent study found that drinking 10 or more cups of coffee a day tripled the risk of heart disease.

What about switching to decaf? There is no evidence, however, that caffeinated coffee is worse for your heart than decaf coffee. In fact, the reverse may be true. A Harvard study of 45,000 men in 1990 found no higher odds of heart disease or stroke from coffee, tea or total caffeine intake. It did find decaf drinkers at slightly higher risk, forcing researchers to see "little merit in switching from caffeinated to decaf coffee" to ward off heart disease.

"For people drinking up to six cups of coffee a day there is no strong reason to give it up, and particularly no strong reason to switch to decaf." – Walter Willett, M.D., Harvard School of Public Health

---

WHAT TO EAT IF YOU HAVE CHEST PAIN (ANGINA)

Chest pain, or angina, is a warning sign that arteries are getting too narrow or partially blocked so oxygen and blood cannot flow through easily. Such narrowing is usually due to atherosclerosis, an accumulation of plaque in the coronary arteries that take oxygen to the heart muscle. It also can result from heart spasms.

Chest pain is linked to low blood levels of the antioxidants vitamin E, vitamin C and beta carotene – and omega-3 fish oil. Thus to alleviate angina, eat more fruits, vegetables, oily fish, cereals, nuts and vegetable oils rich in vitamin E, advises researcher Rudolph A. Riemersma, M.D., at the University of Edinburgh. In a major study of 500 middle-aged men – half with angina – Dr. Riemersma found chest pain least likely in those with higher-than-average blood levels of carotene, vitamin C and particularly vitamin E. Indeed, men with the lowest blood levels of vitamin E were two and a half times more likely to suffer angina than those with the highest levels of vitamin E. Presumably, the vitamin's antioxidant activity discourages arterial damage and clogging. In further research, Dr. Riemersma found that men with higher blood-platelet levels of one type of fish oil, known as EPA, were similarly protected from angina.

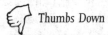 Thumbs Down

ALCOHOL PROMOTES ANGINA

In 1786 the English physician William Heberden recommended alcohol to treat angina and so have many doctors since then but alcohol probably does more harm than good. Current research suggests that alcohol actually brings on angina in patients with pre-existing coronary artery disease.

In one test, Joan Orlando, M.D., and colleagues in Long Beach, California, gave 12 middle-aged men with angina three to four alcoholic drinks (2–5oz (55–140g) of alcohol) and then, an hour later, had them exercise. Chest pain set in much earlier when the men drank the alcohol and exercised than when they drank no alcohol. In fact, they could exercise an average 10–15 minutes longer before angina struck when they did not drink. Drinking also induced an abnormally rapid increase in heart rate and systolic blood pressure in connection with the exercise.

IRREGULAR HEARTBEATS: IS COFFEE A CAUSE?

If you suffer from arrhythmias – irregular heartbeats – it seems wise to restrict caffeine, but you may not need to give it up entirely. Dr. Martin G. Myers, at the University of Toronto, analysed 23 recent studies on the connection between caffeine and heart arrhythmia, and found no evidence that less than 500mg of caffeine – about five cups of coffee a day – increased the frequency or severity of cardiac arrhythmias in normal persons or in patients with heart problems.

Still, some experts think it a good idea to drink only a couple of cups of coffee a day if you have irregular heartbeats. Harvard investigator Thomas B. Graboys gave subjects with life-threatening ventricular arrhythmias caffeine tablets comparable to drinking two cups of coffee and then had them pedal stationary bicycles for five minutes every hour for three hours. Their heart rhythms did not change, whether they had taken the caffeine or placebo pills. Dr. Graboys says: "To categorically proscribe all caffeine for someone with arrhythmia doesn't make sense. There's no reason they can't have one or two cups of coffee."

On the other hand, high doses of caffeine, as found in nine or ten cups of coffee, can aggravate pre-existing ventricular arrhythmias. Further, heartbeat irregularities may be exaggerated in individuals particularly sensitive to caffeine. Recent research at the Oregon Health Sciences University found that the amount of caffeine in two and a half cups of coffee more easily induced severe ventricular arrhythmias in a select population of "caffeine sensitive" individuals. To be extra safe, they advise heart-disease patients to limit coffee to two cups a day.

"At three or more drinks [of alcohol] a day, you don't see adverse coronary effects, but you do see increases in high blood pressure, cirrhosis of the liver, throat cancer, accidents, hospitalizations and mortality." – Arthur L. Klatsky, chief of cardiology, Kaiser Permanente Medical Center, Oakland, California

---

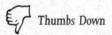 Thumbs Down

HOLIDAY HEART SYNDROME

Can alcohol cause heartbeat disturbances? Decidedly yes, whether you are an alcoholic or casual drinker, say authorities. Alcohol-induced arrhythmias frequently cause sudden cardiac death among alcoholics.

It's so common, for example, in emergency rooms to see people with severe arrhythmias after alcoholic binges on weekends and holidays, particularly between Christmas Eve and New Year's Day, that the problem has been dubbed "holiday heart syndrome". This type of fibrillation or flutter usually vanishes when the alcohol effects wear off, leaving no signs of permanent heart damage. Although it's more common among alcoholics or long-time heavy drinkers, holiday heart syndrome can also strike occasional or moderate drinkers who embark on a drinking binge.

Clearly, heavy drinking boosts your chances of cardiac arrest as well as stroke. One study found that 40 per cent of women who suffered sudden death were diagnosed as alcoholics. According to the well-known Framingham Heart Study, persons who consumed more than five or six drinks a day were more likely to die of sudden death even though they did not show signs of coronary artery disease.

The longer and harder you drink, the more susceptible you are to cardiovascular damage. Cutting down on alcohol consumption often diminishes arrhythmia.

DIET ADVICE TO KEEP THE CARDIOLOGIST AWAY

- The number-one advice to keep heart disease away has to be: eat more fatty fish, high in omega-3 fatty acids – at least 1oz (30g) a day or a fish serving two or three times a week.
- Also go heavy on garlic, onions and all kinds of other vegetables and fruits to keep plenty of antioxidants in the blood, as well as anticoagulants that protect arteries from clogging.
- Shun fatty animal foods, such as high-fat meat and dairy products.
- Use olive oil and rapeseed oil.
- Such advice is doubly important if you have already had a cardiovascular problem. "Second-chance diets" can intervene to prevent further damage to arteries, staving off subsequent heart attacks, strokes and other cardiovascular events.
- If you drink alcohol, a regular dose of a drink or two a day, especially of wine with meals, may act as antidotes to heart disease, but if you do not already use alcohol, do not start drinking, because the dangers can well outweigh the benefits. If you drink more than two drinks a day, cut down. Heavy drinking harms your heart and your general health and boosts chances of death.
- Restrict coffee to a couple of cups a day if you have heartbeat irregularities. There is no known advantage in switching to decaf to prevent heart disease.

CHOLESTEROL

Foods That Can Help Control Cholesterol: Beans • Oats • Apples • Carrots • Olive Oil • Avocados • Almonds • Walnuts • Garlic • Onions • Seafood, Especially Fatty Fish • Fruits and Vegetables Rich in Vitamin C, Beta Carotene • Grains High in Soluble Fibre • Moderate Alcohol

Foods That Can Increase Harmful Cholesterol: High-Saturated-Fat and High-Cholesterol Foods

Cholesterol – that yellow, waxy, fatty stuff – in your blood is one reason your arteries become depositories for biological muck called plaque that narrows the blood vessels and shortens the gap between you and heart disease. Yet cholesterol is not a simple matter. Some components of cholesterol are dangerous to arteries, while others are beneficial. Furthermore, what you eat may actually detoxify detrimental cholesterol so it cannot harm arteries. Regardless of cholesterol's complexities, one thing is undeniable: What you eat can put a striking dent in dangerous cholesterol and, more spectacularly, according to new findings, change its character so it is not so deadly!

This radical new way of controlling cholesterol by detoxifying it, according to new research, promises to slow dramatically the pro–gression of atherosclerosis by 50–70 per cent and even help reverse existing artery clogging by shrinking the clumps of plaque on artery walls, says leading researcher Daniel Steinberg, M.D., at the University of California School of Medicine in San Diego. "We can now attack the disease at the artery wall as well as by simply lowering cholesterol. It's very exciting," he says.

HOW YOU CAN USE FOOD TO CONTROL CHOLESTEROL

Essentially, you should eat in a way to lower one type of cholesterol, called LDL (low-density lipoprotein), and boost another type, known as

HDL (high-density lipoprotein). That's because the LDLs are "bad-guys" that serve as raw material to clog arteries. In contrast, the "good-guy" HDLs gobble up the LDL "villains" and cart them to the liver, where they are annihilated. Obviously, the more HDL and the less LDL you have in your blood, the safer your arteries. Certain foods help bring this about by destroying detrimental LDLs and creating beneficial HDLs.

Now enters an exciting new theory that promises to make it possible to control cholesterol with food in ways unimagined even a few years ago. According to that new theory put forth by Dr. Steinberg and many others, here's how arteries get clogged. Special forms of oxygen known as free radicals in the blood collide with fatty LDL cholesterol molecules, oxidizing them. The LDL then turns rancid, much as unrefrigerated butter does. In this altered form it is quickly gobbled up by cells called macrophages. Stuffed with fat globules, the macrophages enlarge into dreaded "foam cells," which insinuate themselves into artery walls, triggering artery destruction. If you can prevent this toxic transformation, your LDL cholesterol may remain relatively harmless. So the issue is not just how much LDL cholesterol your blood contains, but how much of it is "toxic oxidized LDL," capable of clogging your arteries. Dr. Steinberg and many others now believe that LDL cholesterol is not so dangerous to arteries unless it is converted into a toxic form by oxygen free radicals in your blood.

That's where diet can be a powerful weapon. Mounting evidence shows you can block LDL's toxic transformation, and thus its awesome hazards, by eating foods packed with protective antioxidants. This means you might intervene at the very *genesis of atherosclerosis* at every stage of life, blocking the cascade of arterial events that create clogged arteries, heart attacks and strokes. It is a thrilling prospect.

• BOTTOM LINE • *To combat hazardous blood cholesterol, reduce bad LDL cholesterol, boost good HDL cholesterol, and keep as much as possible of your LDL from becoming toxic to your arteries. Here are your best bets for doing it with diet.*

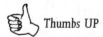 Thumbs UP

MAGIC BEANS

Eat dried beans or legumes. They are one of nature's cheapest, most widely available, fastest-acting and safest cholesterol-fighting drugs. They consistently strike down high cholesterol, studies show. According to James Anderson, M.D., of the University of Kentucky College of Medicine, eating 6oz (170g) of cooked dried beans a day generally suppresses bad cholesterol about 20 per cent. You can expect results in three weeks or so. All types of beans work – pintos, black, navy, kidney, lentils, chickpeas, soya beans – even plain old canned baked beans. In one test 6oz (170g) of Campbell's canned baked beans depressed cholesterol 12 per cent in middle-aged men with high cholesterol who ate a typical high-fat American diet.

6oz (170g) of beans a day (12oz (340g) of baked beans) also drives up good HDLs about 9 per cent, not immediately, but usually after a year or two. Beans improve the critical HDL/LDL cholesterol ratio by 17 per cent, according to one test. Dr. Anderson's advice: For best results spread the beans out during the day: for example, eat 3oz (85g) at lunch, another 3oz (85g) at night. Beans contain at least six cholesterol-cutting compounds; the main one may be soluble fibre.

Don't forget soya beans. They, too, are potent cholesterol-reducers, according to numerous studies done throughout the world. Typical is a recent study by University of Illinois scientist John Erdman showing that cholesterol dropped an average 12 per cent in subjects eating food fortified with soya ingredients. In fact, in Dr. Erdman's study, soya protein was declared the most effective dietary way to suppress cholesterol. The secret is in the soya protein, found in such foods as whole and split soya beans, soya milk, tofu, textured soya protein and tempeh, but not in soya sauce and soya bean oil.

"Most people can lower cholesterol by eating 2oz (55g) of oat bran cereal or 6oz (170g) of beans per day." – James Anderson, M.D., University of Kentucky School of Medicine

---

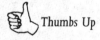Thumbs Up

---

OAT POWER

Eat oats to drive down cholesterol. Dutch scientists discovered the anti-cholesterol power of oats three decades ago, and it's now been confirmed by 23 out of 25 studies, says Michael C. Davidson, M.D., assistant professor of cardiology at Rush-Presbyterian-St Luke's Medical Center in Chicago. Nor does it take fantastic amounts. "A medium-sized bowl of cooked oat bran or a large bowl of oatmeal did the job," Dr. Davidson reported in a recent study. Indeed, he concluded that the biggest dose you ever need to eat is 2oz (55g) of oat bran a day. That amount reduced detrimental cholesterol 16 per cent in those eating a low-fat diet. Half that much – 1oz (30g) cut cholesterol 10 per cent. However, shovelling in 3oz (85g) of oat bran daily *did not lower cholesterol further.*

Oatmeal worked, too, but it takes twice as much oatmeal as oat bran for the same impact. Most telling, says Dr. Davidson, was the fact oats lowered cholesterol enough to save one-third of the group from potent cholesterol-lowering drugs. Even 2oz (55g) of instant oats a day depressed high blood cholesterol by 6 per cent after two months, according to another study.

You can also expect a big bowl of oat bran daily to boost good HDL cholesterol about 15 per cent after two or three months, says Dr. Anderson.

Oats' main cholesterol-busting substance is beta glucans, a soluble gummy fibre that gels in the intestinal tract. This interferes with the absorption and production of cholesterol, so more of it is removed from the bloodstream.

OAT BRAN MYSTERIES: *WHAT YOU NEED TO KNOW*

Oats work better on some people than on others. Some studies find large cholesterol drops of up to 20 per cent, others, a modest three or four per cent. One widely publicized Harvard study declared that oats had zero effect. Here are possible reasons for the variations in research findings.

1.   Commercial oat brans vary widely in their content of soluble fibre namely beta glucans, and thus in pharmacological power. Tests show typical soluble fibre percentages in oat brans range from 8–28 per cent but some have little or no beta glucans – the main active agent, says Gene Spiller, Ph.D., a noted fibre researcher and director of the Health Research and Studies Center in California. Thus they don't work. His advice: If "soluble fibre" content is noted on the label, choose an oat bran with the most or stick with oatmeal; it always contains some beta glucans, he says.

2.   Oat bran, like any pharmacological agent, affects individuals differently. Wendy Demark-Wahnefried, Ph.D., now at Duke University, found that men and women eating 1.7oz (48g) of cooked oat bran or 1.5oz (40g) of Quaker's cold oat-bran cereal daily, had average dips in cholesterol of 10–17 per cent.. Still, 33 per cent of the oat-bran eaters and 27 per cent on low-fat diets had no cholesterol drops at all. In

contrast, cholesterol fell an astonishing 2.08 to 2.6 points in others. The message, says Dr. Demark-Wahnefried, is that oats, like other natural or man-made drugs, are not a universal panacea. If it works for you – it can make a tremendous difference. The only way to find out is to try it.

3. If your cholesterol is high – above 5.98 – the more likely oats are to bring it down. (The same applies to beans and other high-soluble fibre foods.) Oats do not cut cholesterol substantially if it is already normal or fairly low – "in those who don't need it," says Dr. Anderson. Also, oats depress cholesterol even in those eating a typical American high-fat diet. In one study, 2oz (55g) daily of oat bran reduced bad LDL cholesterol 8.5 per cent in men with high cholesterol (5.46–8.45) who ate an extravagant 41 per cent of calories from fat.

4. Oat power may vary with age and gender. Young women sometimes get virtually no cholesterol reduction from oats, while older women often have "a marked drop in cholesterol," concluded a recent review. Men of all ages seem to get intermediate effects.

• BOTTOM LINE • *If your cholesterol is high – over 5.98 – daily oat bran is likely to lower it. If it is already low, oats will probably do zilch. Also you can't expect additional benefits from eating more than 2oz (55g) oat bran or 31/2oz (100g) dry oatmeal a day, according to a review of the evidence by Cynthia M. Ripsin of the University of Minnesota.*

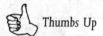 Thumbs Up

A GARLLC CLOVE A DAY

Eat garlic if you are concerned about cholesterol. About 20 published human tests show that fresh garlic and some garlic preparations reduce cholesterol. According to Robert Lin, Ph.D., chairman of a recent international conference on the health aspects of garlic, three fresh garlic cloves a day can lower cholesterol an average 10 per cent and up to 15 per cent in some people. (Of course, less works to a lesser degree.) It does not matter whether the garlic is cooked or raw, he says. It is effective both ways. Fully six compounds in garlic have been identified that lower cholesterol by suppressing the liver's synthesis of cholesterol.

"The humble garlic clove is increasingly being shown to have exciting potential as a safe prophylactic for everyday use against cardiovascular risk factors." – British physician J. Grunwald

---

In a recent controlled test, at L.T.M. Medical College in Bombay, 50 subjects who ate three raw garlic cloves every morning for two months saw their cholesterol drop about 15 per cent – down from an average 5.54 to 4.68. Their blood clotting factors also improved dramatically. In another study, at Bastyr College in Seattle, a daily dose of garlic oil from three fresh garlic cloves drove cholesterol down 7 per cent in a month, but, more important, raised good-type HDL 23 per cent!

NOTE: *Fresh garlic, cooked or raw, as well as pickled garlic can improve cholesterol. Ordinary garlic powder and garlic salt sold in supermarkets are therapeutically worthless.*

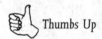 Thumbs Up

HALF AN ONION A DAY

Raw onion is one of the best treatments for boosting beneficial HDL cholesterol. Half a raw onion, or the equivalent in juice, raises HDLs an average 30 per cent in most people with heart disease or cholesterol problems, according to Victor Gurewich, a cardiologist and professor of medicine at Harvard Medical School. Dr. Gurewich got the onion tip from folklore medicine and started testing it in his clinic. It was so successful he advises all his patients to eat onions. The more you cook the onions, however, the more they lose their HDL-raising powers. (Cooked onions fight heart disease in other ways.) Dr. Gurewich does not know which chemicals in onions boost HDLs. He says it could be one or more of hundreds. The onion therapy works in about 70 per cent of patients. If you can't eat half a raw onion a day, eat less. Any amount may help lift all-important HDLs.

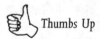 Thumbs Up

HIGH ON SALMON

To boost beneficial HDLs, eat fatty fish, like salmon and mackerel, full of omega-3 fatty acids. They can hike HDLs, even if they are already normal. In a test, men with normal cholesterol feasted on salmon for lunch and dinner for about 40 days. Their HDLs shot up. Most important, according to study director Gary J. Nelson, Ph.D., of the U.S. Department of Agriculture's Western Human Nutrition Research Center in San Francisco, one particular lifesaving fraction of HDL jumped an average 10 per cent. He says this particular HDL fraction is closely linked to thwarting heart disease. Moreover, the HDL hike came within 20 days! The results were surprisingly rapid, says Dr. Nelson, indicating a quick cholesterol and heart dividend from eating fatty fish.

How much salmon? The men ate "the maximum dose" – about 1lb (450g) of fresh salmon a day – high doses are standard to detect an effect but less would also boost HDLs to a lesser degree, says Dr. Nelson. Moreover, if your HDLs are subnormal, you can expect even higher rises from eating fish. Since the active agent is thought to be omega-3 fatty acids, other oil-rich fish (mackerel, herring, sardines, tuna) would similarly drive up HDLs. The salmon also depressed triglycerides, as eating fatty fish usually does.

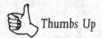 Thumbs Up

OLIVE OIL DOES IT ALL

It's hard to rave enough about the bountiful benefits of olive oil to arteries and cholesterol. It is a triple saviour. Olive oil both cuts bad LDL cholesterol and slightly raises or keeps good HDL the same, improving your heart-saving HDL/LDL ratio. In contrast, oils such as corn, soya bean, safflower and sunflower lower both good HDL and detrimental LDL. A major study even declared olive oil superior to the standard r ecommended low-fat diet in combating cholesterol. When subjects ate 41 per cent of their calories in fat, most of it from olive oil, their bad LDL cholesterol sank more than when they ate a diet with half as much fat. Additionally, good HDLs rose on the olive-oil diet and sank on the low-fat diet.

The clincher is that olive oil also helps defuse bad-type cholesterol, rendering it less capable of destroying arteries. Studies by the University of California's Dr. Daniel Steinberg, as well as by researchers in Israel, find that olive oil dramatically thwarts toxic oxidation of LDL cholesterol. In a landmark study, Dr. Steinberg and colleagues gave one group of healthy volunteers about 40 per cent of their calories in mono– unsaturated fat, equal to about 3 tablespoons of olive oil a day. Others ate regular safflower oil low in monounsaturated fatty acids, then researchers examined the bad-type LDL cholesterol from both groups. Remarkably, the LDL of the monounsaturated oil eaters *was only half as likely to become oxidized and thus able to clog arteries!* This does not mean you should swill down olive oil but it does suggest that when you eat fat, the olive-oil monounsaturated type is a good choice to forestall artery clogging.

"From many surveys on the island of Crete, I have the impression that centenarians are common among farmers, whose breakfast is often only a wineglass of olive oil."
– Dr. Ancel Keys, renowned epidemiologist

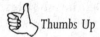 Thumbs Up

RAVES FOR ALMONDS AND WALNUTS

How could nuts be good for cholesterol? Aren't they high in fat? Yes, but, again, it is mostly monounsaturated fat, known to depress cholesterol and discourage LDL from oxidizing. Dr. Gene Spiller had men and women with fairly high cholesterol, averaging around 6.24, eat 3½oz (100g) of almonds a day for three to nine weeks. Others ate equal amounts of fat from cheese or olive oil.

The average cholesterol of the almond eaters sank 10 to 15 per cent compared to that of the cheese eaters. The almonds worked as well as olive oil. This makes sense, says Dr. Spiller, because most of the fat in almonds and olive oil is chemically identical. Thus if olive oil is good for the heart, as much research shows, so is almond oil.

Walnuts work, too, according to new research by Dr. Joan Sabate of Loma Linda University. She studied subjects with normal blood cholesterol. All were on a low-fat diet, but for one month they ate 20 per cent of their calories in walnuts (about 2oz (55g) of walnuts in a daily 1,800 calorie diet). For another month, they ate no nuts. On the no-nuts diet, their cholesterol dropped an average 6 per cent but on the walnut-eating regimen, their cholesterol fell 18 per cent! Average cholesterol dropped 0.57 points. Thus, walnuts added a cholesterol-reducing wallop even to an ordinary low-fat diet. As Dr. William Castelli of the Framingham Heart Study observed: "It looks like folks on nuts will do better than everyone else."

Both Drs. Spiller and Sabate, however, caution you not to eat so many nuts you gain weight. (Nuts have about 170 calories per oz/600 calories per 100g.) The point is to eat a few nuts a day as a substitute for other sources of fat and calories. "It's an easy way to improve cholesterol," says Dr. Sabate.

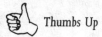 Thumbs Up

AVOCADOS, YES!

It's surprising but true that eating avocados can decidedly lower your cholesterol. Avocados have rich concentrations of the same type cholesterol-improving fat as almonds and olive oil. Israeli investigators recently found that three months of eating avocados, as well as almonds and olive oil, cut detrimental LDL cholesterol about 12 per cent in a group of men. Australian cardiologists at the Wesley Medical Centre in Queensland recently found that eating avocados (one half to one and a half avocados a day) beat out a low-fat diet in reducing cholesterol. In their test, 15 women ate a high-carbohydrate, low-fat diet (20 per cent fat calories) and an avocado high-fat diet (37 per cent fat calories) each for three weeks. The raw avocados were put in salads or spread on bread or crackers.

The results: Average cholesterol dipped 4.9 per cent on the low-fat diet compared with nearly twice as much – 8.2 per cent – on the avocado diet. Most alarming, the low-fat diet wiped out good HDL cholesterol, lowering it a whopping 14 per cent, but did not lower bad LDL cholesterol. Very-low-fat diets often do this. In contrast, the avocados attacked only detrimental LDLs. Investigators noted that avocados also protected arteries against oxidative damage that makes cholesterol dangerous.

• BOTTOM LINE • *Although olive oil, almonds and avocados are high in fat, most of it is monounsaturated fat that tends to improve cholesterol and dramatically protect rather than destroy arteries.*

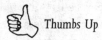 Thumbs Up

CURE YOUR CHOLESTEROL WITH STRAWBERRIES

Give your blood an injection of vitamin C, vitamin E and other antioxidants by eating fruits and vegetables. They are anticholesterol superfoods. Vitamin C combats cholesterol dangers two important ways. It acts as a bodyguard for HDLs that constantly cleanse your arteries of the bad stuff. Both vitamins C and E are potent at blocking transformation of LDL cholesterol that destroys arteries. For example, men and women who ate 180mg of vitamin C a day (the amount in 5oz (140g) of strawberries plus 4oz (115g) of broccoli) had 11 per cent higher HDLs than those who ate one third as much vitamin C, according to Dr. Judith Hallfrisch of the National Institutes of Health. One theory is that vitamin C protects HDLs from attack and destruction by rampaging oxygen free radicals.

You have only to consider the arteries of experimental monkeys to understand how vital vitamin C and E are to preventing artery clogging. Anthony J. Verlangieri, Ph.D., at the University of Mississippi's Atherosclerosis Research Laboratory studied monkeys for six years. When he fed them lard and cholesterol and very little vitamin C and E, their arteries became severely damaged and clogged. He was able to block the arterial deterioration and even reverse it by adding vitamin C and E to the high-fat diet. For example, fat-fed monkeys that got vitamin E had only one-third the artery blockage. More startling, feeding the monkeys relatively low doses of the vitamins for a couple of years actually reversed the arterial blockage by 8–33 per cent!

The antioxidant vitamins work, say experts, by zapping oxygen free radicals that otherwise would turn LDL cholesterol toxic and dangerous. It doesn't take much to mount this defence, says Harvard researcher Balz Frei, Ph.D. He says eating a mere 160mg of vitamin C a day – a couple of large oranges – gives body tissues enough ammunition to block free radicals and cripple LDL's ability to infiltrate arteries. (For foods rich in vitamins C and E, see pages 461–2).

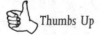 Thumbs Up

TAKE TWO APPLES AND –

Apples and other foods high in a soluble fibre called pectin can help drive down your cholesterol. French researchers had a group of middle-aged healthy men and women add two or three apples a day to their ordinary diet for a month. LDL cholesterol fell in 80 per cent of them – and by more than 10 per cent in half of them. Good HDL also went up. Interestingly, the apples had a greater impact on women. One woman's cholesterol plunged by 30 per cent.

Similarly, David Gee, Ph.D., at Central Washington University, tested high-fibre apple slush left over from making apple juice. He had the apple fibre baked into cookies. When 26 men with fairly high cholesterol ate three apple cookies a day, instead of a placebo cookie, their cholesterol dipped an average 7 per cent. Each apple cookie had 15g of fibre – the amount in four or five apples, he says. Most experts mainly credit pectin in apples, the same stuff used in jam to make it set, with lowering cholesterol, although other apple components also play a part. As Dr. David Kritchevsky of the Wistar Institute in Philadelphia points out, a whole apple lowers cholesterol more than its pectin content predicts. "Something else is at work also," he says.

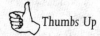 Thumbs Up

CARROTS VS. CHOLESTEROL

Count on carrots to help suppress bad cholesterol and raise good cholesterol. They, too, are full of anticholesterol soluble fibre including pectin, say Philip Pfeffer, Ph.D., and Peter Hoagland, Ph.D., scientists at the U.S. Department of Agriculture's Eastern Regional Research Center. Dr. Pfeffer calculates that the fibre in a couple of carrots a day can lower cholesterol by 10–20 per cent, which would bring many people with moderately high cholesterol into the normal range. After he started eating a couple of carrots a day, his own blood cholesterol dived around 20 per cent. A Canadian test found that men who ate about two and a half raw carrots every day saw their cholesterol sink an average 11 per cent. According to a German study, the amount of beta carotene in one or two carrots also boosted good HDLs significantly.

The carrot fibre remains therapeutic whether the carrots are raw, cooked. frozen, canned, chopped or liquefied, says Dr. Pfeffer.

SUPER SOURCES OF CHOLESTEROL-FIGHTING FIBRE

Some authorities, such as James Anderson, M.D., insist that soluble fibre is the main cholesterol-lowering agent in foods, and that the more of such fibre in a food, the greater its powers to cut cholesterol. Here is Dr. Anderson's rundown of super sources of soluble fibre. He urges eating at least 6g of soluble fibre a day to fight bad cholesterol.

	Soluble Fibre g
Vegetables: 3oz (85g)	
Brussels sprouts, cooked	2.0
Parsnips, cooked	1.8
Turnips, cooked	1.7
Okra, fresh	1.5
Peas, cooked	1.3
Broccoli, cooked	1.2
Onions, cooked	1.1
Carrots, cooked	1.1
Fruit:	
Oranges, flesh only, small	1.8
Apricots, fresh: 4 medium	1.8
Mangos, flesh, 1/2 small	1.7
Cereal:	
Oat bran, cooked: 6oz (170g)	2.2
Oat bran cereal, cold 1oz (30g)	1.5
Oatmeal, uncooked: 2oz (55g)	1.4
Legumes, cooked: 3oz (85g)	
Butter beans	2.7
Baked beans, canned	2.6
Black beans	2.4
Navy beans	2.2
White beans, canned	2.2
Kidney beans, canned	2.0
Chickpeas	1.3

 Thumbs Up

GRAPEFRUIT REMEDY

Eat grapefruit pulp – the segments with membranes and tiny juice sacs. They contain a unique type of soluble fibre called galacturonic acid, that not only helps lower blood cholesterol, but may help dissolve or reverse plaque already clogging your arteries. In one study by

Dr. James Cerda, professor of gastroenterology at the University of Florida, the grapefruit fibre found in about 12oz (340g) of grapefruit segments eaten every day lowered blood cholesterol about 10 per cent. Note: The juice does not contain the fibre or exhibit any cholesterol-lowering effects. Furthermore, in studies on pigs, which have cardiovascular systems similar to ours, Dr. Cerda noted that the grapefruit compound actually resulted in less diseased and narrowed arteries and aortas, somehow sweeping away some of the built-up plaque.

FOODS THAT CAN DETOXIFY BAD CHOLESTEROL

Deliberately eat foods rich in antioxidants that may help keep your LDL cholesterol from becoming oxidized and toxic. So far scientists have zeroed in on five potent antioxidant protectors found in fruits, vegetables, grains and nuts. Here are your best bets for defeating LDL's destructive transformation:

- Eat fruits and vegetables high in vitamin C and beta carotene
- Eat oils, nuts, seeds and grains, notably wheat germ, high in vitamin E
- Eat sardines and mackerel rich in ubiquinol-10, (coenzyme-Q 10), a more recently discovered artery-protecting antioxidant.
- Eat foods high in antioxidant monounsaturated fatty acids, such as olive oil, almonds and avocados, shown to reduce oxidation of LDLs.
- Restrict fats that are easily oxidized. Most easily oxidized are omega-6 vegetable fats, such as corn, safflower and sunflower seed oils.

WHAT TO EAT TO LOWER TRIGLYCERIDES

Another type of blood fat, triglycerides, may be more dangerous than previously thought. New evidence shows high levels can promote heart attacks, especially in women over age 50 and in men with poor LDL/HDL cholesterol ratios. A Finnish study found that men with bad cholesterol ratios and triglycerides over 5.28 had almost quadruple the risk of heart attack but if cholesterol ratios were okay, triglycerides were not a hazard. The problem is that low HDLs and high triglycerides usually go together.

Foods that lower triglycerides

The best dietary therapy is seafood. Studies consistently show that fish oil drives triglycerides down dramatically. In a study at Oregon Health Sciences University, a daily dose of fish oil – comparable to eating about 7oz (200g) of salmon, mackerel or sardines – slashed triglycerides more than 50 per cent. Another test at the University of Washington had men eat shellfish instead of their usual protein (meat, eggs, milk and cheese) twice a day for three weeks. Clams sent their triglycerides down 61 per cent, oysters 51 per cent and crabs 23 per cent.

Other good bets: A daily clove of garlic depressed triglycerides by about 13 per cent in one study and by 25 per cent in another. 3oz (85g) of dried beans depressed triglycerides 17 per cent.

A low-fat diet can also lower triglycerides.

Foods that can raise triglycerides:

Refined sugar, refined flour, fruit juices, dried fruits and excessive alcohol, especially in binge drinking. One or two drinks a day do not generally raise triglycerides, experts say.

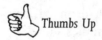 Thumbs Up

GRAPE LORE VINDICATED

Here's the newest addition to foods that can boost all-important HDL cholesterol. It's grapeseed oil, a mild salad oil squeezed from the seeds of grapes, and sold in some specialty food stores. David T. Nash, a cardiologist at the State University of New York Health Science Center in Syracuse, tested grapeseed oil on 23 men and women who had low HDLs – below 1.17. Every day for four weeks, they ate two tablespoons of grapeseed oil in addition to their regular low-fat diet. Their HDLs went up an average 14 per cent! "Some did not respond," says Dr. Nash, "but the HDLs did go up in more than half of them." Generally, those who already had the highest HDLs (above 1.43) were least likely to get further boosts from the grapeseed oil.

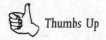 Thumbs Up

A NIP, IF YOU DRINK, IMPROVES CHOLESTEROL

It's a well-established fact that a little beer, wine or alcohol boosts beneficial HDLs. Typical is a British study showing that a glass or two of wine, beer or a mixed drink daily boosted HDLs an average 7 per cent. Another study found that 1.3oz (37g) of alcohol daily boosted HDLs by 17 per cent. Even light drinking brings benefits. A recent study at the Oregon Health Sciences University found that women taking between four and 30 alcoholic drinks a month had higher HDLs than women drinking no more than four drinks a month.

Johns Hopkins investigators also found that men who drank a 12fl oz (340ml) domestic beer a day for two months pushed up blood levels of apolipoprotein A-1, which converts to HDLs. Researchers suggested that drinking a beer a day might well make the difference between health and heart attack.

Beware of binge drinking. Downing seven to 14 drinks a week all on Friday and Saturday night does not benefit cholesterol the same way spreading the alcohol through the week does. Too much alcohol at one time can actually ruin HDL cholesterol and raise LDL, studies show.

• BOTTOM LINE • *Although a little drinking may benefit cholesterol, most researchers oppose recommending drinking as a public health measure to fight heart disease and stress that nobody, particularly people with a personal or family history of alcohol abuse, should take up drinking to try to improve cholesterol.*

SHELLFISH SURPRISE

If you're afraid that eating shellfish will send your cholesterol sky high, don't be. Many experts say it's wrong to avoid shellfish because of such fears. In fact, most shellfish, when substituted for other animal-type protein, actually benefit cholesterol.

In tests by Marian Childs, Ph.D., a lipid expert, formerly at the University of Washington, 18 healthy men with normal cholesterol substituted specific shellfish for three-week periods for their ordinary animal-protein foods like meat and cheese.

FOODS THAT CAN RAISE GOOD HDL CHOLESTEROL

- Olive oil
- Onions,raw
- Garlic
- Salmon, mackerel, sardines, tuna and other fatty fish
- Oysters, mussels
- Grapeseed oil
- Almonds
- Avocados
- Vitamin C-rich foods (sweet peppers, broccoli, oranges)
- Beta-carotene-rich foods (carrots, spinach, broccoli)
- Wine, beer, alcohol in moderation

Caution: Very-low-fat diets (10 per cent or less of calories from fat) depress HDLs.

Not a single one of six common shellfish (oysters, clams, crabs, mussels, prawns, squid) boosted blood cholesterol. Just the opposite – the oyster, clam and crab diets lowered both total cholesterol and detrimental LDL cholesterol. Oysters and mussels improved the good HDL cholesterol ratios.

All around best for cholesterol, says Dr. Childs, were oysters, clams and mussels. Crabs, too, were beneficial. Prawns and squid did not raise cholesterol, but neither did they lower it. Thus, Dr. Childs does not recommend eating prawns or squid to improve cholesterol.

FILTER OUT COFFEE THREAT

If you drink coffee, make it by the drip method in which the brewed coffee goes through a filter. Such coffee does not appear to significantly raise cholesterol, although European-style infused coffee does boost cholesterol, studies show. The probable reason is that the active cholesterol-boosting ingredient in coffee seems to get trapped in the paper filter; about 75 per cent of all the coffee brewed in the United States is filtered.

Dutch researchers solved the puzzle. They extracted a fatty substance, called a lipid factor, from European-type infused coffee. Volunteers who ate the "coffee lipid factor" did experience cholesterol rises of an average 23 per cent – 4.68 to 5.72 – within six weeks, nearly all of it in detrimental LDLs. Apparently, the cholesterol-boosting chemical does not get into filtered coffee. Thus, it appears your cholesterol is safe from elevation by java if you stick to filter coffee. Interestingly, another study at Johns Hopkins University found that even if regular coffee did boost cholesterol slightly, it raised both good HDL and bad LDL equally, making no difference in heart disease risk.

NEW DANGER IN DECAF?

Forget about switching to decaf to control cholesterol. For one thing, research does not condemn caffeine as a cholesterol-booster. In one Dutch test, 45 men and women substituted five daily cups of decaf coffee for their five cups of regular coffee for six weeks. The effect on their blood cholesterol was "essentially zero".

Further, there are increasing hints of hazard in decaf. Investigators at the University of California's Center for Progressive Atherosclerosis Management in Berkeley actually found that detrimental LDL cholesterol rose by roughly 6 per cent in 181 healthy men with normal cholesterol when they switched from regular coffee to decaf. Apolipoprotein B, another heart-disease risk factor, also went up.

However, cholesterol did not change in men who simply stopped drinking coffee, but did not switch to decaf. The Berkeley study's director, H. Robert Superko, calculates that switching to decaf might boost coronary artery disease risk about 10 per cent. That's significant, he says, when you consider that 20 per cent of the 139 billion cups of coffee Americans drink every year is decaf. Dr. Superko believes an unknown chemical in stronger robusta beans, commonly used to make decaf coffee, is at fault. Caffeinated coffee usually comes from weaker arabica beans.

The findings, surprising as they may seem, jibe with other recent studies, such as one at Harvard that detected a marginally higher heart-disease risk in men drinking decaf coffee. The clear message is don't depend on decaf to save you from high cholesterol.

CHOCOLATE, NOT GUILTY

Will eating lots of chocolate raise your cholesterol? Theoretically, yes. In actual fact, maybe not, according to tests at Pennsylvania State University. True, about 60 per cent of the fat in chocolate is saturated but it comes mainly from cocoa butter and cocoa butter's main type of saturated fat is stearic acid, which, oddly, tests show does not elevate cholesterol, and may even lower it.

Penn State researchers checked it out. Investigators had young men with normal cholesterol (under 5.2) pig out on chocolate, cocoa butter or plain old dairy butter for 25 days at a stretch. 31 per cent of their daily calories came from butterfat, chocolate or cocoa butter. That meant 10oz (250g) of <u>pure</u> chocolate a day. "It's like eating seven chocolate bars a day," said researcher Elaine McDonnell.

Still, the men's cholesterol did not rise significantly after eating either the chocolate or the cocoa butter. "Cocoa butter seems to be neutral as far as raising cholesterol," says McDonnell. In contrast, the men's average cholesterol (mostly detrimental LDL) soared 0.468 points during the butterfat binge.

EGGS AND CHOLESTEROL – THE REAL STORY

How hazardous is eating foods such as eggs, liver, caviar and some seafood – all bubbling over with cholesterol? The truth is that high-cholesterol foods are a minor cause of high blood cholesterol; saturated animal fat is the real enemy – fully four times more potent in boosting blood cholesterol levels. In fact, studies at Rockefeller University in New York revealed that a diet rich in cholesterol-laden eggs raised blood cholesterol in only two out of five people. That's because when you eat too much cholesterol, your liver automatically pumps less cholesterol into your bloodstream, so levels remain about the same or do not rise much. Paul N. Hopkins, a cardiologist at the University of Utah in Salt Lake City recently analysed 27 studies on the subject, and concluded that eating high cholesterol foods doesn't make much difference in the blood cholesterol counts of the vast majority of people.

"Saturated fats are four times more likely to raise blood cholesterol levels than dietary cholesterol itself." – John LaRosa, cardiologist, George Washington University

---

Still, overdosing on cholesterol-rich foods is not a good idea for other reasons. For one thing, splurging on high-cholesterol foods can promote heart disease by stimulating the blood to form clots, says Richard Shekelle, Ph.D., professor of epidemiology at the University of Texas Health Science Center in Houston. His recent study also found that high-cholesterol eaters (700mg a day or more) had a shorter life span by an average three years.

On the other hand, fanatically avoiding cholesterol-rich foods altogether could also be hazardous. Surprisingly, if you never or rarely eat high cholesterol foods, you could develop a choline deficiency, leading to liver damage, according to research by Steven Zeisel at the University of North Carolina. Choline is a B-complex vitamin, concentrated in high-cholesterol foods, such as eggs and liver. Dr. Zeisel had healthy males eat a choline-free diet for three weeks; they showed signs of liver dysfunction. A lack of choline in the diet could also impair memory and concentration, suggest other studies. Choline converts to a brain-cell transmitter, acetylcholine; low levels have been linked to poor memory and Alzheimer's disease.

• BOTTOM LINE • *Eat some cholesterol-rich foods to get sufficient choline, but don't overdo it. Generally, heart authorities suggest a limit of 300mg of cholesterol a day – or about four egg yolks a week.*

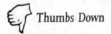 Thumbs Down

THE MOST DANGEROUS FAT

Of all the things you can eat, the most likely to send cholesterol soaring is saturated animal-type fat – the type concentrated in meat, poultry and dairy products. That's been the word since cholesterol was first linked to diet – starting in the 1950s. Unquestionably eating animal fat boosts bad LDL cholesterol in most people to varying degrees, and cutting out such fat usually lowers LDL cholesterol. That's why it's essential to shy away from butter, whole milk, cheese, beef and pork fat and poultry skin to help keep your arteries from clogging.

Study after study shows the same thing: that it is saturated-type fat, not other fats, that boosts bad cholesterol. For example: In one test subjects ate a high-fat diet – 40 per cent of calories from fat – except that one group ate the typical American diet high in saturated fat while the other group ate only 10 per cent of calories in saturated fat. Almost immediately the blood cholesterol in the low-saturated-fat group dropped about 13 per cent. Individuals vary greatly in their responses to saturated fats. Cutting back on saturated fat is most likely to cause the biggest dips in those with fairly high cholesterol.

• BOTTOM LINE • *You should get no more than 10 per cent of your calories from saturated animal-type fat, and less if possible.*

JACK SPRAT'S SALVATION

Can you eat meat and keep your cholesterol down? Yes, several studies suggest, if you trim off all possible fat. Apparently the cholesterol-raising culprit is not the meat itself but the fat that typically comes with the meat. For example, researchers at Deakin University and the Royal Melbourne Hospital in Australia put a group of ten healthy men and women on a high-beef diet – about 1lb (450g) of beef a day for three weeks. The beef was trimmed of all possible fat, making it so lean that the fat content was only 9 per cent of calories. Rather than going up, their blood cholesterol dived an average 20 per cent.

To clinch the case the researchers added beef dripping during the fourth and fifth week of the experiment. The subjects' cholesterol shot up.

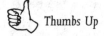 Thumbs Up

FISH OIL VS. A STRANGE TYPE OF CHOLESTEROL

If you have high levels of an odd type of cholesterol known as Lp(a) – pronounced "el pee little a" – you may be vulnerable to clogged arteries and heart attack at an early age, especially if your LDL cholesterol is also high. Some experts blame too much Lp(a) for a quarter of all heart attacks in people under age 60. Ten to 25 per cent of all Americans may have dangerously high Lp(a), which is genetically induced, they say.

A traditional low-fat diet does not curb Lp(a) but there is hope – fish oil. Dr. Jorn Dyerberg, a leading Danish researcher, found that fish oil, taken for nine months, lowered abnormally high levels of Lp(a) by a remarkable 15 per cent in a group of men. The daily dose: 4g – the equivalent of eating 7oz (200g) of mackerel. A recent German study also found that high amounts of fish oil depressed Lp(a) an average 14 per cent in 35 patients with coronary artery disease, although it was not beneficial in a few.

Simple tests are not yet available to detect widely elevated Lp(a). However, the threat provides one more rationale for eating fatty fish two or three times a week just in case you have high Lp(a). This mechanism may be one more mysterious way fish helps prevent heart attacks.

A PERIL OF SUPER-LOW FAT

You may think the less fat you eat, the better for your cholesterol and arteries. Not so. Harvard professor Frank Sacks, M.D., says a very-low-fat diet that restricts calories from fat to 10 per cent or less is likely to ruin your good HDL cholesterol, leaving you as vulnerable to heart disease as before. The reason is that a super low-fat diet drives down both your bad LDL cholesterol *and your good HDL cholesterol*.

Here's what typically happens, says Dr. Sacks. You drastically cut fat in your diet, and your total cholesterol count drops from 6.76 to 5.46 but that is meaningless because your good HDL cholesterol also dives 20 per cent, from 1.04 to 0.83. This means you are left with the same high *ratio* of total cholesterol to HDL of 6:5 as before – a ratio that still puts you at higher risk of heart attack than most Americans. The ratio is a far better predictor of heart disease than total cholesterol. Thus, Dr. Sacks says, after a stringent, demanding diet, you're no better off than before.

In contrast, eating monounsaturated fats like olive oil sinks bad LDLs but not protective HDLs. It makes more sense, says Dr. Sacks, to cut back severely on saturated animal fats which decidedly boost bad LDL cholesterol, and to eat a higher-fat diet, rich in mono–unsaturated fats. He favours a Mediterranean-type diet, that provides 35–40 per cent of calories from fat with most of it coming from monounsaturated fats. If you go on a super-low-fat diet, have your HDLs checked within a few months to be sure you are actually helping, not harming, your cholesterol.

"If I had a cholesterol level in the 4.16 to 4.94 range I would continue to do exactly what I was doing. I would not try to raise or lower it, but if I had a very low cholesterol level, like 3.12, I might actually consider trying to raise it." – Dr. David Jacobs, epidemiologist, University of Michigan

---

CAN CHOLESTEROL EVER BE TOO LOW?

Researchers are increasingly asking that question and the unnerving answer may be yes. Very low levels of cholesterol – under 4.16 – may be dangerous. In one major study of 350,000 middle-aged healthy men, Dr. James Neaton and colleagues of the University of Minnesota found that 6 per cent had very low cholesterol levels and hardly a trace of heart disease. Twelve years later their death rate from heart attacks was half that of men with higher cholesterol counts of 5.2 to 6.214. However, the low-cholesterol men had other problems: they were twice as likely to have a bleeding stroke, to die of chronic obstructive lung disease or commit suicide; they were three times as likely to have liver cancer and five times as likely to die of alcoholism. Another worldwide study of 290,000 men and women, by Dr. David Jacobs at the University of Michigan, found that those with extra-low cholesterol had higher death rates from a variety of causes.

What's going on here? Nobody knows, but in recent years clues have emerged hinting that very low cholesterol may not be safe. Brain haemorrhages in which a weakened vessel "blows out," causing a haemorrhagic or bleeding stroke, appear to be a particular danger from super-low cholesterol, possibly because fragile membranes that cover brain cells need a minimum level of cholesterol to function properly. Interestingly, as average blood cholesterol levels rise among Japanese, their incredibly high rate of haemorrhagic stroke is declining. Low cholesterol has particularly been linked in studies to colon cancer and liver damage.

Then there is new evidence that low cholesterol may somehow help induce depression, at least in elderly men. A study by Elizabeth L. Barrett-Connor, M.D., of the University of California at San Diego, found that such men with low cholesterol levels are strikingly more likely to suffer more symptoms of depression than their peers with moderate or high cholesterol. About 16 per cent of the men 70 and older with low cholesterol of under 4.16 showed signs of mild to severe depression. Only 3–8 per cent of the men with higher cholesterol were depressed.

Why? Dr. Barrett-Connor can only speculate that low cholesterol may somehow lessen concentrations of the brain chemical serotonin, leading to increased depression and aggression.

What is a safe minimum level? Researchers can only guess. It looks as if problems can start when blood cholesterol dips below 4.16, some say.

STRAIGHT TALK ABOUT DIET CURES FOR CHOLESTEROL

Diet therapy usually works best on those with the worst cholesterol – the highest LDLs or lowest HDLs – those who need help the most. It's probably futile and needless to try to use diet to push cholesterol lower if it is already normal or fairly low, under 4.68–5.2.

Also: do not expect all foods to work the same way on all people. Individuals react differently, just as they do to cholesterol-lowering drugs. Experiment to find which foods work best for you. Do not rely on a single food or a few foods. Many different foods have cholesterol-fighting capabilities. Eat a variety of them. Remember, you do not need the super-high doses of each food found effective in studies. You can combine smaller portions of various foods to get similar cholesterol benefits.

Specifically:

- Eat plenty of fruits and vegetables, legumes, high-soluble fibre grains such as oats, and seafood, especially fatty fish like salmon, mackerel, sardines and tuna.
- Cut back on saturated animal fats found in whole milk, cheese, meat fat, poultry skin. This will help reduce your levels of detrimental LDL cholesterol and raise your good-HDL cholesterol.
- Restrict omega-6 type vegetable oils, such as corn and safflower oil, also found in margarine, vegetable shortenings and lots of processed foods. The oils are incorporated into LDL cholesterol particles where they are readily oxidized, converted to a toxic form that can destroy arteries.
- Use oils high in monounsaturated fats, such as olive oil and rapeseed oil.
- Extra important: eat lots of antioxidant compounds concentrated in fruits, vegetables, nuts and olive oil, including vitamin C, vitamin E and beta carotene. They may keep LDL cholesterol safe from toxic changes that threaten arteries and promote heart attacks.
- If you drink alcohol, a daily glass of wine, beer or a drink of spirits may benefit HDL cholesterol. If you don't drink, do not take it up explicitly to try to improve cholesterol.
- Some other foods to eat that studies show can help cut dangerous cholesterol are: shiitake mushrooms, barley, rice bran, kelp (seaweed), skimmed milk and green and black tea.

BLOOD CLOTS

> **Foods That May Discourage Blood Clots:** Garlic • Onions • Hot Peppers • Black Mushrooms • Ginger and Cloves • Vegetables • Olive Oil • Seafood • Tea • Red Wine (Moderate Amounts)
>
> **Foods That May Encourage Blood Clots:** High-Fat Foods • Excessive Alcohol

BLOOD CLOT FACTORS CAN SAVE YOUR LIFE

The surprising fact is that the way your blood clots is probably the single greatest determinant of whether you suffer a heart attack, a stroke or blood vessel damage. Experts now know that thrombotic factors – how the blood flows, its viscosity, its stickiness, the tendency for clots to form and enlarge – are primary in determining such catastrophes. Diet can have enormous influence on blood clotting factors. Indeed, evidence suggests that the major influence of diet on heart disease has more to do with blood clotting factors than with blood cholesterol. The benefits of eating to modify blood clot factors are likely to kick in fairly quickly. A prominent French health official, Dr. Serge C. Renaud, says preventing blood clots can sharply cut your chances of heart attack within a year, whereas it usually takes longer to reduce heart attack risk by lowering cholesterol. However, many foods, such as onions and garlic, do both, so you get double benefits.

"Everybody knows it is not cholesterol that kills you. It's the blood clot that forms on top of the cholesterol-hardened plaque in the arteries that can be deadly." – Dr. David Kritchevsky, Wistar Institute, Philadelphia

Cardiologists once thought the narrowing of arteries from plaque buildup triggered heart attacks by leading to heart rhythm disturbances. It's now widely accepted that a blood clot is the immediate cause of 80–90 per cent of heart attacks as well as strokes. Several factors, strongly affected by diet, are critical to whether or not you form clots. One is how prone your platelets – the smallest of blood cells – are to aggregate or clump together, enabling them to form clots and better cling to vessel walls. Another factor is blood fibrinogen, a protein that is a raw material for clot formation. High circulating levels of fibrinogen are prime predictors of heart disease and stroke.

Also crucial is your "fibrinolytic" system, which breaks up and dissolves unwanted and dangerous clots. The vigour of this clot-dissolving activity along with fibrinogen levels is the "number one determinant of heart disease," says Harvard cardiologist Dr. Victor Gurewich.

HOW FOOD CAN CONTROL BLOOD CLOTTING

Doctors routinely warn against taking aspirin before surgery. The fear is that aspirin can "thin the blood," slowing blood clotting. Therefore, you may bleed longer, causing complications and jeopardizing your recovery, when you need rapid blood clotting to plug the wound made by the scalpel.

Did you ever have a surgeon tell you not to eat Chinese food before an operation or to avoid heavy doses of ginger, garlic, black mushrooms, and fatty fish like salmon and sardines? The truth is that all of these foods are also anticoagulants that may dramatically retard blood-clotting tendencies and often by exactly the same biological mechanism as aspirin – by blocking a substance called thromboxane that clamps down on platelet clumping or aggregation, a crucial step in clot formation.

In contrast, fatty foods like cheese and steak make the blood sluggish by making platelets stickier and more apt to clot.

Additionally, certain foods raise or lower blood clot-essential fibrinogen and rev up or slow down the clot-dissolving activity. Still other foods influence blood viscosity and fluidity, setting the stage for or staving off inappropriate clots that can cause blood vessel blockages in the heart, brain, legs and lungs. Undeniably, foods in very small quantities regularly eaten can have powerful pharmacological effects on the tendency of blood to clot and thus, can help save you from cardiovascular tragedies.

One of your greatest weapons – if not your primary one – against heart attack and stroke is to eat foods that benefit blood clotting factors. Here's what to eat and not to eat.

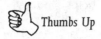 Thumbs Up

GARLIC AND ONIONS: ANCIENT CLOT FIGHTERS

It's an ancient truth: garlic and onions are strong medicines against unwanted blood clots. An early Egyptian papyrus called onions a tonic for the blood. Early American doctors prescribed onions as "blood purifiers". French farmers feed horses garlic and onions to dissolve blood clots in their legs. The Russians claim vodka spiked with garlic improves circulation. It's no longer unsubstantiated folklore. Garlic and onions are full of potent clot-fighting compounds and powers.

Eric Block, Ph.D., head of the chemistry department at the State University of New York at Albany, isolated a garlic compound named ajoene (after *ajo*, the Spanish word for garlic) that has antithrombotic activity, equal to or exceeding that of aspirin, a well-recognized blood clot inhibitor. Indeed, aspirin performs only one way as an anti–coagulant by stifling production of thromboxane. Ajoene does that, and additionally blocks platelet clumping seven other ways – by all pathways known, according to garlic researcher Mahendra K. Jain, Ph.D., professor of chemistry and biochemistry at the University of Delaware. "Garlic's mechanism is unique," he says.

"Clinical studies seem to be pretty much in agreement that there's something in garlic that helps prevent blood clotting." – Eric Block, Ph.D., State University of New York at Albany

---

George Washington University medical researchers have detected three additional anticlotting compounds in garlic and onions, including a major one, adenosine.

Garlic's antithrombotic activity in humans is well documented by numerous studies. Three raw garlic cloves a day recently improved both clotting time and clot-dissolving fibrinolytic activity by about 20 percent in a double-blind study of 50 medical students in India.

Recent German research shows that garlic compounds definitely speed up blood-clot dissolving activity and improve blood fluidity.

Such simultaneous action, researchers at Saarland University in Homburg/Saar say, improves circulation and in fact helps "purify" the blood of unwanted elements.

How much garlic? Only one or two cloves of garlic have a pronounced beneficial effect on clotting activity, says David Roser, a British garlic researcher.

NOTE: *You can eat garlic raw or cooked to discourage blood clots. The bulb's antithrombotic effects are not destroyed by heat; in fact, they can be released by cooking.*

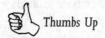 Thumbs Up

ONIONS: A POTENT FAT BLOCKER

To help keep blood free of clots, eat onions, both raw and cooked. Harvard's Dr. Victor Gurewich advises all his patients with coronary heart disease to eat onions daily, partly because their compounds hinder platelet clumping and speed up clot dissolving activity. In fact, onions have a truly astonishing ability to counteract the detrimental clot-promoting effects of eating fatty foods. N. N. Gupta, professor of medicine at K. G. Medical College in Lucknow, India, first fed men a very-high-fat meal, with butter and cream, and documented that their clot-dissolving activity plunged.

Then he gave them the same fatty meal, this time adding 2oz (55g) of onions, raw, boiled or fried. Blood drawn two and four hours after the fatty meal showed that the onions had totally blocked the fat's detrimental blood-clotting proclivities. Indeed less than 3½oz (100g) of onions completely reversed the fat's damaging effects on clot-dissolving activity.

• BOTTOM LINE • *When you eat fatty foods, add some onions. That slice of onion on a hamburger or those onions in your omelette or on your pizza may help counteract the clot promoting powers of the fatty foods.*

DR. JAIN'S BLOOD-THINNING GARLIC TIPS

One of garlic's most powerful and well-tested anticoagulant compounds is called ajoene. Here are some ways to release the most ajoene from garlic, according to garlic researcher Mahendra K. Jain, Ph.D., professor of biochemistry at the University of Delaware.

- Crush garlic instead of chopping it. Crushing releases enzymes and the allicin that converts to ajoene.
- Sauté garlic lightly; cooking releases ajoene.
- Cook garlic with tomatoes or add to other acidic foods. Even a little acid releases ajoene.
- Add just enough vodka to cover crushed garlic, and let steep for several days uncovered. This releases ajoene. Yes, the old Russian folk recipe for this blood-thinning potion really works, Dr. Jain's tests revealed. He also found that mixing crushed garlic with feta cheese and olive oil, which is a reputed Greek remedy for heart disease, produced lots of ajoene.

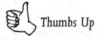 Thumbs Up

HOW ABOUT A LITTLE FISH PATE?

For a clot-blocker and clot-buster, you can't beat fish, high in the marvellous omega-3 fatty acids. Most scientists attribute fish's heart-protecting powers primarily to the oil's remarkable effects on blood coagulation. Studies consistently show that fish oil regulates how the flood flows and clots.

When you eat fatty fish such as salmon, mackerel, herring, sardines, tuna or indeed any fish containing some fat, it launches multiple attacks against clots: the oil tends to thin the blood by suppressing platelet clumping, depressing fibrinogen and revving up clot-dissolving activity. Paul Nestel, Chief of Human Nutrition at the Commonwealth Scientific & Industrial Research Organization in Australia, and his colleagues have found that eating about 5oz (140g) of salmon or sardines a day lowered hazardous fibrinogen an average 16 per cent and prolonged bleeding time by 11 per cent in a group of 31 men. Interestingly, in the same study, fish-oil capsules did *not* affect blood-clotting factors. One explanation, says Dr. Nestel, is that fish have other compounds, besides fat that benefit anticlotting factors.

FISH OIL'S REMARKABLE "BLOOD-THINNING" SECRET

Eating fatty fish literally changes the shape of blood platelets so they can't lock together to form unwanted blood clots. That's what researchers at the U.S. Department of Agriculture discovered. When you eat fish oil, your platelets release much less of the substance called thromboxane that instructs platelets to stick together, according to USDA's Norberta Schoene, Ph.D.

More fascinating, thromboxane creates sticky platelets by stimulating them to swell up into little round balloons and then to grow spikes so that they can interlock with other platelets. In this state they are called "activated" or "sticky," ready and able to clump together to form blood clots.

Thus, fatty fish, by suppressing thromboxane, preserves the healthy normal disc shape of platelets so they can't cling together and form clots to plug up your arteries.

Similarly, Harvard researchers suggested that eating 6½oz (185g) of canned tuna could "thin the blood" as much as taking an aspirin. The anticlotting effects came about four hours after eating the tuna. Also, subjects absorbed more of the oils from tuna than from fish-oil capsules.

• BOTTOM LINE • *You get a favourable antithrombotic effect from eating about 3½oz (100g) of fatty fish – such as mackerel, herring, salmon and sardines – or about 6oz (170g) of canned tuna.*

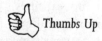 Thumbs Up

RED WINE'S WONDROUS ANTICOAGULANT

A little red wine can often thin your blood, retarding clots. The reason is not just the alcohol but other complex constituents in the red wine.In a classic study, the French scientists Martine Seigneur and Jacques Bonnet, M.D., at the Hospital Cardiologique in Pessac, tested the effects of three alcoholic beverages on blood clotting in 15 healthy men. For two weeks every day they drank 17.5fl oz (500ml) of either a red Bordeaux wine, a white Bordeaux wine or a synthetic wine made with water, alcohol and flavourings. The results: The synthetic wine increased platelet clumping and decreased bad LDL cholesterol. White wine slightly boosted detrimental LDLs and markedly increased benevolent HDLs, but did not change platelets. Red wine was the clear winner! It both depressed platelet clumping and boosted HDL cholesterol. Thus the researchers pronounced red wine's anticoagulant powers unique in protecting the heart. What accounts for its anti-blood clotting effect? The French said they were not sure they wanted to know, nor did they want the compound isolated, insisting that "the medicine is already in a highly palatable form". Cornell University scientists believe that wine's main anti-clotting agent is resveratrol, a chemical in grape skins.

• BOTTOM LINE • *Regular intake of red wine, in moderation with meals, seems to promote antithrombotic activity, discouraging heart disease. Heavier drinking and binge drinking can encourage blood clotting and cardiovascular damage. It's important to drink the red wine with meals so it can directly cancel out clot-promoting factors in the rest of the meal.*

WHY GRAPES MAKE ANTICLOTTING MEDICINE – AND WHERE YOU CAN GET IT

Rejoice in a grape's misfortune. Every time a grape is attacked by fungal infection, it defends itself by spinning out a natural pesticide somewhat the way humans make antibodies to combat infections. This plant pesticide is also a glorious anti-blood-clotting medication. The compound, say Japanese researchers, is the main active ingredient in an ancient Chinese and Japanese folk medicine used to treat blood disorders. Indeed, the Japanese have concentrated this grape compound, called resveratrol, into a drug and, in tests, have found it hinders blood platelet clumping that leads to blood clots and reduces fatty deposits in animal livers.

If you drink red grape juice or red wine you may get some resveratrol, which is concentrated in grape skins, says Leroy Creasy, Ph.D., a professor at Cornell University's College of Agriculture. Dr. Creasy detected high concentrations of the anticlotting substance in red wine, but not in white wine. His explanation: In making red wine, crushed grapes are left to sit with the skins to ferment but in making white wine the grapes are pressed and the resveratrol-rich skins discarded. Dr. Creasy's analysis of 30 types of wine found the most resveratrol in a red French Bordeaux and the least in a white Bordeaux.

Dr. Creasy also found the anticoagulant in purple (but not white) grape juice. It takes about three times as much grape juice as red Bordeaux wine to get equal amounts of the compound, he figures. Table grapes, found in supermarkets, probably contain little of the substance because they are carefully cultivated to prevent fungal infections and blemishes. 1lb (450g) of home-grown grapes, however, can have as much resveratrol as 16fl oz (460ml) of red wine, says Dr. Creasy.

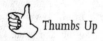 Thumbs Up

DRINK TEA FOR HEALTHY ARTERIES

Curious as it may seem, drinking tea gives your arteries an antithrombotic infusion. In 1967, the British scientific journal *Nature* carried some extraordinary photos of the aortas of rabbits given a high-fat, high-cholesterol diet plus either water or tea to drink. The aortas of the tea-drinking rabbits were much less scarred and ravaged by the high-fat diet. Tea, concluded the researchers from Lawrence-Livermore Labs in California, had prevented much of the arterial damage. They were inspired to do the experiments after noticing that the arteries of Chinese-Americans who regularly drank tea exhibited only two-thirds as much coronary artery damage and only one-third as much cerebral artery damage at autopsy as Caucasian coffee drinkers. Their suggestion that mysterious compounds in tea could keep blood vessels from clogging was ahead of its time.

Science has caught up. Research presented at the first international scientific conference on the physiological and pharmacological effects of tea, held in New York City in 1991, reveals that tea protects arteries by influencing blood-clotting factors. Tea chemicals can reduce blood coagulability, prevent platelet activation and clumping, increase clot-dissolving activity and decrease deposits of cholesterol in artery walls – all of which help fend off artery damage.

A pioneer in tea and atherosclerosis, Lou Fu-qing, M.D. professor and chairman of the Department of Internal Medicine at Zhejiang

Medical University in China, has studied the effect of tea chemicals on heart-attack victims. Dr. Lou told the conference that pigment from common black tea or Asian-style green tea thwarted patients' platelet clumping (also thromboxane production) and improved their clot-dissolving functioning. Surprisingly, he said both ordinary black tea and Asian green tea worked equally well. Scientists at Japan's Ito-en Central Research Institute also noted that a particular type of tannin in green tea, called catechin, blocked the clumping of platelets just as strongly as aspirin did. Tea also appears to help block LDL cholesterol's stimulation of the proliferation of smooth muscle cells on the walls of arteries; such cell growth fosters the buildup of arterial plaque.

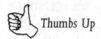 *Thumbs Up*

VEGETABLES ARE CLOT BUSTERS

To discourage unwanted blood clots, eat fruits and vegetables high in vitamin C and fibre. The most prodigious eaters of fruits and vegetables have the most energetic clot-dissolving systems, according to a recent Swedish study of 260 middle-aged adults. Those who ate the least fruits and vegetables had the most sluggish clot-dissolving activity. Other studies show that vitamin C and fibre concentrated in fruits and vegetables, also rev up clot-dissolving mechanisms and help thwart platelet clumping that leads to clots.

Further, the lowest levels of clot-promoting fibrinogen belong to vegetarians, especially vegans who eat no animal products at all, including eggs and milk. The probable reason is that compounds in fruits and vegetables lower fibrinogen, while animal fat and cholesterol push it up. Vegetarians also have lower blood viscosity than meat-eaters; lower viscosity is linked to lower blood pressure. So it's one more way fruits and vegetables ward off heart disease.

 Thumbs Up

THE HOT CHILLI PEPPER EFFECT

Hot chilli peppers are clot busters. Evidence for this comes from

Thailand, where citizens eat capsicum chilli peppers as a seasoning and as an appetizer, infusing their blood with chilli pepper compounds several times a day. Thai researchers reasoned that this may be a primary reason thromboembolisms – life-threatening blood clots – are rare among Thais.

To prove the theory, haematologist Sukon Visudhiphan, M.D., and colleagues at the Siriraj Hospital in Bangkok did a test. They fortified homemade rice noodles with hot pepper, using two teaspoons of fresh ground capsicum jalapeño pepper in every 7oz (200g) of noodles. Then they fed the peppery noodles to 16 healthy medical students. Four other control subjects ate plain noodles. Almost immediately, the clot-dissolving activity of the blood of the eaters of pepper-laced noodles rose but returned to normal in about 30 minutes. Nothing happened to the blood of the plain noodle eaters.

The chilli pepper effect was short-lived. However Dr. Visudhiphan believes the frequent stimulation from hot chillis continually clears the blood of clots, leaving Thais generally less vulnerable to arterial blockage.

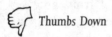 Thumbs Down

SPICY CLOT BUSTERS

Eat common spices to keep your blood free of dangerous clots. Krishna Srivastava, of Odense University in Denmark, screened 11 spices and found that seven discouraged blood platelet clumping. Most potent are cloves, ginger, cumin and turmeric. "Cloves are stronger than aspirin in this respect," says Dr. Srivastava. The primary active agent in cloves is probably eugenol, which also helps protect the structure of platelets even after they have been "aggregated". Dr. Srivastava says the spices work through the prostaglandin system, somewhat the way aspirin, garlic and onions do.

For example, all the spices clamped down on production of thromboxane, which is a potent promoter of platelet clumping. Ginger compounds are a stronger inhibitor of prostaglandin synthesis than the drug indomethacin, known for its potency, says Dr. Srivastava.

Ginger is indeed a proven anticoagulant in humans, as Charles R Dorso, M.D., of the Cornell University Medical College, discovered after eating a large quantity of Crabtree & Evelyn Ginger with Grapefruit Marmalade which was 15 per cent ginger. When his blood did not coagulate as usual, he did a test by mixing some ground ginger with his own blood platelets, and found them less sticky. Dr. Dorso said the active agent is gingerol, a constitutent of ginger, that chemically resembles aspirin.

 Thumbs Up

BLACK MUSHROOMS: A SURE BLOOD THINNER

To ward off clots, infuse your blood with the medicine of the Asian black fungus mushroom known as mo-er or "tree ear". It has a formidable reputation in Chinese traditional medicine for its beneficial effects on blood. Some call it a "longevity tonic". With good reason, according to Dale Hammerschmidt, M.D., a haematologist at the University of Minnesota Medical School. Once after he ate a large quantity of mapo doufu, a spicy Asian bean curd dish, containing the mushrooms, he noticed dramatic changes in how his blood platelets behaved. They were much less apt to clump. He traced the anticoagulant effect to the black mushrooms.

It turns out that the black mushroom (but not ordinary button mushrooms) contains several blood-thinning compounds, including adenosine, also present in garlic and onions. Dr. Hammerschmidt surmises that the combination of so many anticlotting foods in the Chinese diet – such as garlic, onions, black mushrooms and ginger – may help account for their low rates of coronary artery disease.

 Thumbs Up

OLIVE OIL FIGHTS CLOTS

In addition to everything else it does, olive oil even retards the stick–iness of blood platelets, which may help account for olive oil's artery-protecting powers. For example, British researchers at the Royal Free Hospital and School of Medicine in London had volunteers take three-quarters of a tablespoon of olive oil twice a day for eight weeks in addition to their regular diet. Their platelet-clumping scores took a dive. The scientists found that platelet membranes contained more oleic acid (the dominant fatty acid in olive oil), and less arachidonic fatty acid that encourages stickiness.

The olive-oil-fed blood platelets also released less thromboxane A2, a substance that commands platelets to cling together. All told, olive oil benefits platelet function, the researchers concluded, saying it is yet one more explanation of why populations that depend heavily on olive oil – in the Mediterranean area – have less heart disease.

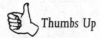Thumbs Up

HIGH FAT – BLOOD CLOT VILLAIN

Go easy on fat if you want to keep your blood clear of clots. Unquestionably, a high-fat diet does bad things to your blood, beyond boosting your blood cholesterol. Too much fat can also buck up the blood's tendency to coagulate and form dangerous clots. A recent study by researchers at South Jutland University Center in Denmark, for example, found that high amounts of both saturated animal-type fat and certain omega-6 polyunsaturated vegetable fats, such as corn oil, promoted clot-forming fibrinogen. In their study, a group of healthy adults who ordinarily ate high-fat diets switched to various lower-fat diets (32 per cent of calories) for two weeks at a time. All the low-fat diets suppressed blood-clotting tendencies by 10–15 per cent. Much research also shows that fat, particularly animal-fat, slows down clot-dissolving activity.

One recent study found that the fat from a fatty meal lingers in the bloodstream, fomenting trouble, for up to four hours.

Thumbs Up

TRY A CLOT-BUSTING BREAKFAST

It's long been a mystery why most heart attacks happen within a few hours after the victim wakes up in the morning. One reason may be that people skip breakfast, suggests research by cardiologist Renata Cifkova of the Memorial University of Newfoundland in St. Johns. She found that skipping breakfast nearly triples your clot-forming potential, leaving you more vulnerable to heart attacks and strokes. Dr. Cifkova explains that blood platelet stickiness is lowest overnight, then climbs rapidly when you wake up but, for mysterious reasons, eating seems to "unstick" the platelets.

As proof, she measured a marker of platelet activity called beta-thromboglobulin (beta-TG) in the blood of 29 normal men and women on days they ate or skipped breakfast. Beta-TG indicates blood platelet potential for clotting. She found that the beta-TG averaged two and a half times higher on the day the group skipped breakfast. However, the beta-TG dropped markedly on the days when they ate breakfast. Thus, it appears that one way to keep your blood platelets from remaining dangerously sticky, and putting you in morning heart-attack territory, is to break your fast when you get up — eat breakfast.

DIET ADVICE TO COMBAT BLOOD CLOTS

Eating to control your blood clotting factors is probably the most important dietary measure you can take to ward off coronary heart disease and strokes — even more important than controlling cholesterol. Here are your best bets:

- Eat fatty fish, garlic, onions, ginger and red wine (in moderation). All may help to thin the blood and keep blood from forming inappropriate clots.
- Restrict fat, notably saturated animal fat and omega-6 type polyunsaturated fats, to discourage blood clots.
- Make it a point to eat clot-discouraging foods at the same time you eat foods that can encourage clotting. Some winning combinations are eggs and onions or lox, red wine and cheese, hot peppers and chilli con carne.

Caution: Don't go overboard. If you are on blood-thinning medications, have bleeding problems or have a family history of "bleeding" or haemorrhagic stroke, you should be moderate about foods that thin the blood.

HIGH BLOOD PRESSURE

> **Foods That May Lower Blood Pressure:** Celery • Garlic • Fatty Fish • Fruits • Vegetables • Olive Oil • High Calcium Foods • High-Potassium Foods
>
> **Foods That May Raise Blood Pressure:** High-Sodium Foods • Alcohol

Your blood pressure is a major marker of heart health, and keeping it normal – not in excess of 140/90 by American standards – unquestionably helps ward off heart attacks and strokes. You can take pharmaceutical drugs, of course; you can also get drugs in foods which possess surprising power to lower blood pressure. Much research shows that foods are laden with blood pressure boosters and reducers. Eating your way out of high blood pressure is increasingly the number-one choice of virtually all experts, in lieu of or in addition to pharmaceutical drugs. Try diet first. The list of foods that may help lower blood pressure is growing longer and capturing the attention and imaginations of ever more mainstream physicians.

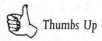 *Thumbs Up*

TRY CELERY, AN ANCIENT MEDICINE

Celery has been used as a folk remedy to lower blood pressure in Asian cultures since 200 B.C, says William J. Elliott, a pharmacologist at the University of Chicago's Pritzker School of Medicine, who recently isolated a blood-pressure-reducing drug in celery. Dr. Elliott became intrigued when Vietnamese graduate student Quang T. Le mentioned that his father's high blood pressure had been successfully treated by a traditional Asian doctor who prescribed celery. After Minh Le, 62-years old, ate two stalks of celery every day for a week, his blood pressure dropped from a high 158/96 to a normal 118/82.

Dr. Elliott made an "educated guess" about what chemical in celery might lower blood pressure. He extracted the compound and gave it to rats with normal blood pressure. It worked. Their systolic (upper number) blood pressure sank an average 12–14 per cent when the animals were given celery extract for a couple of weeks. The doses were comparable to eating four stalks a day. Their blood cholesterol levels also dropped 0.182 points – about 14 per cent. The pressure-lowering chemical is called 3-n-butyl phthalide and gives celery its aroma.

Dr. Elliott says celery may be unique, because "the active blood-pressure lowering compound is found in rather high concentrations in celery, and not in many other vegetables". Dr. Elliott speculates that the celery lowers pressure by reducing blood concentrations of stress hormones that cause blood vessels to constrict. He suggests celery may be most effective in those whose blood pressure is linked to mental stress, which could be up to half of all Americans.

NOTE: Although celery is high in sodium compared with other vegetables, one medium stalk still contains a mere 35mg of sodium. Thus, a two-stalk blood-pressure-lowering dose would add only 70mg daily of sodium, an insignificant amount in a total diet.

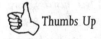 Thumbs Up

GARLIC'S LEGENDARY POWERS

Eat more garlic. It is another legendary folk remedy for high blood pressure, and it is effective, according to recent studies. Long used in China and widely used today in Germany as a blood pressure medication, garlic can have a striking impact. In a recent double blind German test of Kwai, an over-the-counter garlic preparation, doses comparable to a couple of daily garlic cloves pushed diastolic blood pressure down in patients with mild high blood pressure.

The blood pressure in the garlic group sank from an average 171/102 to 152/89 after three months, while the blood pressure of the placebo group stayed the same. Interestingly, garlic's impact grew stronger throughout the test, suggesting that daily infusions of garlic have a cumulative effect.

Garlic probably lowers blood pressure at least partly by relaxing the smooth muscles of the blood vessels, allowing them to dilate. That happens in animals fed garlic juice. Also, both garlic and onions contain a great deal of a compound, adenosine, that is a smooth-muscle relaxant, according to George Washington University researchers. That means eating onions also should help reduce blood pressure. Additionally, onions contain small amounts of prostaglandin A1 and E, substances with blood-pressure-lowering effect.

NOTE: *Both raw and cooked garlic and onions can benefit blood pressure, although raw garlic is thought to be more potent.*

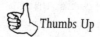Thumbs Up

OH, FOR A TIN OF MACKEREL

Eat fatty fish. "My own blood pressure dropped from 140/90 to 100/70 after I started eating a small can of mackerel fillets every day," says researcher Peter Singer, Ph.D., of Berlin, Germany. Fish's main blood pressure medicine is thought to be omega-3 fatty acids in the oil. A string of studies on fish oil find it helps keep a lid on blood pressure. Dr. Singer, for example, found small doses of fish oil as effective in reducing blood pressure as the beta-blocker Inderal, a commonly prescribed blood pressure medication, as he reported at the 1990 International Conference on Fish Oils in Washington, D.C. He also found that Inderal and fish oil together reduced blood pressure better than either did alone. Thus, if just eating fish does not do the trick, it may still add to the potency of medication, making a lower dose possible.

How much fish is needed to lower blood pressure? University of Cincinnati tests found that blood pressure fell 4.4 points diastolic and 6.5 points systolic in subjects with mild high blood pressure who took 2,000mg of omega-3 fatty acids daily for three months. That's the amount in 3½oz (100g) of fresh Atlantic mackerel, 4oz (115g) of canned pink salmon or 7oz (200g) of canned sardines. The drop was enough to eliminate the need for medication in some people.

Another fascinating Danish study suggests that you need a minimum of three servings of fish a week to control blood pressure. Investigators found that adding fish oil to the diets of those who ate fish three or more times a week *did not reduce blood pressure further*. However, doses of fish oil did depress blood pressure in those who did not eat that much fish. Thus it appears that fish eaten three times a week supplies enough omega-3 oil to control blood pressure in most people, which suggests high blood pressure is partly due to a "fish deficiency". Other components of seafood, such as potassium and selenium, may also contribute to lowering blood pressure.

• BOTTOM LINE • *Eat fish at least three times a week, preferably fatty fish, such as salmon, mackerel, herring, sardines and tuna.*

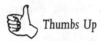 Thumbs Up

MORE FRUITS AND VEGETABLES

Medical fact: There's something magic about a fruit- and vegetable-rich diet that curbs high blood pressure. Vegetarians have strikingly lower blood pressure, and switching to a vegetarian diet typically lowers blood pressure, studies show. Why are fruits and vegetables so powerful? Frank M. Sacks, M.D., an assistant professor of medicine at Harvard Medical School, says there are two obvious possibilities: something in plant foods depresses blood pressure or something in meat forces it up.

At first Dr. Sacks thought meat raised blood pressure, but he scrapped the theory after he tested vegetarians by having them add meat to their diet. In one group of vegetarians who ate 8oz (225g) of lean beef a day for a month, systolic blood pressure rose very slightly, diastolic blood pressure not at all. Neither did a heavy egg diet for three weeks boost blood pressure. Nor could he get blood pressure to budge in response to different kinds of fats. Dr. Sacks concluded that curbing total fat or saturated animal fat does not affect blood pressure at all.

On the other hand, he is convinced that agents in vegetables and fruits have mysterious powers to reduce blood pressure. One blood-pressure lowering drug may be fibre, especially from fruit. A recent Harvard study of nearly 31,000 middle-aged and elderly men found that those who ate very little fruit were 46 per cent more likely to develop high blood pressure over the next four years than men who ate the equivalent fibre in five apples a day. For unknown reasons, fibre in fruit had the strongest anti-hypertensive effect, more so than fibre in vegetables or cereals.

Another possibility is antioxidants in fruits and vegetables that in roundabout fashion increase amounts of a hormone-like substance, prostacyclin, that dilates blood vessels and lowers pressure. Another explanation is vitamin C.

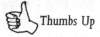 Thumbs Up

VITAMIN C UP, BLOOD PRESSURE DOWN

Eat vitamin C foods. A lack of vitamin C can send blood pressure up. In fact, vitamin C in fruits and vegetables is a powerful preventive medicine against high blood pressure, argues hypertension expert Dr. Christopher J. Bulpitt of the Hammersmith Hospital in London. He points to a string of evidence showing that high blood pressure and stroke fatalities are highest among people who eat the least vitamin C. Researcher Paul F. Jacques, at the U.S. Department of Agriculture's Human Nutrition Research Center on Aging at Tufts University, agrees that a low intake of foods rich in vitamin C predicts high blood pressure. In one study, he found that elderly people who ate the vitamin C in a single orange a day were twice as likely to have high blood pressure as those who ate four times that much. Systolic pressure was eleven points higher and diastolic pressure six points higher among the skimpy vitamin C eaters. In other research, Dr. Jacques concluded that low blood levels of vitamin C raised systolic pressure about 16 per cent and diastolic pressure 9 per cent.

"There is something about not eating enough vitamin C that raises blood pressure," says Dr. Jacques. Thus, if you have high blood pressure, make sure you eat at least the vitamin C in an orange a day. There's also evidence that eating super amounts of vitamin C, in excess of correcting a deficiency, can further depress blood pressure. Dr. Jacques also stresses that other components in such fruits and vegetables, besides vitamin C, may help keep blood pressure in check.

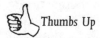 Thumbs Up

POTASSIUM LOWERS PRESSURE

Don't neglect potassium, concentrated in fruits and vegetables and seafood. It, too, is strong hypertension medicine. There's no question that adding potassium to the diet can lower blood pressure and taking it away can raise it. In fact, deliberately eating a low-potassium diet can cause high blood pressure. As proof, in tests at Temple University School of Medicine, ten men with normal blood pressure ate a potassium-adequate diet, then a potassium-restricted diet, each for nine days. Deprived of potassium, the men experienced an average jump in arterial pressure (including both diastolic and systolic pressure) of 4.1 points – up from 90.9 to 95. Their blood pressure shot even higher when the men's diets were loaded with sodium. Thus, potassium also helps keep a high-sodium diet in check, said the study's senior author, G. Gopal Krishna, M.D. He theorizes that too little potassium leads to sodium retention, which over time may trigger high blood pressure.

Getting enough potassium can also lessen the doses of medication you need. A study at the University of Naples in Italy discovered that after a year on a high-potassium diet, 81 per cent of a group of patients needed only half their original dosages of drugs to control their high blood pressure. Further, 38 per cent of the high-potassium group was able to stop medication entirely. They simply ate three to six servings of high-potassium foods a day, boosting their average intake of potassium about 60 per cent. (For a list of foods high in potassium, see page 459).

Thumbs Up

GO FOR CALCIUM-RICH FOODS

A secret weapon against high blood pressure may be high calcium foods. Some experts contend that high blood pressure is more likely due to a deficiency of calcium than to a surplus of sodium, and, in fact, that adequate calcium can cancel the blood-pressure-raising effects of sodium in some people. Dr. David A. McCarron of Oregon Health Sciences University says some individuals simply need more calcium than others to keep blood pressure normal, and quite often those are people who are "salt sensitive," that is, whose blood pressure rises from eating too much sodium. One theory is that such individuals retain water when they eat too much sodium, and that calcium acts like a natural diuretic to help kidneys release sodium and water, thus reducing blood pressure. Another, more complex, explanation is that calcium works by preventing release of the parathyroid hormone that can raise blood pressure.

Unquestionably, in some people calcium does reduce blood pressure. Research at the University of Texas Health Science Center showed that 800mg of calcium a day reduced mild high blood pressure in 20 per cent of subjects by a dramatic 20–30 points. Most, however, had small drops and, oddly, blood pressure went up in about 20 per cent.

Another study found that people under age 40 may cut their chances of developing high blood pressure by eating enough calcium. In fact, the chances of high blood pressure went down an average 20 per cent for each 1,000mg of calcium consumed per day in moderate drinkers (not more than one drink a day) who were not overweight. The risk plunged by 40 per cent in such people who drank less alcohol. Alcohol tends to counteract calcium's powers to lower blood pressure, said study author James H. Dwyer of the University of Southern California School of Medicine in Los Angeles.

NOTE: Milk and dairy foods, of course, are rich in calcium, and there's some evidence that drinking milk may help reduce blood pressure. However, since milk can cause digestive problems and allergies in many people, don't forget that many other foods are high in calcium – such as green leafy vegetables (kale, broccoli, collard greens, turnip greens) as well as canned sardines and salmon with bones. (For a list of foods high in calcium, see pages 457–8).

 Thumbs Up

TRY OLIVE OIL

Putting some olive oil in your diet may help lower blood pressure. A study by researchers at Stanford Medical School of 76 middle-aged men with high blood pressure a few years ago concluded that the amount of monounsaturated fat in three tablespoons of olive oil a day could lower systolic pressure about nine points and diastolic pressure about six points. More remarkable, a University of Kentucky study found that a mere two-thirds of a tablespoon of olive oil daily reduced blood pressure by about five systolic points and four diastolic points in men. In a recent Dutch study, eating high amounts of olive oil drove down blood pressure slightly, even in those with normal pressure.

Further, a major analysis of the diets of nearly 5,000 Italians noted that those eating the most olive oil had lower blood pressure by three or four points, especially men. Among the Italians, those eating lots of butter had higher blood pressure.

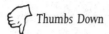 Thumbs Down

TO SALT OR NOT TO SALT?

The first cure most people think of for high blood pressure is to cut down on salt. It may or may not work, depending on your individual biological makeup. Scientists have been arguing for years over the impact of salt on high blood pressure and the debate goes on. It's unlikely that salt is a major *cause* of high blood pressure, concluded a recent Harvard report. Still, Dr. William Castelli, director of the famed Framingham Heart Study, notes that in the few areas of the world where salt intake is low, high blood pressure is rare and does not rise with age as it does among Americans. Also, if you have high blood pressure, restricting salt may help curb it, especially if you are one of the one-third to one-half of those who are particularly sensitive to blood pressure boosts from sodium. Such "salt responders" are most likely to benefit from sodium cutbacks, say most experts but you usually only know if you try it. There's even evidence that restricting sodium can depress normal blood pressure.

How much improvement can you expect? The University of London's Dr. Malcolm Law estimates that eliminating one teaspoon of salt a day from your diet can knock systolic pressure down an average 7 mmHg and diastolic down 3.5 mmHg if you have high blood pressure.

Restricting sodium may also give you younger blood vessels, which can help lower blood pressure, according to Ross D. Feldman of the University of Western Ontario. He and his colleagues noted that ageing vessels lose some dilating ability, which may contribute to high blood pressure; sodium can aggravate the situation. In tests, Dr. Feldman's group found that cutting back on salt helped restore normal functioning in aged blood vessels. They showed that older people on a high salt diet for four days had blood vessels that dilated only half as much as those of younger volunteers. On a low-salt diet the older group's aged blood vessels dilated just as well as those of the younger group. This suggests, says Dr. Feldman, that a low-salt diet may be an antidote to declining blood vessel functions that raise blood pressure.

NOTE: *One big way to cut down on sodium is to limit processed foods, which account for about 75 per cent of the sodium in the food supply.*

SODIUM SURPRISE

Still, sodium restriction may not work for some people. In fact, in a small percentage of people, cutting down on sodium actually has the contrary action of driving blood pressure up, according to Dr. Bernard Lamport of the Albert Einstein College of Medicine. After reviewing the current research, he reported that from 20–25 per cent of those with high blood pressure who moderately restrict their sodium intake, as many doctors recommend, have significant drops in blood pressure. On the other hand, blood pressure rises significantly in 15 per cent of such patients. "In these people, salt restriction is hazardous," he insists.

As a test, Dr. Lamport advises people with high blood pressure to cut down on sodium for a couple of months under a doctor's supervision. If blood pressure goes down, fine, keep on; if it goes up, stop. The point is, he emphasizes, everyone cannot count on sodium restriction to be a panacea for high blood pressure.

The National Institutes of Health advises everyone to eat no more than 6g of sodium a day – the amount in about three teaspoons of salt.

• BOTTOM LINE • *Whether salt restriction controls your blood pressure depends on your individual biological reaction. But, even if you don't have high blood pressure, it's smart to go easy on salt because sodium may promote brain vessel damage and strokes in other ways than by boosting blood pressure, declares Louis Tobian, Jr., M.D., hypertension chief at the University of Minnesota. And if you have kidney or heart problems in addition to high blood pressure, you most certainly should cut back on salt, he cautions.*

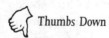 Thumbs Down

WATCH THE ALCOHOL

Undeniably, alcohol can elevate blood pressure, according to over-whelming and consistent research. In a 1992 review of the evidence, physicians at the Royal Perth Hospital in Australia concluded that blood pressure goes up in men and women of all ethnic groups and ages in response to all varieties of alcoholic beverages, including beer, wine and spirits. Further, the more you drink, the higher your blood pressure is expected to go, they found. Studies suggest that each daily drink drives systolic blood pressure up 1 mmHg, and that makes alcohol a greater blood pressure threat than sodium, according to the Australian experts.

In general, they reported that imbibing three or more drinks a day doubles the number of men and women who have high blood pressure of over 160/95.

"Three or more alcoholic drinks a day is the most common cause of reversible or curable hypertension." – N. M. Kaplan, University of Texas Health Science Center, Dallas.

A large-scale Harvard study of women nurses recently found that a couple of beers, two glasses of wine or a shot of spirits a day had no effect on blood pressure. However, drinking more caused a steady, progressive rise in blood pressure. Compared to non-drinkers, women drinking between two and three drinks a day were 40 per cent more likely to have elevated blood pressure. The risk was 90 per cent greater in women drinking more than three drinks a day.

Blood pressure tends to drop when you cut back on alcohol. A study at Kaiser Permanente Hospital found that alcohol-associated high blood pressure dropped to normal within days after cutting out all booze. If you are a heavy drinker, some experts say, going on the wagon may bring blood pressure down as much as twenty-five points. Some reports show that heavy drinking or binge drinking – more than six drinks a day – may boost blood pressure by nearly 50 per cent!

• BOTTOM LINE • *How much can you safely drink without fear of raising blood pressure? No more than two drinks a day, according to the National Institutes of Health. Also be aware that drinking alcohol can cancel out the benefits of both a low-sodium diet and blood pressure medication.*

FEW WORRIES ABOUT COFFEE

Caffeine does not seem to be a prime culprit in chronic high blood pressure. Caffeine can temporarily raise blood pressure in occasional users, and even in regular caffeine users, particularly when they are under mental stress, but in the end, caffeine does not seem to have lasting effects on blood pressure or to shorten life in those with high blood pressure, insist researchers at the University of Texas Health Science Center. In a study of 10,064 Americans diagnosed with high blood pressure, the Texas team found that hypertensives who drank more tea or coffee – brewed, instant or decaffeinated – were not more likely to die of heart disease or any other cause.

Nevertheless, if you are under mental stress, caffeine is more likely to drive up your blood pressure. For example, Dr. Joel Dimsdale, of the University of California at San Diego, had 12 healthy regular coffee drinkers solve arithmetic problems after they had drunk either regular or decaf coffee. In all cases, their blood pressure shot up more (an average 12 points systolic and 9 points diastolic) during the stressful tasks after they had consumed caffeine.

Additionally, the stress-caffeine combination may be more profound in those with high blood pressure or a genetic predisposition to it, according to Dr. Michael F. Wilson, a professor of medicine at the University of Oklahoma. He found that men at high risk of high blood pressure were much more likely to have blood pressure spurts when subjected to stress-producing tests after they had drunk the caffeine in two or three cups of

---

DIET PRESCRIPTION FOR HIGH BLOOD PRESSURE

- The number one thing you can do is eat more fruits and veg–etables of all kinds that are overflowing with known and unknown blood pressure lowering agents, including vitamin C, potassium and calcium. Vegetarians have strikingly low rates of high blood pressure.
- Especially eat garlic and celery.
- Fish is another must for the blood-pressure conscious. Its oil seems essential in keeping blood pressure on a healthy plateau. Eat fatty fish, such as mackerel, sardines, salmon or herring, three times a week.
- Go easy on the salt shaker when cooking and don't add salt at the table. Most of all, be wary of processed foods, which are often loaded with sodium. One study found . that about 70 per cent of all sodium in typical diets came from such processed foods.
- Keep your alcohol intake to a drink or two a day. And avoid binge-drinking, which can drive your blood pressure up markedly.
- If you are overweight, lose weight, which is a sure way to bring blood pressure down.

coffee. Such people, when stressed, have an exaggerated adrenocortical response to caffeine that drives up blood pressure, he says.

• BOTTOM LINE • *Most people with high blood pressure don't need to give up coffee. It usually does not push blood pressure into the "high zone" in healthy individuals, nor aggravate it significantly in those who have high blood pressure. So concluded a special report on high blood pressure by the Harvard Health Letter. On the other hand, if you are commonly stressed out, adding caffeine could be detrimental by helping boost blood pressure, say other experts.*

STROKES

Foods that May Help Prevent Strokes or Lessen Damage:
Fruits • Vegetables • Seafood, Especially Fatty Fish • Tea • A Little
Alcohol

Foods That May Promote Strokes: Salt • Excessive Alcohol
• Saturated Animal Fats

As you grow older, your odds of having a stroke rise steadily. Yet
there is dramatic evidence that what you eat can slash your chances of
stroke as well as the damage it may cause and even help determine
whether it is fatal. About 80 per cent of strokes among Americans are
due to clots in blood vessels of the brain and head. The rest come from
haemorrhages or "bleeding strokes" when vessels rupture, spilling
blood into the brain. Thus foods that help ward off clots, keep blood
vessels flexible and unclogged, and keep blood pressure normal
are good bets for preventing strokes. Even one extra daily portion of
the right stuff may cut an astounding 40–60 per cent or even more
off your chances of having or dying of a stroke. Any drug that promised
to prevent that many strokes a year would be an overnight
sensation, despite its cost and potential side effects. Yet such an effective
and certainly safer and cheaper drug is in everyone's possession right
now.

NATURE'S BRAIN PROTECTORS

The "right stuff" to keep strokes away is fruits and vegetables. More than
a decade ago, researchers discovered that eating fruits and vegetables
prevented strokes and diminished the damage if they occurred. British
researchers at Cambridge University discovered that older people who
ate the most fresh green vegetables and fresh fruits were less likely to

die of strokes. A Norwegian study found that men who ate the most vegetables had a 45 per cent lower risk of stroke. It also found that women who ate lots of fruit were one-third less likely to have a stroke.

 Thumbs Up

STROKE SURVIVAL MEDICINE: AN EXTRA CARROT A DAY

Imagine! Eating carrots five times a week or more could slash your risk of stroke by an astounding two-thirds, or 68 per cent, compared with eating carrots but once a month or less! That's the dramatic finding of a recent large-scale Harvard study that tracked nearly 90,000 women nurses for eight years. Spinach was also a particularly potent stroke deterrent. Part of the protection comes from beta carotene in carrots and spinach. A previous Harvard study found that eating the extra beta carotene in about one and a half carrots, 7oz (200g) of mashed sweet potatoes or 6oz (170g) spinach (weighed raw and then cooked) every day shaved 40 per cent off stroke rates. The drop was evident in those who ate 15–20mg of beta carotene daily versus those who ate only 6mg.

What gives carrots, spinach and other such carotene-rich vegetables antistroke activity is probably their antioxidant activity, speculated lead researcher JoAnn E. Manson, M.D. of Brigham and Women's Hospital and Harvard Medical School. The carotene inhibits cholesterol from becoming toxic and able to form plaque and clots in arteries, she theorized.

More remarkable is new research showing how important it is to have lots of beta carotene and other vitamin A in your blood-stream should you ever suffer a stroke. The vitamin may prevent your death or disability from the stroke, according to Belgian researchers at the University of Brussels, who analysed the blood of 80 patients within 24 hours after they had suffered strokes. They discovered that stroke patients with above-average amounts of vitamin A, including beta carotene, were more likely to survive, to have less neurologic damage and to recover completely! Here's why. When your brain is deprived of oxygen, as in a stroke, cells begin to malfunction, leading to a series of events culminating in oxidative damage to nerve cells, but if you have lots of vitamin A in your blood, researchers speculate, it can interfere at many different stages of this cascade of events, lessening brain damage and chances of death.

Foods rich in beta carotene – also known as vegetable vitamin A because it converts in the body to vitamin A – in addition to carrots are dark green leafy vegetables, such as spinach, collards, and kale, as well as dark orange vegetables such as sweet potatoes and pumpkin. Such foods are also high in potassium, another potent antidote against strokes.

Thumbs Up

THE REMARKABLE CALIFORNIA EXPERLMENT

Eat just one extra serving of a potassium-rich food every day; that too may reduce your risk of stroke by 40 per cent. That's what researchers discovered by analysing the diets of a group of 859 men and women over age 50, living in southern California. The investigators documented that small differences of potassium in the diet predicted who would die of a stroke 12 years later.

Remarkably, nobody with the highest intake of potassium (more than 3,500mg day) died of a stroke. However, those who regularly ate the least potassium (less than 1,950mg per day) had much higher fatal stroke rates than all the others. Among those who skimped the most on potassium, the odds of stroke deaths shot up 2.6 times in men and 4.8 times in women. Further, the more potassium-rich foods the subjects ate, generally, the fewer strokes they had. Indeed, the researchers concluded that with every extra daily 400mg of potassium in food, the odds of a fatal stroke dropped 40 per cent!

That critical margin of 400mg of potassium is so modest you find it in a single piece of most fruits and vegetables, a glass of milk or a small chunk of fish. If you thought it would help protect your brain from that devastating and often irreversible human catastrophe known as stroke or cerebrovascular accident, wouldn't it be worth it to eat every day an extra quarter of a cantaloupe melon, half an avocado, one small baked potato, ten dried apricots, 6oz (170g) of baked beans, or a small tin of sardines?

High potassium foods help lower blood pressure, but potassium exhibits additional powers to prevent stroke directly regardless of blood pressure, says University of Minnesota hypertension expert Dr. Louis Tobian, Jr. In tests, he fed rats that had high blood pressure either a high-potassium diet or a "normal" potassium diet. Forty per cent on the "normal" potassium suffered small strokes, evidenced by bleeding in the brain. No brain haemorrhages occurred in rats on high potassium.

Dr. Tobian's theory is that extra potassium kept artery walls elastic and functioning normally, thus immunizing blood vessels against damage from high blood pressure.

The same thing may happen in humans.

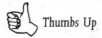 Thumbs Up

FATTY FISH – THE BLOOD FIXERS

Another spectacular thing you can do for blood circulation in your brain is to eat fatty fish. The omega-3 type fatty acids in fish perform several miracles on blood that make strokes less likely to occur. Even if a stroke happens, the damage is likely to be less if you have high levels of such fatty acids in your blood. Even eating a little fish may save you from stroke. Recent Dutch research found that men between the ages of 60 and 69 who ate fish at least once a week were only half as likely to have a stroke during the next 15 years as those who ate no fish.

Further, a series of studies in Japan show that heavy fish eaters are less likely to die if they have a stroke. Researchers found that residents of fishing villages who ate 9oz (250g) of fish daily had 25–40 per cent fewer fatal strokes than farmers who ate only three 3oz (85g) of fish a day.

WHAT PEOPLE EAT WHO DON'T DIE OF STROKES

Each of these foods provides the extra 400mg of daily potassium shown to slash the odds of fatal stroke by 40 per cent:

- 3oz (85g) cooked fresh spinach (423 milligrams)
- 2½oz (70g) cooked fresh beet greens (654 milligrams)
- 1 tsp. blackstrap molasses (400 milligrams)
- 8 floz (225ml) tomato juice (536 milligrams)
- 8 floz (225ml) fresh orange juice (472 milligrams)
- ¼ cantaloupe (412 milligrams)
- 4½oz (130g) acorn squash (446 milligrams)
- 10 dried apricot halves (482 milligrams)
- 2 carrots (466 milligrams)
- 4½oz (130g) cooked sweet potato (455 milligrams)
- 3½oz (100g) cooked green lima beans (484 milligrams)

- 8 floz (225ml) skimmed milk (418 milligrams)
- ½ Florida avocado (742 milligrams)
- 1 banana (451 milligrams)
- 2oz (55g) almonds (440 milligrams)
- 1oz (30g) roasted soya beans (417 milligrams)
- 7oz (200g) baked potato without skin (512 milligrams)
- 7oz (200g) baked potato with skin (844 milligrams)
- 6oz (170g) baked beans (613 milligrams)
- 3oz (85g) (about eight) canned sardines (500 milligrams)
- 3oz (85g) swordfish steak (465 milligrams)

It's also well established that the marvellous omega-3 fat in fish can modify the blood, making it less prone to clotting, obviously dis–couraging blockage in cerebral blood vessels. Some remarkable pioneering studies by William Lands, Ph.D., then at the University of Illinois in Chicago, showed that damage from strokes in animals was con–siderably less if they had previously eaten fish oils. If you are at the age where you fear your capillaries are narrowed by plaque buildup, here is an image to treasure: When you eat fish oil, it settles in the structural mem–branes of your cells. Such cells, when full of fish oil, are less stiff, more fluid and pliable. This means such deformable blood cells are better able to squeeze through constricted blood vessels, supplying brain cells and heart cells with oxygen. Such manoeuvrability could be lifesaving, especially as your arteries age and narrow.

Incidentally, eating saturated animal fat tends to make cell membranes more rigid. It's one more reason for those worried about stroke and cardiovascular disease in general to shun such fat.

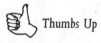 Thumbs Up

SAVED BY TEA

Deflect strokes by drinking tea, especially green tea. A recent four-year study of nearly 6,000 women over age 40, by Japanese physicians at Tohoku University School of Medicine, found that women who drank at least five cups of green tea every day were only half as likely to suffer a stroke as those who drank less. It was also true for women with high salt intake, who typically have increased risk of high blood pressure and stroke. The study is the first of its kind to link green tea directly with stroke prevention, although earlier animal studies in Japan, China and the United States found that green tea decreases blood pressure.

One explanation for the anti-stroke activity may be the high concentration of antioxidants in tea, which might protect blood vessels from damage. One study found green tea chemicals even stronger in antioxidant effect than vitamins E and C, well known for their potent antioxidant powers.

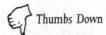 Thumbs Down

NEW SALT DANGER

Beware salt. Even if it does not raise your blood pressure, it may nevertheless be detrimental to brain tissue, helping induce mini-strokes, says Dr. Tobian. He came to this conclusion after tests in which he fed rats either a high-salt or a low-salt diet. The high-salt diet induced deadly strokes in the animals even though it did not raise their blood pressure. Within 15 weeks, an astonishing 100 per cent of the high-salt-fed animals were dead, compared with only 12 per cent of the low-salt animals. The brains of the dead rats on high-salt diets revealed injured arteries and dead tissue, caused by a series of fatal mini-strokes.

Dr. Tobian advises cutting back on salt to avoid stroke even if salt does not boost your blood pressure. This is especially critical for people over age 65 and all of African race, two groups especially vulnerable to salt's damage, he says.

ALCOHOL: GOOD NEWS, BAD NEWS

Light to moderate drinking could help save you from a stroke, but heavy drinking may bring on a stroke, according to new evidence. British researchers recently documented that those consuming a drink or two a day were only 60–70 per cent as vulnerable as, nondrinkers to either a haemorrhagic (bleeding) stroke or clot-induced stroke. On the other hand, heavy drinkers – three to four drinks a day – were three times more prone to strokes than non-drinkers.

Worse, a University of Helsinki study found heavy drinkers six times more susceptible to strokes! Alcohol, the Finnish neurologists remind us, is a brain poison, and in heavy doses promotes brain embolisms, clots and ischemia due to blood changes and contraction of blood vessels – all preludes to strokes. The Finns also found that moderate drinkers were only 6 per cent as likely to suffer strokes as nondrinkers!

• BOTTOM LINE • *A drink or two a day, if you already drink, may be beneficial, but you should not take up drinking to try to avert a stroke. Heavy drinkers should take heed and cut back, for few events are more tragic than a stroke.*

AN ANTISTROKE DIET PRESCRIPTION

It seems urgent and clear: If you are worried about a stroke, do the following five things:
- Eat lots of fruits and vegetables, five or more servings a day. Be sure to include carrots.
- Eat fish, especially fatty fish, at least three times a week.
- Watch your sodium intake.
- Don't drink alcohol excessively – no more than a drink or two a day.
- Consider drinking tea, especially green tea, available in Asian food speciality stores and some large supermarkets.

Remember, such actions could also curb neurological damage and lower your odds of dying if you do have a stroke.

DIGESTIVE SYSTEM

CONSTIPATION

Foods Most Likely to Prevent and Cure Constipation:
Coarse Wheat Bran • Rice Bran • Fruits and Vegetables • Prunes •
Figs • Dates • Coffee • Lots of Fluids

Of Little Value: Rhubarb

HOW FOOD CAN RELIEVE CONSTIPATION AND WHAT IS IT ANYWAY?

Diet is decidedly the "drug of choice" to cure and prevent common constipation, our number-one digestive complaint. So if you are one of the many who suffer from constipation, consult nature for the medicine that long ago was especially designed to keep you regular. Depending on harsh pharmaceuticals can be expensive, unnecessary and potentially harmful, since many laxatives worsen constipation by dulling the nerves of the bowel so it no longer contracts normally.

Not all constipation is due to bad diet. It sometimes comes from physical causes and underlying disease, so if your con–stipation is chronic or is known to result from a medical problem consult a physician before radically changing your diet. On the other hand, you may believe you are constipated when you are not. Lack of a bowel movement every day does not signify constipation. It's normal to have a bowel movement anywhere from three times a week to three times a day, say experts. The most common signs of constipation are straining to pass faeces; hard, dry stools; inability to defecate when desired; abdominal discomfort surrounding bowel movements; and infrequency – usually less than three times a week. Essentially, diet-related constipation means insufficient bulk and mois-ture in the contents of the colon.

"And this I know moreover, that to the human body it makes a great difference whether the bread be fine or coarse; of wheat with or without the hull."
–Hippocrates

Food works as a natural laxative in several complex ways. High-fibre foods such as bran and vegetables add bulk, mostly by absorbing and retaining water, producing softer stools that pass through the colon more quickly and gently. The fibre bulks up the stool because much of it is undigested. Fibre's coarse particles also mechanically activate nerve reflexes in the colon wall, triggering bowel movements. Other foods such as coffee and prunes can chemically stimulate the bowel into action. You also need plenty of fluids to keep faeces soft.

Preventing constipation the natural way also reduces your chances of developing and exacerbating haemorrhoids, varicose veins and diverticular disease – all aggravated by constipation.

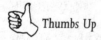 Thumbs Up

GET ON THE BRAN WAGON

If you are concerned about constipation, the best cure is to eat more of nature's magic medicine – roughage. That mainly means more wholemeal bread and whole grains, especially cereal bran, the king of laxatives. Nothing matches bran's purgative stool-bulking capabilities. A little daily bran could restore normal bowel movements in, conservatively, 60 per cent of those who suffer from common constipation, says British authority Nicholas W. Read, M.D., director of the Centre for Human Nutrition at the University of Sheffield. Unquestionably, much constipation comes from a deficiency in high-fibre foods. Dr. Denis Burkitt notes that our ancestors ate about 1¼lb (565g) of whole grain, high-fibre bread a day. We eat only one-fifth as much – a mere 4oz (115g) and most of it made from highly refined white flour that is fibre depleted.

Natural laxatives like bran, which bulk up the stool instead of simply stimulating the bowel nerves as many over-the-counter drugs do, are safer and gentler. "Bran is the safest, cheapest and most physiological method of treating and preventing constipation," agrees W. Grant

Thompson, M.D., gastroenterologist at the University of Ottawa, and author of the book *Gut Reactions.*

"If . . . the average intake of dietary fibre was 40g per day instead of less than 20g, much of the problem of constipation would be eradicated." — Alison M. Stephen, M.D., University of Saskatchewan

---

For a start you can try high-fibre wheat-bran cereals, beginning with ½–1oz (15–30g) a day, adding more as needed, say authorities. Choose heavy, "whole-grain" breads. Look for the words "whole wheat" as the first ingredient on bread labels, or bake your own bread using wholemeal flour. Another quick and easy solution is to add raw unprocessed wheat bran to your favourite cereals or other foods. This bran, also known as miller's bran, because it is the residue from milling white flour, is also commonly available on cereal shelves and in health food stores, and is probably the most scientifically tested remedy for constipation. It is particularly popular in Britain. Classic British studies indicate that eating about 1½oz (45g) of bran a day doubles the weight of the stool. What makes this bran so powerful is its raw, coarsely ground particles. Cereals like All-Bran have been processed, which slightly lessens their laxative powers, meaning you have to eat somewhat more to get an effect. "If the bran is not chewy, it probably won't work," says Dr. Read.

Research shows that bran's rough-edged particles mechanically stimulate the nerves of the bowel lining, promoting colonic movement. The bowel's nerve endings are so exquisitely sensitive that merely touching them with a soft brush induces muscular contractions and secretions, says Dr. Read. Thus, coarse, raw bran flakes have double-laxative activity — by increasing stool bulk and stimulating the colon wall.

HOW MUCH BRAN IS ENOUGH?

To combat constipation, try "a heaping tablespoonful of wheat bran a day," says Dr. Read. He suggests sprinkling the bran on cereal or other foods at each meal. However, there really is no single right "dose" of wheat bran for everyone. Most people need a tablespoon a day to pass soft stools without straining, but others need less and some need several tablespoons. To find out, test it on yourself; wait to see what happens and then raise or lower the dose as needed.

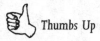 *Thumbs Up*

RICE BRAN – A SUPER SUPERIOR LAXATIVE

For a super laxative, also try rice bran, a foodstuff long used in Asia and now found in some speciality food markets and health food stores. Dr. Read found rice bran surprisingly *superior* even to wheat bran as a laxative. "We didn't expect it," he says. Seeking tastier alternatives to wheat bran, Dr. Read had eight healthy young men eat either 15g of fibre in wheat bran or powdered rice bran or no supplement for ten-day periods. That came to a daily total of about 2½oz (70g) of rice bran and 1⅖oz (40g) of raw wheat bran eaten at mealtime with fluids.

Both brans boosted stool frequency and output of faeces, but rice bran was clearly superior. Rice-bran eaters had about 25 per cent more bowel movements. All had greater stool output. Both wheat and rice bran reduced gut transit time equally well. Neither produced any change in intestinal gas, stool consistency or ease of defecation. Dr. Read speculates that the high starch in rice bran may spur colon bacteria to greater activity, increasing stool bulk. He also says oat bran has some laxative properties.

"A heaping tablespoon of unprocessed wheat bran a day is usually sufficient to combat constipation." – Denis Burkitt, M.D.

GO SLOW AND DRINK PLENTY OF LIQUIDS

If you start eating more high-fibre foods, you can experience some discomfort – bloating and wind initially, says Johns Hopkins professor Marvin Schuster, M.D., although the distress usually disappears in two or three weeks. Add the fibre slowly, increasing it as needed, and cutting back if your discomfort level is high.

You can get into trouble if you suddenly dump too much fibre into your system all at once, and especially if you don't drink enough fluids to soak up this fibre, keeping the bowel contents soft and easy to move. Drinking too little fluid is a classic cause of hard stools and is even more so if you eat a high-fibre diet. Usually six to eight glasses of water a day are enough to prevent hard stools, says Dr. Schuster.

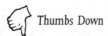 *Thumbs Down*

WHEN THE BRAN CURE IS WORSE THAN THE PROBLEM

Consider one 34-year-old man whose physician told him to eat a large bowl of bran cereal —about 2oz (55g) (with 20g of fibre) every day to cure his constipation. He apparently ate all of that and possibly more on the theory that if some is good, more is better.

Ten days later the fellow was in severe abdominal pain with nausea, vomiting and fever. X rays and exploratory surgery found a large obstruction in the man's small bowel. It was removed by surgery and found to be an 18-inch (45-cm) long mass of fibrous plant material. So reported Daniel Miller, M.D., of the Georgetown University Hospital in the *Journal of the American Medical Association*.

The overdose of fibre was a sudden shock to the man's system, says Dr. Miller. In addition the man did not drink sufficient fluids and was on diuretic medication that pulled fluid from the body. Here's Dr. Miller's advice: Gradually increase your fibre intake over a period of four to six weeks to give your system a chance to adapt. Be sure to drink lots of fluids, especially if you are on diuretic medications. Include a variety of high-fibre grains, fruits and vegetables in your diet.

DR. BURKITT'S BEST BETS TO FIGHT CONSTIPATION – IN ORDER

1. Brans, such as unprocessed coarse wheat bran and rice bran
2. Processed bran cereals such as All-Bran and other whole-grain cereals
3. Wholemeal bread
4. Legumes/peas, beans and nuts
5. Dried fruits and berries
6. Root vegetables, including potatoes and carrots
7. Leafy vegetables such as spinach
8. Apples, oranges and other fruits

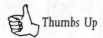 *Thumbs Up*

A CUP OF COFFEE – A FAST-ACTING LAXATIVE

For a quick and mild laxative, try a cup of coffee. Both caffeinated and decaffeinated coffee promote bowel movements in about one-third of the healthy population, says Dr. Read. He did a study after hearing so often from patients that coffee was a laxative. In 14 healthy men and women, Dr. Read documented that the beverage stimulated the urge for a bowel movement in certain coffee "responders". Subjects drank 6fl oz of either regular or decaffeinated coffee, or of plain hot water. Then researchers, using a rectal probe, measured changes in the pressure and movement within the colon.

The coffee had an amazingly fast effect. Surprisingly, distinct con–tractions (motility) in the bowel were detected within just four minutes after drinking the coffee. This suggests, Dr. Read says, that coffee somehow sends an advance message to the colon via hormones in the stomach or some neurological mechanism. There's no way the coffee could reach the colon so fast, he says. The increased motility lasted for at least half an hour. The hot water did nothing unusual.

Coffee is more likely to have a laxative effect in women than in men, Dr. Read found. He also suspects it works best in the morning and perhaps not at all later in the day. As for what the laxative compound in coffee is, Dr. Read does not know. Obviously, contrary to popular belief, it is not the caffeine.

"A cup of strong coffee is a good treatment of occasional acute constipation. But don't rely on coffee constantly as a laxative, because it is addicting." – Andrew Weil, M.D., University of Arizona College of Medicine

---

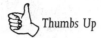 Thumbs Up

YES, PRUNES – BUT WHY IS A MYSTERY

"*Prunes are laxative and nutritious . . . Imparting their laxative properties to boiling water, they serve as a pleasant and useful addition to purgative decoctions. Their pulp is used in the preparation of laxative confections. Too largely taken they are apt to occasion flatulence, griping and indigestion.*" So said the authoritative Dispensatory of the United States, published in 1907, and used by physicians as a prescription guide.

Prune eaters through the ages would agree they are laxatives. But oddly, scientists have never isolated the so-called magic cathartic agent in prunes. Does one exist? Prunes, of course, are high in fibre and Barbara Schneeman, Ph.D., a fibre expert at the University of California at Davis, deems fibre the laxative agent. "There is no other magic in prunes," she insists. In a recent test of 41 men, she found that adding 12 prunes a day to their regular diet increased the bulk of bowel movements an average 20 per cent. (Incidentally, their bad-type LDL cholesterol also fell about 4 per cent). Another possibility is that prunes are extraordinarily high in sorbitol, a natural sugar that is a laxative for many people. Prunes are 15 per cent sorbitol, while most fruits are only 1 per cent sorbitol.

Nevertheless, since 1931, experts have searched for what they believe to be a unique drug like chemical in prunes that, unlike fibre, reportedly stimulates contraction of the intestinal wall and increases secretion of fluid. In 1951, three researchers at Harrower Laboratory, St. Louis, claimed to have cracked the mystery. They reported isolating a chemical called diphenylisatin that resembled an over-the-counter laxative drug. But, try as they might, other scientists could not find this chemical or any other in prunes that acted as a chemical laxative. Numerous tests by the U.S. Department of Agriculture on mice in the 1960s decidedly confirmed prune power, and suggested the mineral magnesium as a possible agent, but isolated, magnesium did not work. "It seems that the famous prune chemical works only when it is in the prunes," researchers concluded. The prune mystery remains unsolved.

LAXATIVE JAM RECIPE

Here's an easy recipe tested on 42 elderly people in a Canadian veterans' hospital in Quebec. Constipated patients who ate about a tablespoon of the jam every day increased their frequency of bowel movements and reduced their consumption of laxatives compared with those who did not get the jam. It was such a success that the hospital has continued to "prescribe" the daily jam as a remedy for constipation.

5oz (140g) stoned dates
5oz (140g) stoned prunes
12 floz (340ml) boiling water. Use slightly less for thicker jam.

Cut dates and prunes into small pieces. Add them to the boiling water and cook until the mixture has thickened. Yield: 20 portions of about one tablespoon.

ANCIENT MIXUP: RHUBARB – THE UNREAL THING

Generations of grandmothers have extolled rhubarb as a laxative, and it has a formidable anticonstipation reputation in folklore, but don't count on it. Actually, common garden rhubarb does not have any significant laxative effects, say experts. True, edible rhubarb contains compounds called anthraquines, common in laxatives such as cascara and senna – but in tiny amounts.

It's all a case of a botanical mixup, explains medicinal plant expert Norman Farnsworth, Ph.D., of the University of Illinois at Chicago. The real laxative, he says, is an ancient variety of rhubarb called tahuang (great yellow) grown high in the mountains of western China and Tibet. The rhizomes (underground stems) of such rhubarb – dried, cut and pulverized into a yellow powder – have been sold for centuries as a powerful purgative. In fact, rhubarb as a laxative was first mentioned in a Chinese herbal dated about 2700 B.C. and was a prized drug, carried by trading caravans to ancient Greece, Turkey and Persia. Some commercial laxatives may still contain these rhubarb extracts, says Dr. Farnsworth.

Our rhubarb is a distant cousin and pale imitation of the traditional medicinal rhubarb of the Orient. Our edible rhubarb stems have no measurable laxative properties, says Dr. Farnsworth. The leaves may have purgative powers, but it would be unwise to use them because they are poisonous.

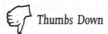 Thumbs Down

FOODS TO WATCH OUT FOR

Caffeine. Although coffee can be a laxative, caffeine can also contribute to constipation in some. One survey of 15,000 men and women by University of North Carolina researchers noted that those who were often constipated drank more tea and coffee. A possible reason: the nerves of the colon may come to tolerate the constant stimulant effect of coffee and caffeine, and thus become sluggish, just as they often do when people become overdependent on over-the-counter stimulant-type laxatives. Another possibility, according to Scandinavian investigators: caffeine acts as a diuretic, disturbing the body fluid balance by drawing fluids out of the gut where they are needed to soften the stool. Thus the stool stays hard and becomes difficult to expel.

If coffee makes you constipated, it's time to let up on it.

Milk and calcium. In some people milk and cheese can be extremely constipating, probably because of the calcium, cautions Dr. Schuster.

DIET ADVICE FOR REGULARITY

• To prevent and relieve simple uncomplicated constipation, eat more high-fibre foods, including fruits and vegetables and mainly bran cereals. Unprocessed wheat bran and rice bran are the most powerful.

• Add fibre gradually to your diet, and drink lots of liquids. There is really no reason for so many people to be on harsh, potentially dangerous pharmaceutical laxatives, when a natural, safe food remedy is so readily available.

Caution: Although the same general advice for combating constipation in adults applies to children, it is not a good idea to add wheat bran or rice bran directly to a child's diet because of their high potency. Concentrate on giving a constipated child lots of fibre-rich wholemeal breads and cereals, fruits and vegetables and fluids. If that does not cure the problem, see your doctor.

DIARRHOEA

Foods That Can Trigger Diarrhoea: Milk • Fruit Juices • Sorbitol • Coffee

Foods That Relieve or Prevent Diarrhoea: Starchy Soups and Cereals • Yoghurt

Foods That Can Delay Recovery: Caffeine • High-Sugar Juices and Soft Drinks • "Rest the Bowel" Diets

---

Diarrhoea plagues us all periodically from birth to death. Infants are particularly vulnerable. For most people diarrhoea is a swift attack of short duration. For others, it is a habitual, chronic problem with seemingly no detectable cause. Also, few visitors to other parts of the globe escape that common malady known as *turista* or "traveller's diarrhoea".

Simply defined, diarrhoea is too much water excreted in the faeces, resulting in frequent watery bowel movements. It happens because of a decrease in water absorption in the intestinal tract, because of increased water secretion, or a combination of both. Bacteria such as E. coli and staphylococcus bring on diarrhoea by stimulating water secretion, which explains why food- and water-borne infections commonly cause diarrhoea, including "traveller's diarrhoea". Some laxatives work the same way. The most common causes of diarrhoea are gastro-intestinal bacterial, viral and parasitic infections; intolerance, allergies or sensitivities to certain foods or food compounds, and disease conditions such as irritable bowel syndrome or coeliac disease. Anyone suffering chronic diarrhoea, lasting weeks or months, could have a serious underlying medical problem and should consult a doctor.

Unquestionably, diet can bring on, aggravate and alleviate diarrhoea. Food triggers can provoke diarrhoea through complex intolerance mechanisms. The foods you eat can definitely prolong or cut short the duration of occasional episodes of diarrhoea. In fact by eating the right stuff, you can shorten by one-third to one-half the recovery time from a bout of diarrhoea.

CAUTIONS ABOUT INFANT DIARRHOEA

Important: An infant with diarrhoea must be treated differently from an older child or an adult with diarrhoea. The hazard is greater. What is usually a mere inconvenience and discomfort in an adult can be serious, even potentially deadly, in an infant. The main immediate danger to an infant is losing too much fluid and important minerals and becoming dehydrated. Although infant dehydration is far less common in industrialized nations than in Third World countries, it does happen. Dehydration can occur suddenly, within a few hours in an infant. Thus, the first action is to replace fluids but do inform your doctor.

By far the most foolproof rehydration answer for infants is scientifically formulated oral rehydration therapy (ORT) solutions such as Dioralyte, sold in chemists shops. These formulas take all the guesswork out of determining the nutrients and electrolytes needed to keep tiny bodies safe from dehydration and are the number-one choice of experts in treating infant diarrhoea.

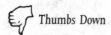 Thumbs Down

LET THE BOWEL REST? WRONG!

Most important, don't stop eating. It's critical to continue eating when you have diarrhoea – at any age. Nature's medicine helps cure diarrhoea. Yet the pervasive mythology that it is better to stop eating and "let the bowel rest" persists around the world.

The truth is, you are more likely to recover faster from diarrhoea if you keep eating – even though you don't feel like it, says William B. Greenough III, M.D., professor of medicine, Johns Hopkins University and president of the International Child Health Foundation. "Don't stop eating," he urges. "Simply shift to foods that will shorten the diarrhoea – high-bulk foods like rice or carrot soups, tapioca puddings, and not too much sugar." Eat frequently, and slowly; gulping down food can promote nausea.

The so-called BRAT diet – bananas, rice, stewed apples and toast – commonly recommended for youngsters is fine, says Dr. Greenough.

Encourage children with diarrhoea to eat frequently as much as they want – about five to seven times a day or every three to four hours, he advises. The American Academy of Pediatrics cautions against letting youngsters with acute diarrhoea fast for more than 24 hours.

DRINK THE RIGHT STUFF – IT'S NOT CLEAR LIQUIDS

Lately, researchers have become more precise about the best thing to eat if you have diarrhoea. "Clear liquids" are out. So are sugary fluids. Starchy "cloudy" fluids are in. First, contrary to popular opinion, confining yourself to insubstantial broths, teas and other beverages while your colon is weaned gradually back onto a solid diet is generally needless, restricts nutrients (which are important in growing infants and children) and prolongs diarrhoea, according to recent findings. Another reason clear liquids are far from ideal in treating diarrhoea is that most contain too much sodium (for example, beef and chicken broths) or not enough sodium (soft drinks and tea). Other home remedies lack critical potassium (Lucozade and jelly) or are too high in sugar (juices, and sugary soft drinks). "Such household beverages are inappropriate in the treatment of diarrhoea, especially in infants," concluded Helen B. Casteel, M.D., associate professor of paediatrics at the University of Arkansas for Medical Sciences, after comparing such commonly used "clear liquids" with meticulously designed commercial "rehydration" solutions.

"Do not give a baby with diarrhoea soft drinks, sweetened fruit juices or sports drinks. They can make the diarrhoea worse!" – William B. Greenough III, M.D., Johns Hopkins University

---

The "major villain in many home remedies is sugar," says Dr. Greenough. "Sugar passes right through you and draws water and salts out of the body, leading to vomiting," he warns. In fact, solutions with excessive sugar have caused deaths in infants with diarrhoea. That's why sugary fizzy drinks and sweetened juices are poor choices to replace fluids lost in diarrhoea, especially in babies. Additionally, sugar-based solutions do not cut the duration of diarrhoea, as cereal-based solutions do, he says.

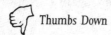 *Thumbs Down*

A CASE OF DIARRHOEA AND DIET POP

If someone suggests clear liquids for your child's diarrhoea, the last thing he or she means is diet fizzy drinks. "Not even regular soft drinks are acceptable," says Paul Lewis, M.D., a paediatrician at the University of Washington, "but diet drinks are worst of all." Dr. Lewis recently treated a five-year-old boy who was hospitalized with diarrhoea. Blood tests showed him to be literally "starving". Perplexed, Dr. Lewis on a hunch asked the parents if they had given the boy diet lemonade thinking it was a good "clear liquid". They had.

Diet drinks are particularly dangerous, warns Dr. Lewis, because they contain no nutritional value and but a single calorie. Thus, they leave the child starved at a vulnerable time when he needs nourishment to fight the diarrhoeal disease.

Nor is tap water acceptable, says Dr. Lewis. For an older child Lucozade though not ideal, is better than tap water or any other kind of fizzy drink.

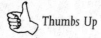 *Thumbs Up*

OLD REMEDIES VINDICATED

The best cure for diarrhoea is a starchy fluid. A thick soup or drink made from any starchy food, such as rice, corn, wheat or potatoes, is therapeutic. Such foods have long been used in many cultures as antidiarrhoea remedies. Favourites around the world are lentil soup, rice porridge, carrot soup, tapioca pudding, coconut juice and chicken noodle soup. Starchy liquids, unlike sugary ones, tend to diminish vomiting, reduce the amount of fluid lost and speed recovery time.

Indeed, studies have validated folk wisdom that calls for staple starchy foods. Recently, scientists compared the therapeutic power of such traditional foods with a modern lactose-free infant formula. For example, in Peru, a group of diarrhoea-suffering children got mixtures of wheat flour (or white potato), pea flour, carrots and oil. In Nigeria they ate a mixture of fermented maize pap, toasted cowpea flour, sugar and palm oil. After the first couple of days, the youngsters on the food mixtures often had less diarrhoea and experienced a return to normal stools earlier than the formula-fed children.

Most striking, the duration of the diarrhoea was "dramatically shorter" in the staple-eating kids than in those getting the formulas. For example, in Peru, kids fed local staples recovered 70 per cent faster from diarrhoea — in one and a half days compared with five days for kids fed a soya-based infant formula. Why? Experts can't really explain this "consistent phenomenon" they see repeated in numerous studies. They speculate that "some unabsorbed component of the diet, such as fibre or resistant starch," returns the stool to normal consistency and hastens an end to the diarrhoea.

A DIET TO CUT DIARRHOEA SHORT

Foods to Eat If You Have Diarrhoea
- Cereals, bananas, rice, tapioca, root vegetables such as carrots and potatoes.

Foods That Can Aggravate Diarrhoea
- Gaseous foods, such as beans, cabbage and onions, which cause discomfort, cramps and bloating.
- High-fibre bulky foods, such as coarse fruits and vegetables, fruit and vegetable peels, and whole-grain cereals that are hard to digest.
- Milk, notably if you have any intolerance to milk-sugar (lactose).
- High-sugar liquids, including soft drinks and juices.
- Coffee and other caffeine-containing beverages. Caffeine robs the body of needed fluids.
- Very diluted soups. Although often recommended as fluids, they are not nutritionally sufficient and are usually too high in sodium.

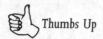 Thumbs Up

DR. GREENOUGH'S CEREAL SOUP

Here's a home remedy that may cut your diarrhoea short. For best results take it as soon as signs of diarrhoea appear. In cases of extreme diarrhoea, this cereal soup could reduce diarrhoea by 50 per cent in about three hours, says Dr. Greenough. "In ordinary cases, the diarrhoea might stop in two days instead of three or one day instead of two." Indeed, tests confirm this cereal "soup" is just as effective in curtailing diarrhoea as commercial oral rehydration formulas, he adds.

ANTI-DIARRHOEA CEREAL SOUP RECIPE

¾ pint (425ml) dry precooked unsweetened baby rice cereal*
¾ pint (425ml) water
¼ level teaspoon table salt

Stir all ingredients together until well mixed.

Caution: There's no danger in using too much cereal. Make the solution as thick as you can but still drinkable. However, *do not use more than a level ¼ teaspoon of salt*. More salt could be harmful Do not add sugar!

*In a pinch you can also use cereals, such as oats and instant porridge, but if they are not pre-cooked, you must cook them first and thin them down until they are "drinkable."

Do not gulp the porridge down all at once. Infants and youngsters should take a teaspoonful every minute or so. Give it as often and as much as the child will take. If a baby spits it out, try feeding smaller amounts and giving it more often. Adults can take more, but also at intervals. Usually, your thirst will dictate how much you need unless you are nauseated or vomiting.

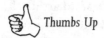 Thumbs Up

SPICY DIARRHOEA FIGHTER

Here is another folklore remedy for diarrhoea that has scientific validity. For adults – not children – one-half teaspoon of fenugreek seeds with water three times a day often produces quick and "marked" relief, usually after the second dose, says Dr. Krishna C. Srivastava at Odense University in Denmark. Fenugreek, a spice used in Indian and Middle Eastern cooking, has long been a natural medicine for diarrhoea and gastrointestinal spasms, he notes.

CAN EATING PEPPER PROMOTE DIARRHOEA?

Both popular and medical dogma have long warned people with bowel problems, including diarrhoea, away from eating pepper. The theory is that red and black pepper aggravates diarrhoea by speeding up peristalsis, the rhythmic bowel movements that propel contents along. According to new research by gastroenterologists at Our Lady of Mercy Medical Center in the Bronx, New York, this does not seem to be true. In fact, they found that pepper tends to slow down a tendency to bowel movements. In their tests, normal, healthy individuals ate pepper – about one teaspoon of red cayenne pepper or three-quarters of a teaspoon of black pepper in capsules. Measurements of intestinal activity showed that the pepper did not stimulate peristalsis and the urge for bowel movements in any of the sixteen subjects. In most, pepper actually delayed the passage of contents through the bowel. This does not mean you should take pepper to relieve diarrhoea, but neither does it appear to be harmful.

 Thumbs Up

IN SWEDEN, IT'S BLUEBERRY SOUP

Swedish doctors and grandmothers have long prescribed dried blueberries, usually made into a soup, to treat childhood diarrhoea. The common therapeutic dose: about ⅓ oz (10g) dried blueberries. Blueberries are rich in anthocyanosides, which kill bacteria, including E. coli, a common cause of diarrhoea. Also rich in the antidiarrhoeal compounds are blackcurrants. In fact, a black currant extract made from the dried skins is sold in Sweden under the name Pecarin as an anti–diarrhoeal drug. It has proved effective in human tests in combating gastrointestinal infections.

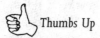 Thumbs Up

YOGHURT: "THE SAFE FOOD"

What's the safest food you can eat to help prevent diarrhoea? Yoghurt, according to tests by Drs. Dennis Savaiano and Michael Levitt of the University of Minnesota. Yoghurt is safe because it is unlikely to harbour the bugs that cause diarrhoea. When the two researchers put yoghurt cultures in test tubes with the number-one instigator of traveller's diarrhoea – various strains of E. coli bacteria – the infectious bugs either died or did not grow, but they thrived like crazy in ordinary milk or broth. As the authors note, the fact that yoghurt is used instead of milk in many underdeveloped areas probably comes from long experience demonstrating that eating yoghurt does not cause diarrhoea – but drinking milk does.

Even in Western countries, eating yoghurt regularly can prevent diarrhoea, according to studies at the University of California at Davis. Dr. Georges Halpern found that healthy people who ate 6oz (170g) of ordinary yoghurt a day had fewer bouts of diarrhoea throughout the year.

Eating yoghurt may also help you recover faster from diarrhoeal infections, according to Dr. Levitt. The bacterial cultures in yoghurt produce lactic acid in the intestine. This makes the intestine more acidic, inhibiting the ability of infectious bacteria to survive and thrive.

How potent yoghurt is against diarrhoea depends on the nature of its bacterial cultures; some are better than others. For example, Tufts University professors Sherwood Gorbach and Barry Goldin have used a special strain of bacteria called Lactobacillus GG to make a new yoghurt designed expressly to cure and prevent diarrhoea. The yoghurt has been tested and marketed in Finland. Studies showed that infants hospitalized with severe diarrhoea who got the yoghurt recovered 30 per cent faster.

In one study of tourists in Turkey, yoghurt made with *Lactobacillus GG* was 40 per cent protective against traveller's diarrhoea.

Patients on the antibiotic erythromycin also had less diarrhoea, stomach pain, wind and other abdominal distress when they ate 4oz (115g) yoghurt a day. Dr. Gorbach says that unlike some other yoghurt cultures, *Lactobacillus GG* survives for several days in human intestinal tracts and produces an antimicrobial substance that performs much like an antibiotic. Dr. Gorbach expects the yoghurt to be sold throughout the world.

Note: If yoghurt is heated, it no longer kills *E. coli* bacteria although it still can stop them from multiplying.

TRAVELLER'S DIARRHOEA: A SPECIAL EVENT

It's nasty business that can cut short the happiness of a trip to a foreign country – so-called traveller's diarrhoea. It strikes 30–50 per cent of visitors to developing countries, notably in Latin America, Africa, the Middle East and Asia. The diarrhoea comes quickly, usually during the first week of arrival, often bringing abdominal cramps with nausea and malaise. By far the most prevalent bacterial cause of this international health scandal is *Escherichia coli*, or *E. coli*, responsible for at least half of all cases.

You pick up the bacteria from eating faecally contaminated water or food, commonly fresh, uncooked leafy greens, unpeeled fruits and raw vegetables, uncooked or poorly stored meat and raw seafood.

To prevent traveller's diarrhoea, drink only bottled beverages; drinks made with boiled water such as tea and coffee; cooked food and fruits that are peeled. Avoid unpasteurized dairy products, tap water, ice cubes and food from street vendors and raw salads. Yoghurt is okay. If you drink the local water, do so only after purifying it by boiling for five minutes, or adding iodine or chlorine preparations.

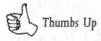 Thumbs Up

INCIDENT IN PORTUGAL: SAVED BY CARBONATED WATER

When travelling in foreign countries, choose carbonated bottled water over plain bottled water. Carbonation makes water acidic enough to kill most microorganisms, including those that cause diarrhoea. That's why carbonated water can help save you from infectious diarrhoea, says David Sack, M.D., associate professor of medicine at Johns Hopkins University.

To illustrate: Dr. Sack tells of an outbreak of cholera in the mid-1970s in Portugal that was traced to a bottling plant. The plant bottled both noncarbonated and carbonated water. A subsequent investigation revealed that cholera struck only those who had drunk the non–carbonated bottled water. The carbonation apparently protected the others.

If you get traveller's diarrhoea, do the same as you would for any other diarrhoea: Keep eating. Drink liquids such as caffeine-free, sugar-free carbonated drinks, and eat local starchy foods, such as potato, rice and lentil soups. Chicken-noodle soup, if it's not too salty, is a good choice, says Dr. Sack. Also okay are salted crackers, bananas, rice and toast. Stay away from milk, caffeine, fatty foods and any form of roughage.

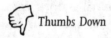 Thumbs Down

MILK GONE SOUR

Be sure diarrhoea is not caused by cow's milk; it is a common and often hidden cause of diarrhoea for people of all ages. "Allergy to cow's milk is a major cause of chronic diarrhoea and failure to thrive in infancy," says Richard A. Schreiber, M.D., a paediatric gastroenterologist at Massachusetts General Hospital in Boston.

Diarrhoea at all ages can be due to an inability to digest milk sugar, known as lactose intolerance. Infants, also, commonly are sensitive to proteins in milk that can trigger diarrhoea. This includes yoghurt. Be especially suspicious of milk-induced diarrhoea in "highrisk" infants, those with close family members who have allergies. One test found that 36 per cent of such infants fed milk-based formulas had allergies, including diarrhoea and other gastrointestinal upset, as well as wheezing and skin rashes. Just as many infants suffered diarrhoea and allergies from soya-based formula. There are a couple of solutions: breast-feeding and infant milk formulas devoid of offending proteins. Your baby is much less likely to have diarrhoea, as well as allergies in general, if you breast-feed. This shields the infant from diarrhoea-causing pathogens and allergens in milk. Next best are specially formulated so-called casein hydrolysate formulas, in which the troublesome proteins are disarmed.

QUICK TIPS FOR KIDS WITH DIARRHOEA

- Continue breast-feeding an infant who has an acute attack of diarrhoea.
- Watch milk-formula babies carefully for signs of lactose intolerance due to the diarrhoea. Consider switching to a special formula, such as Nutramigen, in which the protein has been neutralized. Consult your doctor.
- Give infants and children under age five a commercial re–hydration fluid, such as Dioralyte sold in chemists. You can substitute the cereal soup, page 112.
- Keep kids with diarrhoea eating starchy bland foods like rice soups and diluted cooked cereals.

WHAT TO DO IF YOU SUSPECT MILK DIARRHOEA

- For infants on cow's milk formulas, stop giving the milk for about a week. You can substitute soya formula, but many babies are also intolerant of soya foods. It's more reliable to substitute commercially available casein hydrolysate formula in which the diarrhoea-causing milk protein has been neutralized.
- If you are nursing a baby with diarrhoea, stop drinking milk temporarily (you can take supplements for calcium), because your own breast milk can carry and pass on to the nursing infant the diarrhoea-inducing agents. It happens frequently. Studies show that when the nursing mother gives up all dairy products, the infant's diarrhoea and other gastrointestinal symptoms often totally disappear.
- Children and adults with chronic diarrhoea can go on a lactose-free diet for a couple of weeks or so. Primarily, avoid milk, cheese and ice cream. Yoghurt is okay, but not if frozen. If the diarrhoea subsides, it was probably at least partly caused by an intolerance to milk. (See the chapter on lactose intolerance, pages 132–4.)

NO YOGHURT FOR INFANTS

Eating yoghurt may help prevent and possibly treat diarrhoea, especially traveller's diarrhoea in older children and adults, but experts advise against feeding yoghurt to babies under age one. Although this is common practice in some Middle-European and Mediterranean countries, the proteins in yoghurt, as in milk, may trigger reactions, causing diarrhoea, as well as sleeplessness and colic, and even skin and breathing allergies later in life.

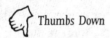 Thumbs Down

TODDLERS' DOWNFALL: FRUIT JUICES

If your toddler or infant has persistent diarrhoea (lasting more than 14 days) suspect fruit juice. About 15 per cent of all toddlers have "chronic nonspecific diarrhoea," also known as "the irritable colon of childhood". Many miraculously recover when they don't drink fruit juice, namely apple, pear and grape juice. In a Dutch study, children aged 14–25 months were immediately cured of chronic diarrhoea when they were taken off apple juice. Dr. Jeffrey Hyams and colleagues at the University of Connecticut Health Center found essentially the same thing for pear and grape juice.

Such juices contain high concentrations of fruit sugars, namely sorbitol and fructose that promote diarrhoea in susceptible youngsters who can't totally digest them. Studies show that about two out of three youngsters have trouble absorbing such fruit sugars. Consequently, the sugars hang around the large intestine where they are attacked by bacteria, creating fermentation, diarrhoea, wind and crampy abdominal pain.

The worst culprit, say experts, is apple juice because it is extra high in both fructose and sorbitol. Next in line – pear and white grape juice. Ironically, apple juice accounts for about half of all juice consumed by youngsters under age six. The safest juice – least likely to cause chronic diarrhoea in an infant or toddler – is orange juice, according to a committee of paediatric professors writing in the Journal of Pediatrics. Orange juice is low in fructose and has no sorbitol.

The good news is that cutting out or down on the offending fruit juice solves the problem. Normal bowel movements usually come back within a couple of weeks. And most kids outgrow the tendency to diarrhoea by age four.

COMMON CULPRITS IN DIARRHOEA

- Cow's milk
- Coffee
- Sorbitol sweetener
- Fruit juices

 Thumbs Down

ONE TOO MANY DIET SWEETS

Attention, dieters and diabetics. If you have unexplained diarrhoea, it could be too much sorbitol, a natural sugar substitute in diet sweets, sugarless gum and processed foods. Sorbitol is a medically recognized laxative. So no wonder a few sorbitol-sweetened candies can wreak havoc in the intestinal tract of those who cannot properly absorb it — which according to one study, is 41 per cent of healthy adults.

And it doesn't take much. In one test, a sorbitol dose equal to four or five sorbitol-sweetened mints caused abdominal pain, bloating and diarrhoea in 75 per cent of those who ate it. The distress came on within 30 minutes to three and a half hours after downing a sorbitol-sweetened drink. The problem was discovered in 1966 when a physician first noticed that an infant was stricken with diarrhoea after eating diet sweets.

Sorbitol also occurs in fruits, notably cherries, pears and plums, but it's usually not concentrated enough to be cathartic. It takes about 3½oz (100g) of cherries to provide as much sorbitol as that found in a single sorbitol-sweetened mint, according to one expert.

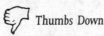 Thumbs Down

COFFEE TROUBLES

If you have chronic diarrhoea, give up drinking coffee for a few days and see if your diarrhoea clears up. Coffee is a common cause of diarrhoea in some with "sensitive colons". As little as a single cup of coffee, either caffeinated or decaffeinated, can stimulate muscle contractions in the bowel in at least one-third of the population, according to British tests. Further, caffeine is a diuretic that tends to rob the body of fluids that are much needed when you have diarrhoea. Thus, drinking coffee may induce or aggravate diarrhoea.

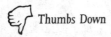 Thumbs Down

WATCH OUT FOR MUFFIN OVERLOAD

Fibre is a terrific remedy for much that ails you, but you can create a bad case of diarrhoea if you go overboard, as noted in the *New England Journal of Medicine*. A 64-year-old physician, after a lifetime of regular once-a-day bowel movements, began to have episodes of explosive diarrhoea that were embarrassing and virtually unpredictable — occurring randomly two or three times throughout the day. Normal stools dropped to once a week. It turned out the diarrhoea had begun when the doctor started eating "high potency" bran muffins provided at staff meetings by the hospital.

He stopped eating the high-fibre bran muffins, and within two or three days his diarrhoea had cleared up.

DIET PRESCRIPTION TO CURB DIARRHOEA

- If diarrhoea is chronic, the cause, whether in infants, children or adults, could be a reaction to something in the diet.

To find a cause of chronic diarrhoea

- First, give up milk and dairy products to see if the diarrhoea ceases.
- Rid the diet of the natural sweetener sorbitol.
- If that doesn't work, give up coffee, both caffeinated and decaf.
- Avoid gaseous foods.
- In toddlers, cut back on fruit juices, especially apple juice.

To treat diarrhoea

- Keep hydrated with lots of low-sugar, low-sodium fluids.
- Try cereal soup (see page 112) or a commercial rehydration solution.
- Continue to eat regular foods, such as soft starchy foods like cooked carrots, potatoes and tapioca.
- Do not institute a diet of "clear liquids" or go on a fast to "rest the bowel".
- Avoid irritating high-fibre grains, gaseous foods and certainly milk if you are lactose intolerant.
- Shun high-sugar fluids like fruit juices and sugar-sweetened carbonated drinks. Do not give youngsters diet drinks.
- Eat and take fluids, a few sips at a time, even if you feel nauseated and are vomiting. It will help shorten the course of the diarrhoea. Always drink small amounts of fluids instead of lots at one time. Too much at once is more likely to cause vomiting. Essentially, you should drink enough fluids to replace those you have lost.

UPSET STOMACH

Everybody has an upset stomach occasionally – acid stomach, nausea, motion sickness or intestinal parasites. The pain and discomfort are usually short-lived and not serious. Since stomach complaints are so common, folk medicine has a long list of soothing cures, dating back to ancient China and Babylonia. For example, the ancient drug of choice for nausea was ginger and it is still the number one natural medication for nausea today.

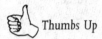 Thumbs Up

COFFEE CURSE BANANA CURE

It feels like an ulcer, but tests show it's not. You might call it indigestion, but doctors have another name for it, non-ulcer dyspepsia. That means you have persistent episodes of stomach distress, sometimes with abdominal pain and nausea – often after eating, but nobody knows what causes it. The latest evidence chalks it up to an extraordinarily "sensitive" stomach.

Bananas may help. This longtime folk remedy for upset stomach specifically relieves dyspepsia, according to a study of 46 patients by Indian researchers. Half the sufferers took banana powder in capsules every day for eight weeks. Of these, 50 per cent got *complete* relief, 25 per cent partial relief and 25 per cent no relief from the bananas. In contrast, only 20 per cent of the group taking placebo capsules said their stomachs felt better. The bananas were four times more effective than the placebo. "So if your stomach's bothering you, a banana a day may keep the doctor away!" says Ronald Hoffman, M.D., author of *Seven Weeks to a Settled Stomach*.

On the other hand, go easy on coffee, with or without caffeine. Coffee can bring on dyspepsia, according to researchers at the University of Michigan. Their study of 55 people with the problem revealed that half suffered digestive distress after drinking at least two cups of coffee a day. Even drinking decaf caused indigestion. "It may be acid in the coffee," the researchers suggested.

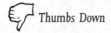 Thumbs Down

STOMACHACHES AND PAINS: LIKELY FOOD CULPRITS

What food is most apt to give you a stomachache or pain or just plain discomfort? German researchers at a hospital in Munich asked that question and here's what they found. Normal healthy people were most likely to react with stomach pain to eating mayonnaise, cabbage, fried and salted foods. Those with dyspepsia (without ulcers) suffered stomach pain from coffee, meat, fried foods, carbonated beverages and fruit juices. Those diagnosed with ulcers had the most painful reactions to coffee, carbonated beverages, mayonnaise and fruit juice.

ACID STOMACH: WHAT TO EAT AND AVOID

If you have an acid stomach, try 3½oz (100g) of cooked rice as an antacid, suggests Ara H. DerMarderosian, Ph.D., professor of pharmacognosy and medicinal chemistry, Philadelphia College of Pharmacy and Science. Rice is a complex carbohydrate that ties up excess stomach acid, and is particularly easy on the stomach.

Other studies find that dried beans, particularly white and red beans, as well as corn in modest amounts also tend to neutralize stomach acid. Tofu (soya bean curd) got high marks in combating stomach acid, according to research.

Other complex carbohydrate foods, like bread, can also help calm acid stomachs, says Dr. DerMarderosian. But don't go overboard, he cautions. Eating too much of any food stimulates the stomach to produce more acid, needed for digestion.

In contrast, here are beverages to avoid if you are bothered by acid stomach. All have the wicked ability to stimulate the production of stomach acid, according to tests: beer, wine, milk, coffee (both caffeinated and decaffeinated), tea with caffeine, 7-Up, Coca-Cola. Worst of all, according to German studies, is beer. Drinking beer nearly doubled stomach acid within an hour. Milk is deceptive; it may seem to ease stomach pain, but it actually has a rebound action, encouraging secretion of more stomach acid.

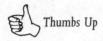 Thumbs Up

GINGER: A SUPER DRUG FOR NAUSEA

It really works. The amazing fact is that when researchers put ginger to the test, it came out as well or better than some modern pharmaceuticals in fighting motion sickness, seasickness, post-surgery nausea, morning sickness and plain old nausea. Unlike drugs, it does not produce side effects, even drowsiness, because ginger does not work through the nervous system. That ginger is an excellent antinausea medicine has now been proved by at least three controlled scientific studies.

The first classic study, by Daniel B. Mowrey, Ph.D., a Utah psychologist, discovered that ginger worked better than the common motion-sickness drug Dramamine when subjects were put into twirling chairs until they became nauseated. No one given 100 milligrams of Dramamine was able to stay past six minutes in the spinning chair without becoming sick and vomiting. Fully half of those who took about half a teaspoon of powdered ginger survived more than six minutes of stomach-turning activity.

A test of 80 Danish naval cadets on the rough seas showed that those who took ginger capsules – equal to a scant one-half teaspoon of ground ginger – were better able to stave off seasickness than those taking a placebo. The researchers found that ginger suppressed vomiting by 72 per cent and overall, was about 38 per cent protective against seasickness. The protection took effect within 25 minutes of taking the ginger and lasted about four hours.

Ginger even ranks high at suppressing nausea that often comes with recovery from anesthesia after surgery. Postoperative nausea has persisted at about the same rate (30 per cent of patients) for half a century, despite the continued introduction of new drugs to try to curb it, says British physician M. E. Bone at St. Bartholomew's Hospital in London. He and colleagues tried ginger in a double-blind randomized test of 60 women who had had major gynecological surgery. In this test, the drug, ginger or a placebo was given prior to surgery to specific groups of patients. Dr. Bone concluded that oral doses of 0.5g of ginger (one-third teaspoon) "produced better results than 10mg of injected metoclopramide," a common antiemetic.

Ginger's great attraction is its lack of side effects. Dr. Bone says surgeons are discouraged from using modern pharmaceuticals to curb post-op nausea because of their dire side effects. "Ginger may be the answer," he says. Since ginger has no recorded side effects, it might even be used prophylactically on a wide scale in patients prior to surgery, some experts suggest.

There's also enough ginger in ginger snaps and ginger ale to work against mild nausea, says U.S. Department of Agriculture's medicinal botanist Dr. Jim Duke.

DR. KOCH'S ANTINAUSEA FOOD REMEDIES

Kenneth L. Koch, M.D., a gastroenterologist and nausea researcher at the Hershey Medical Center and professor of medicine at Pennsylvania State University, sees hundreds of patients suffering from chronic nausea. "We find that what you eat or drink is very important if you have nausea or vomiting," he says. Here are his recommendations based on his extensive research and clinical experience.

It's okay to drink clear liquids to help settle your stomach. The first rule is to sip them slowly, taking 2–3fl oz (55–85ml) at a time; don't gulp them. Dr. Koch's two favourites, which he commonly recommends to nauseated patients, are warm and salty bouillon and Lucozade sports drinks which also has some salt and sugar. "Both are very easy on the stomach. The salt is especially good to restore electrolytes after vomiting, so you don't get dehydrated."

Avoid juices, especially citrus juices. "If your stomach is unsettled because of nausea or motion sickness, I would not put citric acid in the stomach. It is too irritating," Dr. Koch advises.

Warm or cold liquids? Many people opt for warm beverages as more soothing when their stomach is out of sorts, but "It probably doesn't matter, because it has been shown that when you drink something cold it very quickly reaches body temperature, says Dr. Koch. So the choice is up to you – whatever makes you more comfortable.

If you drink carbonated beverages, like Coke and 7-Up, let them go flat first. The gassiness may distend the stomach, further irritating it. The fizz may also induce belching, possibly giving you acid reflux and heartburn. "Carbonation is just another potentially aggravating factor," says Dr. Koch.

Is there any magic in Coca-Cola syrup, a longtime home remedy for nausea? Dr. Koch has done a controlled test of an over-the-counter

Coke-based syrup called Emetrol. He gave it to people with nausea, including those with morning sickness during pregnancy. "It did not settle nausea down in any significant way. In fact, we found, it often made nausea worse," he concluded, possibly because it is so heavily sugar. However, Dr. Koch thinks Coke syrup might help relieve vomiting because the heavy sugars might relax the stomach.

Should you drink tea? Absolutely. "Tea seems to be very soothing to many, many people. I don't know if it is the warmth or something in the tea," says Dr. Koch.

Coffee? "No. I think most people with nausea would have trouble with that." Plain tap water also makes many people with upset stomach feel worse.

WIND

Everybody has wind. If you don't have wind – the normal healthy person passes wind fourteen times a day – you're not alive. Excessive accumulation of wind in the intestinal tract – or flatulence (from the Latin *flatus* – a blowing) is an ancient universal complaint that has spawned lots of natural remedies, called "carminatives," such as peppermint, that help expel wind. Usually, they are the same foods that make you belch. Too much wind can be uncomfortable, sometimes painful and socially embarrassing, but it's rarely a sign of a serious disease, says Dr. Michael Levitt, University of Minnesota, whose research has gained him an international reputation as an authority on flatulence. But, if wind seems troublesome to you, the best way to control it is by diet.

HOW FOOD CAUSES WIND

When you eat carbohydrates – sugars, starches and fibre – much of them are not completely absorbed or digested in the stomach or small intestine. The residue then ends up in the large intestine, the home of hungry, harmless colonies of bacteria that feast upon the leftovers. This fermentation process spews off mixed gases; most of these are odourless, but a few are so odoriferous they can be detected by the human nose in a mere 100 parts per million of air.

How much gas you produce varies greatly from person to person.

Here are the most copious gas producers in most people:

• The most notorious universal gas producer is the family of oligosaccharide sugars, notably raffinose, highly concentrated in beans and much less so in other vegetables. These reach the large intestine in massive amounts because humans lack the enzyme (alpha-galactosidase) to digest them properly. Eating baked beans, one study found, increased the amount of gas released by twelve times.

• Lactose, a sugar in milk, is another big gas generator for the many people who are deficient in the enzyme lactase, needed to digest the milk sugar. Such people are deemed "lactose intolerant". Drinking two glasses of milk boosted gas release by eight times in a study of persons with lactose intolerance.

• Soluble fibre like that in oat bran (beta-glucans) and apples (pectin), also often passes into the large intestine, becoming fodder for gas-producing bacteria. Drinking around 1½ pints (850ml) of apple juice increased gas output about four times, in one test.

• Small amounts of starch can escape intact from the stomach and small intestine to become food for large bowel bacteria. This means that virtually all starchy foods – wheat, oats, potatoes, corn and even plain bread and pasta made with white flour, can sometimes be gaseous, says Dr. John Bond, another flatulence researcher at the University of Minnesota. Among carbohydrates, rice is least likely to cause gas, he says.

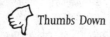 Thumbs Down

GREAT WIND FROM THE COW

Looking for a wind culprit? Focus on milk and dairy products (except yoghurt). Surprisingly, dairy foods, not beans, are the number-one cause of flatulence in America, says Dr. Levitt. The reason is simple – varying degrees of lactose intolerance, much of it unsuspected. You can have from mild to severe lactose intolerance and not even know it, but one sign is excessive wind after drinking milk or eating certain dairy products. Yoghurt is exempt. It does not produce gas, Dr. Levitt's tests show. (For more details, see the chapter on lactose intolerance, pages 132–34.)

HOW TO FIND YOUR WIND NEMESIS:

If you have the patience and persistence, and enough incentive, you can probably identify all the foods that give you wind. Consider one man who, at age 28, had suffered for five years from excessive flatulence and had consulted seven different doctors, who probed his intestinal tract with endoscopic examinations, always finding him normal. Told his

---

INFAMOUS GAS PRODUCERS

Although individuals vary, here are the foods most likely to produce gas, as reported in *Environmental Nutrition*:

HIGHLY GASSY

Broccoli, Brussels sprouts, cabbage, cauliflower, dried beans and peas, milk and dairy products (for people who have difficulty digesting the natural sugar in milk), onions, swedes, soya beans, turnips.

MODERATELY GASSY

Apples, bananas, bread and bread products (including bagels), carrots, celery, aubergines

NOT SO GASSY

Eggs, fish, meat, oils, poultry, rice

---

problem was that he swallowed air, he was counselled to eat slowly with his mouth closed and to reduce the pace of his life. No luck. Nor did a variety of medications help. Finally he was given that ultimate medical diagnosis signifying a doctor's defeat: He was told his problem was psychogenic – all in his head. He didn't buy it.

Instead, he decided to keep a record of every time he released gas and the food he had eaten. Over a year's time he averaged 34 passages of gas in a day – 250 per cent more than similar men his age. By this time he had come under the care of Dr. Levitt, who, suspecting a milk problem, proposed a test.

For two days the fellow ate nothing but milk – 3½ pints (2 litres) per day. Sure enough, the gas incidents jumped to a daily 141, including 70 in a single four-hour period. He also produced lots of gas when he drank two glasses of milk with a meal. He was pronounced lactose intolerant. When he cut out milk, the flatulence decreased dramatically but still not enough to suit him. He kept up his investigation, and finally linked his problem to milk, onions, beans, celery, raisins, bacon and Brussels sprouts.

YOUR GAS TIMETABLE

How long does it take for a food to produce gas? A healthy individual who eats beans is likely to produce no extra gas for the first three hours, say experts. After that, gas begins and you can expect the maximum output after five hours. Gas levels then start to decline and should be back to normal within seven hours.

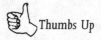Thumbs Up

BLOCK GAS WITH GINGER AND GARLIC

Add a little garlic and/or ginger to your pot of beans or other gaseous vegetables. Both are reputed in folk medicine to be anti-flatulent. Recently researchers at India's G. B. Pant University documented their effectiveness. After finding green peas to be a major producer of gas in animal experiments, the investigators did a test on dogs by adding a little ginger or garlic — amounts generally used in cooking — to the peas to see what would happen. Indeed, the herbs were potent gas blockers, taking nearly all the gas-producing power out of peas. When the dogs got peas with either ginger or garlic, gas production was no greater than it was from a wheat cereal, which was the least gaseous food tested. The researchers pronounced the tradition of adding spices to legumes and vegetables to be based on "sound principles".

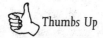Thumbs Up

DE-GAS YOUR BEANS

You can rob beans of their "flatulence factor" by soaking them, according to U.S. Department of Agriculture researchers, who cooked nine varieties of dried beans, using a special "blanch and soak" method. The de-gassed beans lost about 50 per cent of their gaseous powers. Here's how to do it, according to USDA researchers:

Rinse beans. Add them to boiling water and boil in a covered pot for three minutes. Let stand for two hours. Pour off the water, add new water at room temperature to just cover the beans. After two hours, pour this water off: Add more water and let soak overnight. Rinse again with room-temperature water. (Actually, researchers rinsed five times, but once or twice is enough, they say.) Then add water to cover and cook until done, about 1¼–1½ hours.

ANTIWIND DIET PRESCRIPTION

- If you have excessive wind suspect lactose intolerance from milk and dairy products; the exception is yoghurt.
- Beware sorbitol, the low-calorie sweetener, another ferocious gas producer.
- Observe your diet to determine which foods produce gas.
- Use cooking methods that minimize gas production from beans.
- Add garlic and ginger to gaseous foods.
- If the problem is troublesome, cut down on eating foods you know cause wind.

LACTOSE INTOLERANCE

Dairy Foods That Cause Distress: Plain milk • Buttermilk •
Acidophilus Milk • Cheese • Butter • Frozen Yoghurt • Whey •
All Dairy Products Added to Processed Foods

Dairy Foods That Are Okay: Yoghurt • Chocolate Milk

About 70 per cent of the world's population just can't drink milk or
eat dairy products (except yoghurt) without getting an upset stomach.
It's genetic and happens most often in people of African, Asian
and Mediterranean descent. It's caused by a deficiency of lactase, an
enzyme needed to absorb and digest the milk sugar, lactose. Un–
digested, the milk sugar lingers in the colon and ferments, creating
intestinal distress – abdominal pain, bloating, wind and diarrhoea – that
sometimes defies diagnosis or is misdiagnosed as serious bowel
disease.

"I know hundreds of people who have spent years and thousands of
dollars on tests looking for ulcers or spastic bowels, and who have been
told they're crazy. I tell them to lay off all dairy products for two weeks.
The results are usually so striking that it changes their lives," says David
Jacobs, M.D., a Washington, D. C., internist certified in nutrition,
allergy and immunology.

So don't believe you have a serious bowel disorder until you are sure
milk is not at fault.

How much upset milk causes depends on the severity of your lactase
deficiency. From 60–80 per cent of those with lactose intolerance can
still drink a single glass of milk without distress and about half can drink
two glasses of milk, says noted researcher Dr. Dennis Savaiano of the
University of Minnesota. One study found that normal people absorbed
92 per cent of milk's lactose; those with lactose intolerance absorbed
only 58 per cent.

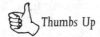 Thumbs Up

THE YOGHURT SALVATION

Yoghurt is safe because it comes predigested. In one of nature's small miracles, the bacteria in yoghurt take over for the missing enzyme and digest much of the milk sugar for you. According to tests by Dr. Savaiano, two bacterial cultures, *Streptococcus thermophilus* and especially *Lactobacillus bulgaricus*, that transform milk into yoghurt gobble up much of milk's lactose during fermentation, and once in the intestine eat much of the remaining lactose. Be sure the yoghurt has live bacterial cultures, as nearly all commercial yoghurts do; killed bacteria do not work so avoid long-life or pasteurized yoghurt. Plain yoghurts have more anti-lactose activity than flavoured yoghurts. Buttermilk and acidophilus milk, although fermented, still cause as much distress in

---

THE INTOLERANCE TEST: HOW TO TELL IF THE COW IS UNFRIENDLY

If you suspect you may be lactose intolerant, stop drinking any milk or eating any dairy products for at least two weeks. Be sure to check processed foods for hidden sources of dairy products. Whey, for example, has more lactose than any other food and it is frequently added to processed foods. So is dry milk.

If you feel better – and the gastrointestinal symptoms have diminished – you can do a "challenge" or "reintroduction" test to try to determine how much of which dairy foods you need to avoid. Drink a little milk or eat a little cheese and wait for two or three days to see what happens. It may take that long for symptoms of lactose intolerance to show up, say experts.

Your physician can also give you more definitive tests to diagnose lactose intolerance, including blood tests and a simple breath-hydrogen test.

---

most people as plain milk.

Beware of frozen yoghurt. When yoghurt is commercially frozen, it is sometimes repasteurized (reheated) and this kills the bacteria. Dr. Savaiano once tested all the brands of frozen yoghurts sold in

Minneapolis and St. Paul. He found that "none had significant enzyme activity," and thus were worthless against lactose intolerance. Even though some frozen yoghurt claimed to contain "live active cultures," there were not enough to do the job.

 Thumbs Up

DR. LEE'S CHOCOLATE TREATMENT

Try chocolate milk. It does not cause distress in most lactose-intolerant people, says Chong M. Lee, Ph.D., professor of food science and nutrition at the University of Rhode Island. In tests, adding one and a half teaspoons of cocoa to 8fl oz (225ml) of milk blocked cramping, bloating and other signs of lactose intolerance in 51 per cent of 35 subjects. Most likely, cocoa stimulates enzyme activity. In test tubes, cocoa increased lactase activity by 500–600 per cent, Dr. Lee found.

To make Dr. Lee's chocolate milk:

1. Stir one and a half teaspoons of pure cocoa and a little sugar (optional) or three and a half tablespoons of commercial sweetened chocolate mix into a mug of milk.

2. Wait two or three days after drinking it to see if there is a reaction. If there is, drink less of the chocolate milk until you find your own tolerable level. Some people who can't drink a whole glass at one time can drink half a glass, he says. Don't add more cocoa. Surprisingly, Dr. Lee found in animal tests that low levels of cocoa actually worked better in stimulating lactase activity than high amounts.

IF YOU ARE LACTOSE INTOLERANT – WHAT TO EAT

The consequences are likely to be less if you:
- Drink smaller quantities of milk at one time.
- Drink milk with meals.
- Drink whole rather than skimmed milk.
- Drink chocolate milk.
- Stay away from buttermilk and acidophilus milk and frozen yoghurt.

You can also add Lactaid or other similar tablets to milk, which supply the missing enzyme, or use special milk products, in which the lactose is reduced.

HEARTBURN

The Top Ten Heartburn Scoundrels: Chocolate • Fats
• Peppermint • Garlic • Onions • Orange Juice • Red-Hot Sauce
• Tomatoes • Coffee • Alcohol

It's sometimes called acid indigestion, sour stomach, regurgitation or "acid reflux". It's best known as heartburn – a fiery and painful sensation in the chest that plagues about 10 per cent of Americans every day.

Actually heartburn primarily results from "gastroesophageal reflux" in which the stomach's digestive juices – hydrochloric acid and an enzyme called pepsin – slosh back up into the lowest part of the oesophagus where they don't belong, causing smoldering sensations and pressure beneath the breastbone. (In some cases the crushing sensation is so great it is mistaken for heart attack.) The tender lining of the oesophagus, unlike that of the stomach, was not made to endure contact with such caustic substances, and thus reacts with irritation and pain.

Unquestionably, what you eat is a prime – and perhaps the prime – factor in whether heartburn strikes, how severe it is and whether it worsens through the years. Some people may be born anatomically more vulnerable to heartburn, but most often the predisposing culprit is your dietary pattern, says Donald Castell, M.D., a professor of medicine at the University of Pennsylvania School of Medicine and an eminent authority on the matter. He blames diet greatly for both bringing on and aggravating heartburn. Nor is heartburn necessarily a consequence of ageing. "Most of the patients I see with heartburn are in their twenties, thirties and forties," he says. "However, once you have reflux, like diabetes and hypertension, it does not go away." Anyone can have occasional heartburn from overindulging. The idea is to keep a rare or occasional bout with heartburn from becoming chronic.

Thus if you do not have recurring heartburn, diet is critical in keeping it away, and if you do have it, diet is even more important in keeping it from striking and/or progressing.

HOW HEARTBURN HAPPENS

Initially to blame is a failure of the lower oesophageal sphincter, a small muscular ring that separates the oesophagus from the stomach. The sphincter's job is to keep the stomach contents down where they belong. Ordinarily, when you swallow, this muscle relaxes to allow food to pass into the stomach. It should then quickly close tightly but, like an old rubber band, the muscular ring can become weakened and stretched so it no longer snaps tightly shut, or it may relax and spring open at the wrong time. In either case, it allows an opening for stomach acid and partially digested food to backwash into the oesophagus, touching sensitive cells and producing burning pain along with a bitter acid taste in the mouth.

FOUR WAYS FOOD ENCOURAGES HEARTBURN

1.   Specific foods can relax the sphincter muscle, causing it to open and allow stomach acid to backwash into the oesophagus. These are: chocolate, peppermint, spearmint, fatty foods, alcohol, probably onions. Clue: some of the same foods that make you belch can give you heartburn.

2.   Food can increase acidity of stomach juices, making them more painful when they wash up into the oesophagus. Foods that commonly spur stomach acid secretion are coffee (regular and decaf), colas, beer and milk.

3.   Such foods as citrus and tomatoes, hot spicy foods and coffee, when swallowed can directly contact an already damaged oesophagus, causing irritation and burning.

4.   Eating too fast and too much can overload the stomach, making it overfull, pressuring a weakened sphincter muscle to pop open. Lying down, especially on your right side, too soon after eating also thwarts gravity, pushing food up against the muscle, encouraging it to open. Carrying too much weight around the abdomen can also put pressure on the sphincter muscle, weakening it and promoting reflux. In that case, losing weight often alleviates heartburn attacks.

Undeniably, certain foods actually act as muscle relaxants, enticing the elastic ring to get lazy and open up. Since the pressure is greater inside the stomach than out, such a relaxation of that ring causes a spurt of stomach contents and acid upward into the oesophagus. If this happens enough, the oesophagus may become inflamed by the repeated exposures to acid. Then, even swallowing certain irritating foods can trigger spasms of pain. So the pain of heartburn can be caused by food going down as well as by a reflux action sending caustic stomach juices back up. Obviously, the more acidic the stomach juices, the greater the burning sensation and potential damage to the oesophageal wall.

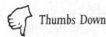 Thumbs Down

A DOCTOR'S CHOCOLATE-CHIP HEARTBURN

Beware chocolate. It is one of the most common culprits in heartburn. "I can bring on heartburn any time I want," says Dr. Castell, who has spent more than 20 years probing the exact mechanisms by which various foods precipitate heartburn. His own nemesis? "It's chocolate-chip cookies," he says. He does it rarely, but if he eats a big batch of such cookies, he has heartburn all night long, he says. That's not uncommon. Dr. Castell started investigating the villainy of chocolate because so many of his patients complained of heartburn after eating chocolate-chip cookies and fudge brownies.

Dr. Castell discovered that chocolate acts like a tranquillizer on the sphincter muscle that's supposed to guard against invasions of stomach acid. What makes the muscle mellow-out on the job, he thinks, is contact with a family of chemicals in chocolate called methylxanthines. Three of these chemicals are suspected of luring the muscle to relax: caffeine, theophylline and theobromine. Of these, Dr. Castell calls theobromine the strongest; chocolate has higher concentrations of smooth-muscle-relaxing theobromine than any other common food.

To prove how chocolate behaved, Dr. Castell had people drink about 4fl oz (115ml) of chocolate syrup; then he measured the pressure of their lower oesophageal sphincter muscle; it lapsed into a flabby lethargy that lasted an average 50 minutes. Further, he found the acid footprints of damage in the oesophagus from eating chocolate. He tested both ordinary people and patients who already had oesophageal inflammation from recurring heartburn attacks. On alternate days, after meals, the volunteers drank either a glass of water mixed with about 5 tablespoons (75ml) of chocolate syrup or a plain sugar-water solution. Within an hour after downing the chocolate drink, those with frequent heartburn showed detectable increases of stomach acid in their oesophagi, but no effect from sugar-water.

However, chocolate did not provoke an acid backflow in those who rarely or never had heartburn. Thus, Dr. Castell warns that chocolate is a special threat to those known to suffer from heartburn.

CHOCOLATE'S QUADRUPLE THREAT

Chocolate, especially milk chocolate, which is most common in this country, is a multiple threat in heartburn because it contains at least four substances (caffeine, theobromines, theophylline and fat) that can loosen the tight grip of the lower oesophageal sphincter, letting burning stomach acid escape up into the oesophagus, causing heartburn.

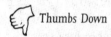 Thumbs Down

FAT – BIG DANGER

To avoid becoming a victim of heartburn and its attacks, cut down on fatty foods. Fried foods, milkshakes, cheese, hamburgers or any kind of fatty food dramatically lifts the chances of heartburn, says Dr. Castell. In fact, fatty foods are nearly twice as likely to aggravate heartburn in susceptible people as chocolate alone. About 76 per cent of such people are stricken with heartburn after eating high-fat foods, compared with 40 per cent after eating chocolate. More alarming, regularly eating lots of fat is apt to push you over the edge into chronic heartburn.

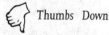 Thumbs Down

THE McMUFFIN EPISODE

Documenting the heartburn happening from eating fat required a trip to McDonald's. On one day a group of ten men and women with intermittent signs of heartburn and ten with severe heartburn ate a low-fat meal – mainly, McDonald's hotcakes with syrup and 8fl oz (225ml) of skimmed milk. The next day, they ate a high-fat meal – McDonald's sausage-and-egg muffin. Calories in both meals were the same, but the low-fat meal got 16 per cent of its calories from fat; the high-fat meal derived 61 per cent of its calories from fat. For three hours after the meals, Dr. Castell and colleagues monitored the acid in each subject's oesophagus.

As expected, acid was detected in the oesophagi of the habitual heartburn sufferers after the high-fat meal and, surprisingly, even after the low-fat meal. The high-fat meal was also more detrimental when the subjects lay down too soon after eating – within three hours. More striking was proof of the hazard of too much fat to occasional heartburn victims. The test sounded a warning for healthy individuals who have only intermittent signs of heartburn. Their exposure to acid shot up about four times more after they ate the high-fat meal than the low-fat meal. Further, the acid backwash into the oesophagus lasted for three hours after eating!

Fat-rich foods do lower sphincter muscle pressure, allowing acid backwash, probably because fat encourages the release of certain hormones, particularly cholecystokinin, from the lining of the stomach that regulates muscle control. Fat also delays emptying of the stomach, so high levels of acid and food hang around longer, giving them more opportunity to gush back upwards.

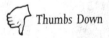 Thumbs Down

SPARE THE SPICY STUFF

It's true that pungent, spicy foods can aggravate heartburn. Take raw onions, for example. Gastroenterologists at the Oklahoma Foundation for Digestive Research and Presbyterian Hospital in Oklahoma City heard so many patients complain of heartburn after eating spicy meals with onions that they decided to test onions. They had 16 heartburn patients (heartburn episodes an average 4.4 times a week) and 16 normal subjects (heartburn less than once a week) eat a plain hamburger on one day. On another day they topped the hamburger with 1½oz (40g) slice of raw yellow onion. The doctors monitored the acid levels in the oesophagus and counted the number of reflux episodes.

The results: The onions caused no heartburn or other distress whatsoever in the normal men and women. About 40–50 per cent of the heartburn subjects suffered reflux episodes, increased acid in the oesophagus and the painful, burning sensations known as heartburn, says investigator Mark Mellow, M.D. Those with frequent heartburn also tallied up more belches.

One surprise, according to Dr. Mellow: The acid exposure in the oesophagus grew steadily worse in the two hours after eating the onions. This shows onions are potent and long-lasting in promoting heartburn, he says. Dr. Mellow speculates that onions in Mexican and Italian dishes are at least partly to blame for heartburn attributed to such "spicy" dishes. On the other hand, the onions used in the study were raw. Whether cooking onions reduces the risk of heartburn is unclear, he says. Although it is assumed that onions cause the sphincter muscle to relax, it's possible, says Dr. Mellow, that onions also directly irritate the oesophagus.

Once the oesophagus is damaged by assaults of upwardly mobile stomach acid, certain foods tend to irritate the oesophagus as they pass through, causing burning and painful sensations. Heartburn patients most often complain about citrus juices and hot spicy tomato-based foods. Tests indeed show that these foods don't feel good going down if you have a sensitive oesophagus induced by frequent attacks of heartburn. Whether spicy and pungent foods bring on heartburn sometimes depends on how much of it you eat. One prominent gastroenterologist says he can bring on heartburn by eating four – but not three – slices of pepperoni pizza.

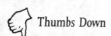 Thumbs Down

ALCOHOL: THE SILENT CULPRIT

Alcohol, especially if you drink it shortly before going to bed, can trigger heartburn attacks, notably in those with frequent reflux problems, but even in ordinary healthy folk. During the night, alcohol tends to relax the crucial sphincter muscle, allowing acid to seep up into your oesophagus without your knowing it. That's what Scottish researchers at the University of Dundee found in a test of 17 men and women who did not have reflux or heartburn symptoms.

The volunteers drank 4fl oz (115ml) (a little more than two doubles) of Scotch whisky (40 per cent alcohol) neat or with 4fl oz (115ml) of water. They usually had the Scotch at least three hours after eating the evening meal, at about 10 P.M. and then went to bed within two hours. On other nights they drank a placebo drink, which was mainly tap water.

During the night, investigators monitored the acid levels in the oesophagi of the subjects. Fully seven of the seventeen, or 41 per cent, experienced prolonged reflux events as they slept that spewed acid back up into the oesophagus, although they did not feel any heartburn pain. The acid attacks most frequently occurred three and a half hours after drinking the alcohol. The acid remained in the oesophagus for an average forty-seven minutes, and in some cases more than an hour and a half. The subjects did not have reflux events on the nights when they drank plain water.

DIET PRESCRIPTIONS TO ESCAPE HEARTBURN

If you don't have a history of frequent heartburn, go easy on fat; it's the dietary villain most likely to convert you from a sometime heartburn victim to a frequent sufferer. Also hazardous in making heartburn a constant companion are large meals, alcohol, eating late and lying down soon afterward.

If heartburn is a recurring condition, you can reduce the frequency and severity of the attacks by doing the following:

• Cut back on fatty foods and eat more complex carbohydrates and protein.

• Restrict or avoid chocolate, peppermint, coffee, alcohol and raw onions which can relax the sphincter muscle and induce acid-backwash.

• If you suspect your oesophagus is sensitive to citrus juices and hot spicy foods, stay away from them. If you have heartburn after eating such irritants, immediately drink water (or other nonacidic liquid) to wash the offending substance out of the oesophagus.

• If overweight, lose weight. Losing 10–15lb (4.5–6.8 kg) can cause symptoms to improve, says Dr. Castell. The extra weight apparently presses on the sphincter muscle.

• Don't lie down for three hours after eating. When you sit or stand, gravity helps prevent reflux, but you lose that advantage by lying down. Sleeping with your head elevated also helps avoid heartburn.

• Lie on your left side rather than on your right side to avoid heartburn. It's because the oesophagus enters the stomach from the right. So when you lie on your right side, the oesophagus is below the stomach opening, making it easier for acid to flow downward and into the oesophagus. Research definitely shows that people are less likely to have heartburn attacks when they lie on their left sides.

• Beware of drinking alcohol and then going to bed too soon. Such actions frequently trigger reflux incidents even in people with no history of heartburn.

COLIC

Food That May Cause Colic: Milk.
Food That May Alleviate Colic: Sugar Water

Diet is by no means always implicated in infant colic, but it should ways be a serious suspect. That colicky infants could be in such agony because of something they ate seems almost beyond belief. Yet some researchers believe that the *majority* of infants with colic – or some five hundred thousand newborns a year in the United States – suffer dreadfully and inflict overwhelming distress on their parents mainly because their food disagrees with them. The number-one culprit: milk.

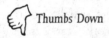 Thumbs Down

CRYING TILL THE COWS GO HOME

If a newborn has colic, immediately suspect milk. The idea that colic might be tied to a food reaction dates back to 1927, but not until the 1970s did the widespread incrimination of cow's milk gain credibility. Now about a dozen studies indict cow's milk as a colic instigator in susceptible infants. In fact, three recent studies show that about 70 per cent of colicky infants have an aversion to cow's milk.

Take away an infant's milk bottle and colic often totally disappears. For example: Swedish physicians discovered that 43 of 60 babies hospitalized for colic quickly recovered when switched from cow's milk formula to either soya milk formula or a special commercial casein hydrolysate formula in which milk's offending proteins are destroyed.

Researchers at the University of Edinburgh had almost identical success in a double blind study of 19 babies with colic. Fully 68 per cent were almost completely "cured" within a week when they were taken off infant formulas made with cow's milk. Some also could not tolerate soya milk.

Recently, Italian scientists got a 71 per cent colic cure rate in 70 infants, with an average age of one month, by taking away their cow's milk formulas. As a "challenge" test to be sure, the researchers gave the babies milk again on two occasions. The symptoms of severe colic returned in *all of them*.

HOW TO TELL COLIC FROM ORDINARY CRYING

All babies cry, but colicky crying is decidedly distinct from normal infant crying, and is a torment unique unto itself, say physicians. Medically, it's colic when an infant cries inexplicably and inconsolably for a total of three hours a day, three days a week for three weeks or more.

Colic is the frustrating fate of 15–40 per cent of infants around the world, affecting about a million newborns in the United States every year. It can be agonizing for both parent and child. Here's how Dr. Alexander K. C. Leung, assistant professor of paediatrics at the University of Calgary, Alberta, described it: "Typically infants with colic scream, draw their knees up against the abdomen and appear to be in great pain. They may pass some flatus, be quiet for a few moments and then begin crying again. These episodes usually occur late in the day or in the evening, and they may last from a few hours to many hours."

Such "spells of unexplained irritability, agitation, fussiness or crying" usually start in the first two weeks after birth, become most intense at four to six weeks, and may persist through the third and fourth months of age, Dr. Leung says.

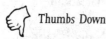 Thumbs Down

TROUBLE IN MOTHER'S MILK

Even mothers who breast-feed infants must be on guard against colic-inducing cow's milk. Mother's milk, too, can carry the colic hazard if the mother drinks milk or eats dairy products. The colic-creating substances in dairy foods can survive digestion, become concentrated in breast milk and flow right into a baby's system, causing just as much havoc as if the baby had taken them directly. A pioneering study by Swedish paediatrician Irène Jakobsson found that 12 of 19 breast-fed babies were jubilantly free of colic when their mothers cut out cow's milk.

In another test Dr. Jakobsson put the mothers of 85 breast-fed colicky infants on milk-free diets for about a week. Colic vanished in 48 of the infants, (56 per cent) and came quickly back in 35 of them as soon as their mothers took up drinking milk again. Just drinking one glass of milk put a mother's milk in the colic hazard zone, says Dr. Jakobsson.

"About one-third of breast-fed infants with colic will be free of symptoms when the mother is placed on a cow's milk-free diet." – Irène Jakobsson, M.D., Department of Pediatrics, Malmö General Hospital, Malmö, Sweden

---

CRACKING THE MILK MYSTERY

What agent in cow's milk could send an infant into colicky wails of protest? That has long baffled scientists. Now Anthony Kulcyzcki, M.D., an immunologist and associate professor of medicine at Washington University School of Medicine in St. Louis, thinks he and colleague Patrick S. Clyne, M.D., have found it. It is a pesky protein – a specific cow antibody that gets from the bovine's bloodstream into its milk.

Yes, cows, like humans, develop antibodies to fight off infections from various bacteria and viruses. Obviously, this is one antibody some infants, for unknown reasons, find drastically disturbing. Dr. Kulcyzcki detected the antibody in both cow's milk formula and breast milk. "Most mothers have an incredible amount of cow antibodies in their milk," he says. Further, he found that the more milk antibodies there were the more colic the babies had. Mothers with colicky babies had 31 per cent more cow antibodies in their milk than mothers without colicky babies. Mothers with the least antibodies in their breast milk had no colicky infants at all.

However, not all infants fed the antibody-laced milk got colic. Dr. Kulcyzcki surmises that stricken infants must also have some special susceptibility, perhaps an underdeveloped digestive system that balks at handling the foreign antibodies. In any event, Dr. Kulcyzcki is convinced these antibodies are "the major cause of colic". He adds: "It could even be the only cause".

Important: The colic-inciting antibodies hang around in breast milk and in the infant's tissue for an extraordinarily long time – a week or even longer in some cases – before being flushed out, he says. That gives them lots of time to cause pain and distress. It also means you will probably not see quick relief when you stop feeding an infant cow's milk. It's usually not enough to wait two or three days to see if colic subsides, although it does in some cases. In more than half of mothers it takes at least a week for the no-milk therapy to kick in, says Dr. Kulcyzcki.

THE COLIC MILK TEST

It can be tricky to determine if cow's milk is provoking colic in your infant, because keeping track of fussiness and crying is tedious and inexact. Here are some guidelines:

• If you are breastfeeding a baby with colic, stop drinking milk and eating dairy products for at least a week. If you are worried about calcium, take supplements.

• If your infant is on cow's milk formula, discontinue it and substitute casein hydrolysate formula (for example, Nutramigen or Pregestimil) for a week or so. This type of formula is considered safest for infants with reactions to cow's milk because the offending proteins have been obliterated. Nutramigen is only available on prescription. Pregestimil is available over the counter but is about four times the cost of ordinary formula. You can also try less expensive soya-based formula, but many infants also find it intolerable.

• After you stop the cow's milk, keep a daily record of your infant's colicky symptoms for a couple of weeks. If the infant experiences fewer or less severe colicky episodes, you have good reason to suspect milk. Sometimes the colic ceases entirely. Another less time-consuming test is to notice how often the baby wakes up at night for a couple of weeks. If the awakenings diminish after milk is discontinued, you may have found your culprit.

• If you want to risk a return of colic, you can test the theory by returning to cow's milk for a day or two. If colic comes back, you have even more proof.

• Give each change time and check with your health visitor. Rapidly swapping formulas will not help.

• BOTTOM LINE • *To find out whether cow antibodies are colic culprits, keep an infant and nursing mother away from exposure to cow's milk and other dairy products for at least a week, advises Dr. Kulcyzcki. It takes that long for the colic-causing cow antibodies to be eliminated from an infant's system and mother's milk.*

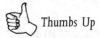 Thumbs Up

A SWEET CURE FOR CRYING

A newborn crying infant nearly always calms down immediately when given a little sugar water, confirming an old folk remedy of letting crying babies suck on a "sugar teat," a spoonful of table sugar wrapped in cloth. So found Dr. Elliott Blass, professor of psychology at Cornell University in Ithaca, New York. Using a syringe, researchers gave the crying infants a drop of either plain water or a water solution of 14 per cent sugar once every minute for five minutes. The babies getting the sugar water instantly stopped crying and remained quiet for about ten minutes. Their crying time dropped from about 40 per cent to 3 per cent.

Moreover, their heart rate fell from a fast 155 beats per minute to a normal 125–130 beats a minute. "The infants were less agitated and much more relaxed, but they were still very much alert," said Dr. Blass. "They were not drowsy. The sugar water worked in about 85 per cent of the newborns, he found. Sugar water was also three to five times more likely to subdue infant crying than a dummy.

Additionally, sugar water blocked pain in the infants. When subjected to painful medical tests or circumcision, newborns given sugar water cried about half as long as those not getting sugar water. "It increased their pain threshold," according to Dr. Blass. Dr. Blass speculates that such tiny amounts of sugar activate "opioid" chemicals in the brain that reduce pain and distress. In other words, the sugar acts directly on the brain as a painkiller. Both plain table sugar (sucrose) and fruit sugar (fructose) worked. Milk sugar (lactose) was useless.

A few drops of sugar water could therefore be a valuable aid in pacifying babies but no one would suggest using a sugar-dipped teat or cloth for prolonged contact because of the great harm likely to be caused to developing teeth.

WHAT ABOUT STRONG STUFF IN MOTHER'S MILK?

If you are breast feeding an infant, should you cut back on caffeine and spicy and pungent foods, for fear the substances will irritate the infant or contribute to colic? "There's no evidence such foods are a major problem in colic," says Morris Green, M.D., chairman of the Department of Pediatrics at Indiana University School of Medicine.

Actually, suckling infants seem to like it when mothers eat strongly flavoured odoriferous foods. A good whiff of garlic in mother's milk caused infants to take more of it and suck longer at the breast, according to new research. A little alcohol in mother's milk, however, put the babies off, depressing their appetites.

Still, nursing mothers may want to cut out chocolate, says Dr. Kulcyzcki, because chocolate usually contains a lot of milk – which could carry the offending proteins. As for caffeine, its well known it gets into mother's milk, and possibly could affect a baby.

COLIC-CURING DIET PRESCRIPTION

• If a bottle-fed baby won't stop crying, try switching the formula from a cow's milk base to a soya base or casein hydrolysate cow's milk formula. Wait at least a week to see if there is improvement.

• If you are breast-feeding an infant with colic, stop drinking milk and eating dairy products for a week. To get calcium, take supplements.

• Try giving the infant a little sugar water, after checking with a doctor to be sure the cause of crying and colic is not tied to an undetected physical problem. It's important to determine that colic is not due to some other-than-dietary cause. Don't give sugar in a form where it will be in prolonged contact with developing teeth, such as on a teat or in a dinky feeder.

SPASTIC COLON

> **Foods That May Aggravate:** Milk • Sorbitol • Fructose • Coffee • Cereals and Other "Allergic" Triggers
>
> **Food That May Relieve:** High-fibre Bran

If you are among the many who suffer from that mysterious and virtually untreatable disorder known medically as "irritable bowel syndrome" and commonly as "spastic colon," you should know that there could be some dietary relief. The same food culprits incriminated in persistent diarrhoea may be a primary cause of IBS. Indeed, such food intolerances, or "gut reactions," often masquerade as irritable bowel syndrome. Some experts even say the distress in most IBS sufferers could be alleviated or eliminated by changes in the diet. New evidence, mostly from here in Britain, suggests that food reactions are, indeed, a prime cause of spastic colon. Discovering, and restricting or eliminating the offending foods may clear up the problem entirely. It's a remedy worth considering for a condition that otherwise appears incurable.

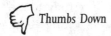 Thumbs Down

FIRST, SUSPECT MILK

Before you surrender to the diagnosis of irritable bowel syndrome, be sure your problem is not in your milk bottle. Before doctors knew about milk "allergy" or lactose intolerance, the inability to digest milk sugar, the problem was routinely misdiagnosed as IBS. All too often, it still is. The symptoms of the two disorders are in-distinguishable. Thus, when Italian physicians took a look at 77 hospitalized patients with long-standing complaints of IBS-like abdominal distress, they found that an astonishing 74 per cent had some degree of milk intolerance. When the patients were put on a milk-free diet for three weeks, their distress diminished or disappeared. When they went back to drinking milk for three weeks, their symptoms flared up again.

If you have long-standing abdominal distress, pain and diarrhoea, always rule out milk before accepting a diagnosis of irritable bowel syndrome, the researchers advise.

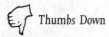 Thumbs Down

RULE OUT "DIETETIC" SUGARS

Dietetic sugars can produce a good imitation of irritable bowel syndrome, notably the natural sugar sorbitol. One study of 42 healthy adults detected sorbitol intolerance in a surprising 43 per cent of whites and 55 per cent of nonwhites after they ate a mere 10g of sorbitol – the amount in five sticks of sugarless gum, five sugar-free mints or a tablespoon of dietetic jam. In fact, 17 per cent of the group had *severe* IBS-like symptoms from eating such tiny amounts of sorbitol. Gastroenterologists at New York Medical College in Valhalla, who reported the study, said they had treated 15 patients in two years who had "sorbitol intolerance masquerading as irritable bowel syndrome". They concluded that such sorbitol-induced spastic colon and diarrhoea is common, poorly recognized and often precipitates expensive, futile "diagnostic procedures and a lifelong diagnosis of irritable bowel syndrome".

Another natural sugar, fructose, alone or combined with sorbitol can also produce a good imitation of IBS in many people. One study found that half of all IBS patients suffered intestinal distress after eating about 1oz (30g) of fructose.

If you have symptoms of IBS, especially chronic diarrhoea, cut out or reduce high-sorbitol foods in your diet, urges Gerald Friedman, M.D., associate professor of gastroenterology at Mount Sinai School of Medicine in New York. Such high-sorbitol foods, he says, include peaches, apple juice, pears, plums, prunes, sugarless gums, dietetic jams and chocolate.

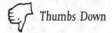 *Thumbs Down*

GO EASY ON COFFEE

Coffee may just be too harsh on the sensitive colons of people with IBS. In any event, about 30 per cent of 65 patients with irritable bowel syndrome said that coffee made them feel worse, according to British research.

"Eat a couple of handfuls of wheat bran every day, plus one orange and one apple. It helps defeat irritable bowel syndrome, constipation and diverticular diseases." — Martin A. Eastwood, M.D., a gastroenterologist-researcher at the University of Edinburgh Medical School

---

 Thumbs Up

EAT MORE FIBRE

A mere decade or two ago, the "medicine of choice" for irritable bowel syndrome was the same as for diverticular bowel diseases — a bland, low-fibre diet. Today, it's exactly the opposite. Doctors are high on fibre. Mount Sinai's Dr. Friedman says dietary fibre, eaten over an extended period of time, can actually "correct" some of the abnormal motor patterns of the colon common in functional bowel problems. For example, he says, fibre may help slow down or speed up contractions, helping in constipation or diarrhoea.

If a main problem of IBS is diarrhoea, the best remedy again is a high-bulk diet with bran or psyllium, according to W. Grant Thompson, M.D., a gastroenterologist and professor of medicine at the University of Ottawa, Canada "It's cheap and safe," he says. "Bran may solidify liquid stool and improve gut function generally." He recommends one table-spoonful of wheat bran three times daily on a trial basis for two to three months to see if it clears up diarrhoea due to irritable bowel syndrome. If it does, he calls it "the best solution" to a vexing, benign disorder.

WHEN IBS IS A STRANGE FOOD REACTION
___

People diagnosed with IBS may simply be allergic to a variety of foods, including milk, according to another theory, advocated by a group of British physicians. Gerard E. Mullin, M.D., an immunologist at The Johns Hopkins University School of Medicine, agrees "there is clear evidence that certain IBS patients do have allergic-type reactions and get better when they stop eating certain foods". Although medical opinion holds that this is true in a small minority of IBS sufferers, some startling statistics suggest otherwise.

A change in diet helped at least *half of all those diagnosed with IBS*, concluded British investigators at the Radcliffe Infirmary in Oxford. They recently found that 48 per cent of 189 people with IBS who excluded certain foods from their diet for three weeks had "marked improvement". Half of them identified two to five foods that upset them. Most commonly incriminated were dairy products (41 per cent) and grains (39 per cent).

TOP FOOD VILLAINS

Here are the foods that caused distress in more than 20 per cent of patients with irritable bowel syndrome in studies by British authorities John O. Hunter, M.D., and V. Alun Jones, M.D. They advise individuals with IBS to give up eating these foods for at least three weeks to see if they feel better:

- Cereals, mainly wheat and corn

- Dairy products

- Coffee

- Tea

- Chocolate

- Potatoes

- Onions

- Citrus fruits

After a year, the doctors reported that those who avoided the foods were still doing well. "The difference in symptoms between the two groups was striking," they wrote. "Of those responding to the diet, 73 were continuing with some dietary restrictions and all but one were well. Of 18 who reverted to former ways of eating, 6 were not well."

Even more striking are the findings of V. Alun Jones, M.D., and John O. Hunter, M.D., gastroenterologists at Addenbrookes Hospital in Cambridge, and leading pioneers of the theory. In a 1982 landmark study published in *The Lancet*, they found that 67 per cent of a group of IBS patients had food intolerances as confirmed by food challenges, and were symptom-free when they avoided the foods. Further, 42 per cent had relapses when they went back to their former diets.

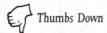 Thumbs Down

CHECK FOR *A WHEAT* CONNECTION

Ironically, the top offending food in the Jones-Hunter study was wheat – the very remedy most physicians prescribe to relieve IBS symptoms! In fact, the researchers said they were prompted to do the study by complaints from some patients saying they felt worse after eating the recommended bran. However, Dr. Hunter points out sufferers often can't spot their nemesis because it is so familiar. "We never ask patients, 'Do you think any food upsets you?', because if you ask that they will always say something that is fairly exotic. The foods we find most important are the cereals and the dairy products, but most people do not make the link between the foods and their symptoms because they are eating these foods every day." Other prominent offenders in the study were corn, dairy products, coffee, tea and citrus fruits.

The original Jones-Hunter studies were so successful that the doctors continued to treat IBS with restricted diets. Follow-up studies of patients after two years showed that 87 per cent stuck to their diets and were free of symptoms. Also, reactions to a particular food were fairly consistent; if a food caused IBS symptoms at one time, it was likely to do so at other times.

As a test, Hunter and Jones simply suggest cutting out foods they know have caused gut-wrenching reactions in at least 20 per cent of IBS patients. (See Top Food Villains, page 152.) Then you can add back the foods little by little, in search of the culprit or culprits. The person most likely to benefit from a restricted diet is the one with diarrhoea and pain. "It is usually a patient who is complaining of three or more loose stools a day on at least four days a week," says Dr. Hunter. "They may also complain of abdominal pain, headache and tiredness." People with constipation are not likely to benefit as much from the restricted diet, he says.

"If your colon kicks up from eating wheat, be wary of rye and corn also. People who react to wheat usually cannot eat rye or corn either. Barley is middling as a provocateur of irritable colons. On the other hand, rice is the safest. It rarely upsets sensitive colons." – Dr. John O. Hunter

---

WHY FOOD-TRIGGERED GUT REACTIONS HAPPEN

IBS-induced food reactions are not typical allergies, involving the immune system. Rather, they are delayed reactions that according to Dr. Hunter's theory, occur literally in the gut. He believes the problem stems from an abnormal imbalance of bacteria in the gut, triggered by eating certain foods, as well as by taking antibiotics. Normally, there are twice as many anaerobes – bacteria that don't need air to survive – in healthy colons. But Dr. Hunter found excessively high numbers of aerobes (bacteria that require air) in faecal samples of IBS patients after they ate an offending food. In two people with severe food intolerances, the number of aerobes jumped a hundredfold. Thus certain foods tend to wreck normal bacterial activity, Dr. Hunter argues, triggering the disturbances in the colon leading to the constipation, diarrhoea, pain and bloating known as IBS.

DIET STRATEGIES TO DEFEAT SPASTIC COLON

• Be sure your irritable bowel or spastic colon is not due to a reaction to or intolerance of common foods, mainly milk, sorbitol, wheat, corn and coffee.

• To find out if diet and IBS are linked, keep a detailed dietary history for at least seven days. Write down exactly what you eat and how much. Write down any symptoms that occur after you eat the food and write down the frequency and consistency of bowel movements. The idea is to try to see if there is a pattern of distress and intestinal upset after eating certain foods as opposed to others. You may spot a pattern.

• If you suspect your bowel problems are linked to diet, you can eliminate this food for three weeks and see if the IBS improves. If it does and you want to be sure of a connection, you can start eating the food again and see if there is a flare-up. You should also report your observations to your doctor.

• If constipation or diarrhoea are problems, try eating more fibre such as wheat bran, for relief but if this is not agreeable, be aware that you might be allergic to wheat. A good high-fibre substitute, not likely to produce a reaction, is rice bran.

DIVERTICULAR DISEASE

You won't find remedies for this common condition in ancient medical texts – no advice from the great physicians of the ages, Hippocrates, Galen and Maimonides. Why? Because it was nonexistent. It is unique to Western cultures of this century. Before 1900, diverticulosis – the presence of tiny grapelike pouches or sacs called diverticula, along the outer wall of the colon – was a medical curiosity, rarely seen. Now it is the most common disorder of the colon in Western populations, existing in one-third to one-half of all such people over age 60, many of whom are not aware of it. Further, about 10 per cent will develop more serious diverticulitis – a painful inflammation, leading to episodes of cramping, lower abdominal pain, and constipation or diarrhoea. Yet, diverticular disease is still rare in primitive communities, such as African villages, that have not adopted Western eating habits – and are still eating like our Stone Age ancestors.

The same thing that cures and prevents ordinary constipation is also considered the key to combating this disagreeable digestive disease: high-fibre foods, notably bran. In fact, relieving constipation itself also helps combat diverticulosis, for straining during bowel movements tends to expand the tiny diverticula along the muscle walls of the colon, causing discomfort.

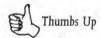 Thumbs Up

A "BRAN-NEW" IDEA

Imagine. For nearly 50 years, doctors treated diverticular diseases with a low-fibre diet. The theory was that "roughage irritates the gut". Ironically, this misguided practice was a cause, not a cure for the problem, says the man who helped change it all, Neil S. Painter, a surgeon at Manor House Hospital in London. Dr. Painter released his landmark study in a 1972 issue of the *British Medical Journal*, showing that diverticulosis was caused by a fibre-deficient diet. Knowing that such patients ate only half as much fibre as people with healthy colons, he persuaded seventy diverticulosis sufferers to go on a high-fibre diet. It was a near total success. After a 22-month follow-up period, he found that the diet had alleviated or abolished the symptoms (pain, nausea, flatulence, distension, constipation, etc.) associated with diverticular disease – in 89 per cent of them! Bowel habits were normalized; all but a few gave up laxatives.

What did they eat? One-hundred-per cent whole-wheat bread, cereals high in bran, plenty of fruits and vegetables. They also added unprocessed wheat bran to every meal and gradually upped the dose until they passed one or two soft stools a day without straining. This bran has about five times the fibre of ordinary whole wheat, says Dr. Painter.

RECIPE FOR RECOVERY

How much bran they needed was determined by "trial and error". Dr. Painter pointed out there was no single correct "dose" of bran to help such bowel problems. It varied greatly, ranging from a mere one dessertspoon daily (3g) to three tablespoons three times a day (12–14g). "Most required two teaspoons of bran three times a day, to render the stools soft and easy to pass," he said.

Dr. Painter's advice: Start with two teaspoons of unprocessed bran three times a day. After two weeks increase (or decrease) this dose if necessary and until you can move your bowels once or twice a day without straining. Since the bran is difficult to eat dry, Dr. Painter's subjects sprinkled it on cereal, mixed it with porridge, added it to soup or took it with milk or water. A few patients were able to overcome their symptoms simply by eating processed bran cereals, such as All-Bran, instead of unprocessed wheat bran.

Dr. Painter explains that a deficiency of dietary fibre alters the consistency of the faeces so that the sigmoid part of the colon has to generate high pressures to propel the faeces more vigorously. This causes the herniation of the walls of the colon, characteristic of diverticular disease.

NEW ADVICE ON PIPS AND SEEDS

At one time experts cautioned people with diverticulosis against eating foods with seeds and hulls, such as tomatoes, strawberries and popcorn. It was feared such matter could become trapped in the diverticular pouch and promote inflammation and a painful acute attack. In actuality, such pips and seeds are not much of a worry, many experts now say, and have reversed their ban on them.

———————

"There is no dose of bran that is correct for every patient any more than there is a standard dose of insulin. Each patient must find the amount of bran required by trial and error over a period of at least 3 months." – Neil Painter, M.D., British surgeon

———————

ULCERS

Foods That May Help Heal Ulcers: Bananas • Plantains • Cabbage Juice • Liquorice • Tea • Hot Chilli Peppers

Foods That May Aggravate Ulcers: Milk • Beer • Coffee • Caffeine

---

In the first century A.D., the celebrated Roman medical encyclopaedist Aurelius Celsus warned: "If the stomach is infested with an ulcer, light and glutinous food must be used . . . . Everything acrid and acid is to be avoided." A seventh-century physician, Madhavkar, from West Bengal, blamed fried and hot food, alcohol and irritating and sour foods for the pain of peptic ulcer. In this century, for nearly seventy years (from 1911 to 1980), ulcer therapy was dominated by the Sippy milk diet, named for its inventor, American physician Bertram Welton Sippy (1866–1924). It mandated drinking cream and milk at regular intervals all day long for at least six weeks. For nearly two thousand years, a bland diet has been the drug of choice for ulcer sufferers. No longer. Modern science has turned that concept topsy-turvy.

HOW FOOD CAN AFFECT ULCERS

The immediate cause of peptic ulcers is fairly simple. The stomach secretes more corrosive acid and digestive enzymes than the lining of the stomach and duodenum (first part of the small intestine) can tolerate. Consequently, the acid-enzyme mixture eats away, actually digesting tissue that would resist digestion if it had the strength. The attacks create inflammation, sores, tiny holes, sometimes bleeding and often a great deal of gnawing, burning abdominal pain. Thus, ulcers are an imbalance between acid's misguided attacks and the stomach lining's (mucosa) ability to resist being chewed up.

The underlying cause of ulcers is still controversial, although extensive new evidence blames a bacterial infection from a germ called *Helicobacter pylori*. Speculation is that the infection releases acid in the stomach, promoting ulceration. Thus many physicians now use antibiotics to try to keep ulcers from recurring.

Regardless, food and drink journeying through the stomach and intestines infringe intimately on ulcer territory and can ease or worsen symptoms. Your choices of food and drink can help control the amount and destructive quality of acid secretion, build up stomach cell defences, making them less vulnerable to attack; and perhaps help nip ulcers by attacking bacteria. Many foods, long used to treat ulcers, have anti–biotic effects which may help explain their success. Certainly what you eat can worsen or alleviate your stomach pain and contribute to or detract from the healing of the ulcer wound.

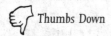 Thumbs Down

THE MILK MYTH

If anyone today says, "Drink lots of milk to soothe your ulcer," clutch your abdomen and escape quickly. The commonsense belief that milk "neutralizes" or buffers stomach acid and helps heal ulcers is myth. As early as the 1950s researchers began to suspect milk was a dud remedy when they could not confirm that it neutralized stomach acid. In fact, milk's neutralization of acid is woefully transient, often lasting a mere 20 minutes. Then acid levels rebound even higher, because milk strikes back with a vengeance by encouraging secretion of the hormone gastrin, which triggers release of even more acid.

A 1976 landmark study, at the University of California at Los Angeles School of Medicine, proved the point by having normal people and patients with duodenal ulcers drink whole, low-fat and nonfat milk. In all cases stomach acid levels jumped far above normal levels, and rose highest in ulcer sufferers. (Ulcer patients apparently are especially sensitive to milk's acid-stimulating effects.) Further, milk continued to stimulate stomach acid production for about three hours.

The clincher came in 1986 when Indian researchers, writing in the *British Medical Journal*, reported that milk actually blocked ulcer healing, making it much worse than an ordinary diet. Investigators randomly assigned 65 duodenal ulcer patients to a regular hospital diet or an all-milk diet – eight cups a day. (All were also on the antiulcer drug cimetidine.) After a month, doctors using a fibre optic device known as an endoscope directly inspected each ulcer. In those eating a regular diet, 78 per cent of the ulcers had healed. Only 50 per cent had healed in the milk drinkers!

Yet, interestingly, both ulcer groups had experienced identical *relief* of *pain*. Thus, milk made the stomach feel better even as it promoted damage. Milk's ability to ease pain while wreaking destruction may account for its long-time misguided use as an ulcer remedy, the researchers concluded.

"*No controlled study has ever shown the superiority of a bland diet or a strict peptic ulcer diet over a regular diet.*" – S. K. Sarin, G. B. Pant Hospital, New Delhi, India

---

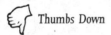 Thumbs Down

FAREWELL TO BLAND DIETS

Beware a bland diet. There is little or no proof that the long-recommended low-fibre bland diet relieves or prevents ulcers. Just the opposite, according to current thinking. A lack of roughage, far from discouraging ulcers, encourages them, especially duodenal ulcers that were rare before 1900 and have skyrocketed in this century, argues Frank I. Tovey, M.D., a surgeon at the University College of London and a prominent researcher on diet and ulcers.

As evidence, Dr. Tovey points out that the Japanese, who eat a heavy diet of polished rice, have the highest peptic-ulcer rate in the world. Ulcers are also a major problem in the rice-eating areas of Southern India. But guess what? They are rare in North India where chapattis are the staple food, those pancake-like rounds of unleavened bread made from unrefined wheat. It's about the same in China, where ulcers are prevalent in the southern rice-growing areas and less so in the northern wheat-raising lands, he says. He can make a good case for the same variations in Africa, where processed foods equal higher rates of ulcer, and high-fibre unprocessed foods are linked to lower ulcer rates. Further, shifting to a high-fibre diet seems to help heal ulcers and prevent relapses. In Bombay, Dr. S. L. Malhotra took a group of 42 patients with healed ulcers who were regular rice eaters. He had half of them convert to a Punjabi type unrefined-wheat diet. He followed them for five years. During that time, fully 81 per cent of the rice-eaters had relapses – their ulcers flared up again. In comparison, only 14 per cent of the high-fibre wheat eaters had a recurrence of ulcers. The same thing happened among a group of healed ulcer patients in Oslo, Norway. Within six months, 80 per cent of those on a low- fibre diet had ulcer relapses compared with only 45 per cent on a high-fibre diet.

How fibre might work is unclear. One theory is fibre has a buffering effect; it reduces gastric acid concentrations. Fibre might irritate the stomach lining, toughening it up.

• BOTTOM LINE • *High-fibre carbohydrate fools are good for ulcers; a low-fibre diet is detrimental, say experts.*

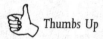 Thumbs Up

BANANAS BUILD STRONG STOMACHS

To protect your stomach against acid and ulcers, eat bananas and plantains, the large banana-like fruits that are a staple in many tropical countries. These fruits are definitely antiulcerogenic, and have long been used in folk medicine to treat ulcers. The evidence is so persuasive that Indian physicians often prescribe Musapep, a dried powder made from green plantains, to treat ulcers; reportedly the success rate is 70 per cent.

Bananas work in a most remarkable way – not by neutralizing stomach acid, as once thought. Instead, according to British pharm– acist Dr. Ralph Best at the University of Aston in Birmingham, bananas stimulate proliferation of cells and mucus that form a stronger barrier between the stomach lining and corrosive acid. In fact, when animals are fed banana powder, researchers can observe a visible thickening of the stomach wall. In one Australian test, rats fed bananas and then fed high amounts of acid to induce ulcers suffered very little stomach damage. The bananas prevented 75 per cent of the expected ulceration.

NOTE: *Plantains must be cooked before eating because they are too hard and tough to eat raw. Green plantains are considered more potent medicine for healing ulcers than ripe ones.*

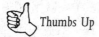 Thumbs Up

THE *AMAZING CABBAGE* EXPERIMENTS

There are natural antiulcer drugs in cabbage. That cabbage can help heal ulcers was shown by the pioneering experiments of Garnett Cheney, M.D., a professor of medicine at Stanford University School of Medicine, in the 1950s. He demonstrated that just over 1½ pints (850ml) of fresh cabbage juice every day relieved pain and healed both gastric and duodenal ulcers better and faster than standard treatments did. In a test of 55 patients who drank cabbage juice, 95 per cent felt better within two to five days. X rays and gastroscopy revealed a rapid healing of gastric ulcers in only one-quarter of the average time. The duodenal ulcers of patients fed cabbage also healed in one-third the usual time.

In a double blind study of 45 inmates at San Quentin Prison in California, 93 per cent of the ulcers in prisoners taking cabbage juice concentrate in capsules – the equivalent of just over 1½ pints (850ml) of fresh cabbage juice every day – were healed after three weeks. Only 32 per cent of the ulcers healed in those taking a dummy capsule.

How could cabbage work? Seemingly by strengthening the stomach lining's resistance to acid attacks. Cabbage contains gefarnate, a compound used as an antiulcer drug, as well as a chemical that resembles carbenoxolone, another infrequently used antiulcer drug. Essentially, the drugs incite cells to spin out a thin mucus barrier as a shield against acid attacks. Indeed, G. B. Singh, of India's Central Drug Research Institute in Lucknow, induced ulcers in guinea pigs and cured them with cabbage juice. During the healing he took extensive microscopic photos of the cell changes, documenting that cabbage juice generated increased mucus activity that rejuvenated ulcerated cells leading to healing.

Another possibility is that cabbage is an antibiotic. It can destroy a variety of bacteria in test tubes, perhaps including H. pylori bacteria, now implicated as a cause of ulcers.

DR. CHENEY'S ANTIULCER CABBAGE RECIPE

Make juice from fresh, raw green cabbage. (It's easier today because you can use a juicer.) Chill. Drink just over 1½ pints (850ml) a day. You should notice results in three weeks, said Dr. Cheney. Spring and summer cabbages are therapeutically superior and the freshest are best. "The quicker the trip from garden to stomach, the better," according to Dr. Cheney. Long storage saps their powers. The cabbage must be raw; heating or processing destroys cabbage's active antiulcer agents.

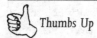 Thumbs Up

THE LIQUORICE CURE

"If I had an ulcer, the first thing I'd go for is liquorice," says James Duke, Ph.D., botanist at the U.S. Department of Agriculture. Dozens of studies, he says, endow liquorice root with formidable antiulcer properties. For example, Scandinavian scientists found that liquorice compounds reduced acid, stimulated mucus secretion and helped stomach wall cells repair themselves.

Pharmaceutical companies have even developed a drug called Caved-S − which is essentially liquorice without its most troublesome ingredient, glycyrrhizin. In a British test of one hundred ulcer patients the liquorice drug, which is chewed, was just as effective as the commonly used ulcer drug Tagamet in healing ulcers.

NOTE: *Some liquorice sweets are not the real thing; they may be flavoured with anise, which does not have liquorice's therapeutic effects. Liquorice sticks are the real thing and are often available in health food stores. However, be cautious about eating too much liquorice, especially if you have high blood pressure or are pregnant. Potential side effects are fluid retention and potassium depletion with a consequent rise in blood pressure. Eating two to three sticks of true liquorice raised one man's blood pressure from 120/70 to 240/160.*

BEAN BUFFERING

In studies published in the *Scandinavian Journal of Gastroenterology*, researchers looking for foods with high buffering capacity against stomach acid found the best to be red and white beans. The legumes mopped up the most acid. Also good were corn and unpolished rice. The researchers urged ulcer patients to eat more beans, especially red beans, which exhibited the most antacid activity.

 Thumbs Up

HOW JAPANESE MICE AVOID ULCERS: THEY DRINK TEA, OF COURSE

Give tea a chance; it may also discourage ulcers. The Japanese have a lot of peptic ulcers, but the rate might be even higher if they didn't drink green tea, surmises Dr. Yukihoko Hara, a food researcher in Japan. Green tea is rich in antibacterial, antioxidant polyphenols, called catechins.

"It's very clear these tea polyphenols reduce ulcers in mice," says Dr. Hara. In tests, the mice drinking green tea developed fewer and smaller ulcers after being given ulcer-causing chemicals. Indeed, the higher the concentration of tea compounds, the less the ulcer damage. Lower catechin doses reduced ulcers 22 per cent; moderate doses, 47 per cent and the highest doses of tea compounds wiped out the development of ulcers 100 per cent!

Dr. Hara deems the tea drugs powerful enough to fight ulcers in humans. "The doses we used are very low, comparable to what people ordinarily drink in Japan," he says. The probable mechanism is catechin's antibacterial powers, although the compounds might also help neutralize pepsin activity, he speculates. Because tea has some caffeine, which could stimulate acid secretion, Dr. Hara says it's better to drink decaffeinated tea. Black and oolong tea also possess catechins, but in lesser amounts than Asian green tea.

TOP STOMACH ACID MAKERS

Ulcer sufferers are commonly told to lay off coffee, cola and alcohol. The purported reason is that they tend to rev up stomach acid production, but researchers at the University of California at San Diego discovered that other beverages were just as bad or worse. They had normal healthy subjects drink 12fl oz (340ml) of several popular beverages, as well as water for comparison. Then they measured stomach acidity. It shot up, usually within a half hour after drinking all the beverages; investigators concluded that "each of the beverages is a potent stimulus of gastric acid secretion."

Here are the acid-producing culprits in order of potency:

1. Milk
2. Beer
3. Kava (low-acid coffee)
4. 7-Up
5. Sanka (decaf coffee)
6. Coffee (with caffeine)
7. Tea (with caffeine)
8. Coca-Cola

NOTE: Obviously, caffeine was not at fault. Decaf Sanka was more potent than regular coffee. And 7-Up was a particular surprise, since it has no caffeine or other agents thought to spur acid secretion. Beer also caused an unexpected surge in acid, and not solely because of the alcohol. In fact, researchers said it was doubtful that alcohol per se spurred the acid production. Topping the list as the champion acid stimulator was milk – no surprise. The researchers did not test wine, which has been found in other studies to stimulate acid.

 Thumbs Up

TEX MEX AND HOT SPICES MAY HELP, NOT HARM

Contrary to popular belief, spicy food does not cause ulcers or retard their healing or harm normal stomachs in any way, according to David Y. Graham, M.D., professor of medicine at Baylor College of Medicine in Houston, who has the pictures to prove it. He and colleagues had volunteers eat test meals at different times: a bland meal of steak and french fries; a pepperoni pizza; and a Mexican meal of enchiladas, beans and rice topped with hot sauce and 1oz (30g) of chopped jalapeño green peppers.

Then doctors used videoendoscopy – close-up photos of the subjects' stomachs and duodena – to search for damage. They found none. To be extra sure, the investigators put 1oz (30g) of ground-up jalapeño pepper directly into the stomach through a tube: still no sign of bleeding or erosion of the stomach lining. Concluded Dr. Graham, "Spicy food seems safe. We found no gastric or mucosal abnormalities after ingestion of highly spiced foods, and previous studies have shown that the administration of large amounts of red peppers does not reduce the rate of healing of duodenal ulcers."

Crazy as it seems, hot peppers may help protect the stomach lining. The hot stuff in peppers is capsaicin, and animal studies show that capsaicin limits damage ordinarily caused by aspirin or alcohol.

DR. WEIL'S HOT PEPPER TEA FOR ULCERS

"Experiment with cayenne pepper. This may sound absurd, but in fact spicy foods do not aggravate ulcers, and red pepper specifically can help them. It has a good local anesthetic effect and also brings blood to the surface of the tissue. Try sips of red pepper tea (one-quarter teaspoon of cayenne pepper steeped in a cup of hot water) or a small capsule of the powder if taste is too strong."
— Andrew Weil, M.D., University of Arizona College of Medicine

---

In one experiment, Dr. Peter Holzer, at the University of Graz in Austria, gave rats an aspirin solution that, as expected, damaged tissue of the stomach lining, producing bleeding. However, rats that got capsaicin along with the aspirin had 92 per cent less bleeding. Experts suspect capsaicin protects by stimulating nerves in the stomach wall, dilating blood vessels and improving blood flow.

There are some reports that ulcer patients who ordinarily eat spicy foods — Indians who eat hot curry and Latin Americans who eat fiery peppers — do not complain as much of ulcer symptoms as do people on bland diets.

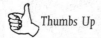 Thumbs Up

GARLIC — GOOD FOR YOUR STOMACH

Don't shun garlic; the pungent condiment may also retard stomach damage and ulcers. So found researchers at Catholic University Medical College in Seoul, Korea. They fed rats doses of alcohol designed to harm the stomach lining. Some animals also got pure garlic or garlic compounds — diallyl disulphide and allicin. The rats downing the garlic and components had much less stomach damage, especially less haemorrhaging and cell destruction beneath the surface of the lining.

Researchers attributed the protection not to the inhibiting of gastric acid secretion, but to mild irritation that stirred up production of protective hormone-like substances (prostaglandins) that strengthened stomach lining resistance.

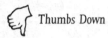 Thumbs Down

COFFEE SPURS ACID

Go easy on coffee, regular and decaf, if you have an ulcer or acid stomach. There's no evidence that coffee causes ulcers, but it does incite stomach acid secretion. The caffeine in three to six cups of coffee stimulates both gastric acid and pepsin production studies show. Interestingly, even without caffeine, coffee is just as powerful an acid instigator. Thus, either regular or decaf coffee can aggravate ulcers.

Theoretically, coffee, by pumping up acid secretion, should increase ulcer pain; in fact, it often does not. When researchers ask patients if they have discomfort after drinking coffee, a surprising number say no. A study at the University of Michigan found that coffee drinkers with ulcers had no more complaints of ulcer pain than non-coffee-drinking ulcer patients.

THE ALCOHOL PUZZLE

Worried that a little alcohol can produce ulcers or cause your ulcer to kick up? It's unclear, although most physicians advise ulcer patients to go easy on alcohol. Alcohol and alcoholic beverages, studies consistently show, inflict damage, including ulcerations and bleeding, on the stomach lining. However, evidence that drinking causes ulcers, delays healing or causes relapses is not consistent. After a comprehensive review of the medical literature on ulcers and diet in 1985, Dr. S. K. Sarin, a gastroenterology professor at the G. B. Pant Hospital in New Delhi, India, wrote: "There is no evidence to suggest that the use of alcohol is associated with an increased frequency of duodenal ulcer. . . . A recent study has even shown that moderate drinking appears to promote ulcer healing."

Indeed, German researchers at the University of Dusseldorf followed 66 ulcer patients for a year and discovered to their surprise that moderate drinking – roughly the amount of alcohol in a shot of spirits a day – hastened ulcer healing. Their theory is that the repeated hits by mild irritants, such as low concentrations of alcohol, toughen up the resistance of the stomach lining so it can better stand up to attacks by subsequent strong irritants, including acid.

Still, it doesn't make sense to try to build a tougher stomach by drinking alcohol, when you can do it in other safer ways. And alcoholic beverages do churn out disagreeable amounts of acid, not entirely because of their alcohol content. Beer is a case in point.

"It seems reasonable for patients with peptic ulcer disease to avoid alcohol, at least alcohol in a concentrated form, such as 80° proof alcohol." – Martin H. Floch, M.D., Yale University School of Medicine

---

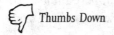 Thumbs Down

BEWARE BEER: THE ACID FACTORY

Beer is a particularly potent prod of stomach acid, according to studies by professor Martin V. Singer, at the University of Heidelberg in Germany. Dr. Singer and colleagues found that drinking beer nearly doubled the stomach acid secretion in subjects within an hour. White wine also increased acid output by 60 per cent in the same time. It's noteworthy that neither whisky nor cognac boosted stomach acid.

The investigators concluded that constituents of beer other than alcohol were the main instigators of the surges in stomach acid. Most responsible was fermentation caused by adding yeast.

This study suggests it may be a good idea to single out beer as something to be especially avoided by people with ulcers, heartburn and other stomach acid problems. White wine for unknown reasons seems to be another avoidable nemesis for stomach acid worriers.

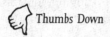 Thumbs Down

SOME LIKE IT TOO HOT

Don't drink boiling hot liquids. Even if spicy foods do not hurt your stomach, foods hot in temperature can. Some people, believe it or not, drink liquids so hot that if it were spilled on their skin, it would produce burns. Although it stands to reason that pouring really hot water down your throat could produce burns and ulcerations along the way, some people don't think about it. Such individuals are more likely to have diseases of the oesophagus, stomach and duodenum. As early as 1922, a physician reported that most of his ulcer patients preferred hot drinks. Current thinking is that drinking very hot liquids, notably tea, can even instigate oesophageal cancer. Hot liquids may also damage the lining of the stomach. It's well-known from animal studies, say investigators, that drinking water hotter than 60° C can cause extensive damage to the stomach lining and can induce gastritis

Surgeons at the Manchester Royal Infirmary recently became interested in the subject. As a test, they asked volunteers to drink tea and coffee at "comfortable temperature". Half of the test-group had ulcers. The others did not. Guess who drank the hottest tea or coffee? Yes, the ulcer patients, who preferred their drinks at a near-scalding 62° C. The non-ulcer group liked their beverages 6°C cooler, at 56°C. Interestingly, those who drank the burning hot liquids did not notice discomfort or pain.

It makes sense that people with ulcers should not drink superhot liquids, nor should anyone else. (Drinking boiling hot tea has been declared a cause of oesophageal cancer in Japan.)

DIET PRESCRIPTION TO PREVENT AND HEAL ULCERS

• Obviously, the bland diet of yesteryear is not necessary to placate ulcers and in fact appears detrimental. This does not mean ulcer patients can never drink milk – many doctors allow a couple of glasses a day – but deliberately drinking lots of milk as a cure for ulcers is unwise. You should also go easy on other acid-stimulating beverages, especially beer.

• On the positive side, it makes sense to eat foods with antiulcer activity, including cabbage juice, bananas, especially plantains, green tea, especially decaffeinated tea, liquorice in moderation, high-fibre foods and red beans.

• Hot peppers and garlic can be good medicine for ulcers, contrary to popular belief, but don't continue eating them if you suffer any pain or other discomfort.

• Another common bit of advice – to eat small frequent meals instead of three meals a day – has no ulcer-healing benefits, according to diet recommendations from the Mayo Clinic. In fact, such frequent eating could be detrimental by increasing acid secretion, say experts at the clinic. On the other hand, it's also not good to eat large quantities of food that distend the stomach.

GALLSTONES

> **Foods That May Prevent Gallstones:** Lots of Vegetables • Soya beans • A Little Alcohol • Olive Oil
> **Food That May Promote Gallstone Attacks:** Coffee • Sugar

HOW GALLBLADDER ATTACKS HAPPEN – AND HOW FOOD CAN PREVENT THEM

It's been described as fingers of pain that radiate from the upper right of the abdomen reaching up into the lower right chest and sometimes over the shoulder and spreading down the back. Such a gallstone attack can last minutes or hours with much anguish and no relief, and sometimes with nausea or vomiting.

The gallbladder is a little pear-shaped pouch tucked under the liver; it is full of bile that squirts into the intestine to help digestion. Ninety per cent of stones in Westerners form when the bile becomes supersaturated with cholesterol that crystallizes into hard pellets as small as grains of sand or as big as an inch (2.5cm) in diameter. Eighty per cent of the time the stones are harmless, often undetected; but sometimes, when the gallbladder contracts to release bile, a stone shoots out and plugs the opening of the duct leading to the liver and small intestine. That's when the pain comes. The attack may end when the stone falls back into the gallbladder or complications, such as inflammation of the gallbladder, can become so serious as to necessitate removal of the stone and the gallbladder: Gallstones come with age, strike women, especially obese women, three times as often as men, and run in families.

Some individuals are just more prone to gallstones but diet can make a decided difference. What you eat can thwart formation of stones by lessening or increasing the degree of saturation of the bile with cholesterol – the prime contributor to gallstone formation. Certain foods can also provide more "detergent" to keep the cholesterol safely dissolved. Diet can also regulate contractions that expel stones into the duct, bringing on a painful gallbladder attack.

 Thumbs Up

VEGETABLE ANTIDOTES

A good bet to help prevent both gallstones and attacks is to eat more vegetables. An unidentified ingredient in vegetables appears to ward off gallstones. Vegetable lovers and, certainly, vegetarians have fewer gallstones. A British study found vegetarian women only half as apt to have gallstones as meat-eating women, regardless of age or weight.

A recent large-scale Harvard study of some 88,000 middle-aged women of normal weight found that women with the highest intake of vegetables were only 60–70 per cent as likely to have gallstone symptoms as women who ate the least vegetables. Women who ate the most nuts, beans, lentils, peas, lima beans and oranges, specifically, were especially resistant to gallbladder attacks.

What is the gallstone-fighting ingredient in vegetables? Maybe fibre, but most likely vegetable protein, researchers theorize. Feeding animals vegetable protein, including soya bean protein, consistently blocks gallstones by reducing the saturation of cholesterol in the bile. Researchers suspect the same thing happens in humans. Remarkably, studies at Wistar Institute in Philadelphia showed that eating lots of soya protein even caused small gallstones in hamsters to dissolve.

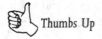 Thumbs Up

LIGHT DRINKING MAY HELP

A little alcohol discourages gallstones. Half a glass of wine or beer a day or one third of a shot of whisky reduced gallstone incidence about 40 per cent in the recent Harvard study. However, drinking more than that did not offer more protection, says study director Dr. Malcolm Maclure, assistant professor of epidemiology at Harvard.

Theoretically, a little alcohol increases the breakdown of cholesterol, making less of it available to form gallstones.

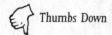 *Thumbs Down*

TOO MUCH SUGAR – TOO LITTLE FIBRE

Beware a typical modern fibre-depleted, sugar-rich diet. Fibre helps immunize against gallstones. In one British test, a group prone to gallstones ate either a high-fibre or low-fibre diet for six weeks at a time. The low-fibre diet contained only 13g of dietary fibre and nearly 4oz (115g) of sugar a day, plus white flour and white rice. The high-fibre diet called for 27g of fibre, lots of vegetables and fruits, whole grains and no sugar.

Decidedly, the cholesterol content of bile shot up (super-saturated bile forms gallstones) on the low-fibre high-sugar diets. Thus, the researchers advised those susceptible to gallstones to lay off sugar and eat lots of whole grains and fruits and vegetables. Other experts agree.

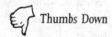 *Thumbs Down*

COFFEE CALAMITY

If you know you have gallstones, beware of coffee. So advise researchers Bruce R. Douglas and colleagues at the University Hospital in Leiden, the Netherlands. Coffee straight up, with no cream or sugar, and with or without caffeine, can stimulate the gallbladder to contract, possibly bringing on a gallbladder attack, they discovered.

In tests of healthy normal men and women, the Dutch invest-igators found that drinking as little as 4fl oz (115ml) of either regular or decaf coffee stimulated gallbladder contractions. In comparison, plain salt water had no effect. Obviously, the unknown substance in coffee that stimulated higher levels of blood cholecystokinin – an intestinal hormone – and consequent contractions is not caffeine. The researchers advise people prone to gallstones to avoid all types of coffee.

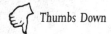 Thumbs Down

AVOID THE BREAKFAST GAP

Going for long periods without eating – as in fasting – or even skipping breakfast helps bring on gallstones, according to James Everhart, M.D., a scientist at the National Institute of Diabetes and Digestive and Kidney Diseases. He tracked 4,730 women over a ten-year period and found gallstones highest in women who fasted overnight for fourteen hours or more, presumably skipping breakfast. Least likely to have gallstones were women who fasted fewer than eight hours. Furthermore, the longer the fast, the greater the gallstone risk. Dr. Everhart says that without the stimulation of food, the gall– bladder does not put out enough "solubilizing" bile acids that keep cholesterol dissolved and unable to form stones. His advice: To help prevent gallstones, eat breakfast and beware of long periods of fasting.

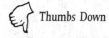 Thumbs Down

TEN POUNDS TO GO

Being even a little overweight is a gallstone hazard, notably in middle-aged women, according to much evidence. The risk rises dramatically with weight gain, according to the recent large-scale Harvard study. Obese women were six times as prone to gallstones as women of normal weight. More surprising, the study found that women only 10lb (4.5 kg) overweight had nearly double the chance of developing gallstones.

For unknown metabolic reasons, it is thought that excessive fat leads to production of more internal cholesterol, which is then secreted into the bile to become potential stones. If you have high triglycerides and low HDL cholesterol, your susceptibility to gallstones also rises.

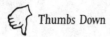 Thumbs Down

QUICK WEIGHT-LOSS DANGER

Obviously, if carrying excess fat promotes gallstones, the logical solution is to lose weight but there is a paradox. One of the surest ways to bring on gallstones is to lose weight rapidly. Indeed, several studies show that rapid weight loss from low-fat, low-calorie diets (under 600 calories and less than 3g of fat a day) can cause gallstones in up to 50 per cent of dieters. Those who are heaviest and lose the most quickest are at highest risk. Further, says Dr. C. Wayne Callaway of George Washington University, dieters often have gallstones but never experience symptoms until they get off a drastic weight-loss diet and then try to eat normally.

You may be able to overcome some of the hazard by including at least 5–10g of fat in one meal each day, according to Steven Heymsfield, M.D., of the Obesity Research Center at St. Lukes-Roosevelt Hospital in New York. For example, you can add a couple of teaspoons of olive oil every day.

This fat is necessary to stimulate the gallbladder to empty bile completely at least once a day, retarding gallstones. When you drastically cut fat intake, the gallbladder does not contract as often to expel bile into the intestine, says Dr. Heymsfield. Thus, bile builds up and can trigger formation of gallstones.

Many experts think it is unsafe to lose more than ½–1lb (225–450g) a week.

FAT MISUNDERSTANDINGS

Will eating less fat save you from gallstones? Eating too much fat can make you fat, and therefore more vulnerable to gallstones. And overindulging in saturated animal fat and cholesterol may aid the formation of gallstones. Greek researchers recently documented that people who ate lots of animal fat, such as fatty meat and butter, were more apt to develop gallstones. Interestingly, they found that a high consumption of olive oil actually discouraged formation of gallstones.

Its doubtful however that cutting down on fatty foods after you have gallstones can help stem the painful attacks.

According to a once-popular theory, high-fat meals incite a release of the hormone cholecystokinin, which tells the gallbladder to contract, forcing gallstones into the duct. New evidence holds that the stones are passed at random and have nothing to do with the amount of fat eaten. A landmark study at Georgetown University School of Medicine found that a gallstone attack was just as likely to occur after a fat-free or low-fat meal as after a high-fat meal.

In the test, 15 subjects on four separate days ate either a breakfast with less than 15g of fat, more than 30g of fat or no fat at all. Using ultrasound, the researchers measured the gallbladder contractions every fifteen minutes for an hour. They concluded that the contractions were totally unrelated to the intake of fat. Surprisingly, contractions occurred as often after a fat-free meal as after a high-fat one. The Georgetown investigators contended that a low-fat diet specifically to fend off gallbladder attacks is generally not warranted, although a low-fat diet is good for health in general.

WHAT TO EAT TO PREVENT GALLSTONES

- Eat lots of vegetables, especially legumes.

- Go easy on sugar.

- If you already drink moderately, this may help.

- Do not fast for long periods, and be sure to eat breakfast.

- Lose excess weight slowly. Quick weight loss can bring on gallstones. Eat some olive oil every day.

KIDNEY STONES

Foods That May Help Block Kidney Stones: Fruits • Vegetables • High-fibre Grains (such as Rice Bran) • Fluids, Mainly Water

Foods That May Promote Kidney Stones: High-protein Foods, Notably Meat • Sodium • High-oxalate Foods, Like Spinach and Rhubarb

HOW FOOD MAKES KIDNEY STONES

One of humankind's oldest maladies, kidney stones are rock-hard accumulations of crystal deposits, usually composed of calcium and oxalates, that can grow and obstruct the flow of urine through the kidneys. Men are three times as susceptible to kidney stones as women. Once you have kidney stones, the chances of a recurring stone are about 40 per cent in the next five years, and 80 per cent in the next 25 years.

Whether you develop stones depends on many factors, including heredity, metabolic abnormalities, infections, medications – and diet. How do stones form and why can diet intervene? Crystals of minerals, including food supplies of calcium and oxalates, are dissolved in the urine that passes through the kidneys. When the urine becomes supersaturated, the crystals fall out and collect into tiny masses that accumulate into hard stones. What you eat helps determine the crystal content and crystal saturation of your urine. The answer is to eat in a way that keeps high levels of cal–cium and oxalate out of the urine. About 80 per cent of all stones afflicting people in industrialized nations are made of calcium oxalate.

Kidney stones, like other modern chronic diseases, appear to be another fallout from a Westernized diet of affluence, too rich for some susceptible individuals. In Western countries kidney stones are ten times more common today than in 1900.

TRY THE DIET CURE FIRST

If you have recurring kidney stones, diet should be the "drug of choice" – the first therapy to try to ward of the stones. Why submit to a lifelong drug regimen with many potential side effects when you can often get the same marked benefit from diet without the hazards? That is the view of experts like Stanley Goldfarb, M.D., professor of medicine at the University of Pennsylvania School of Medicine in Philadelphia. He says changes in diet can eliminate more than half of all stone recurrences. Mayo Clinic researchers once showed that a whopping 58 per cent of 108 patients with recurring kidney stones who came to Mayo's stone clinic and received broad dietary advice, mainly to drink more fluids, had no signs of new kidney stone growth over the next five years!

Important: Diet works for *active stone-formers* – those who are pass–ing recently formed stones or have stones that are growing larger, as determined by X ray. Which dietary restrictions work best depends on whether the urine is high in calcium, oxalates or other minerals, and can best be determined by a 24-hour urine test of volume and minerals. Generally, however, stone formers need to pay attention to five factors: protein, sodium, oxalate, calcium and fluids.

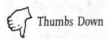 Thumbs Down

MEAT FOR THE STONE AGES

If you are prone to kidney stones, cut back on meat, especially if you eat more than 7oz (200g) a day. Much of that animal protein eventually turns to stone. The reason is that eating animal protein can drive up urine levels of the stones' raw materials – calcium, oxalate and uric acid – multiplying the chances of stone formation. Some stone formers are gluttons for protein, often eating nearly twice as much as dietary recommendations advise. On the other hand, even normal amounts of animal protein can stimulate abnormally high levels of uri-nary calcium in some individuals, for unknown reasons. Men who eat the most protein boost their chances of kidney stones by one-third, according to a new Harvard study.

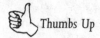 *Thumbs Up*

THE *VEGETARIAN DEFENCE*

Here is additional proof of meat's encouragement – and vegetables' discouragement – of kidney stones: vegetarians are much less likely to have kidney stones. In Britain, for example, vegetarians have only one-third as many kidney stones as meat eaters. Such vegetarians also eat twice as much fibre recognized as an antidote to kidney stones, and they excrete less calcium. Studies show that vegetarians, when put on meat diets, have increases of calcium in their urine.

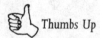 Thumbs Up

THE JAPANESE EXPERIMENT

In Japan, the rate of kidney stones has tripled since World War II, reportedly because the Japanese are eating more like Americans. Researchers at Kinki University in Osaka found that a change in diet did have remarkable impact on retarding stones. Among a group of 370 men, some were simply asked to increase their fluid intake and others were instructed to eat vegetables at every meal and cut back on meat. They also ate three meals a day, avoided large dinners and allowed more time between dinner and bedtime.

The low-meat, high-vegetable diet was a great success. Over four years, such men were from 40–60 per cent less likely to have recurring kidney stones than the men who merely drank more fluids. The diet worked in men both on and off medication, and was most effective in those with high urinary calcium. The investigators concluded that diet should be the first line of prevention against kidney stone disease in Japan.

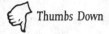 Thumbs Down

CUT DOWN ON SALT

Cut down on sodium. "It's one of the most effective things you can do," says Alan G. Wasserstein, M.D., director of the Stone Evaluation Clinic at the Hospital of the University of Pennsylvania, "especially if you eat a lot of salt." Restricting sodium, he says, slashes the amount of calcium in the urine, notably in those who excrete large amounts of calcium. In tests when Dr. Wasserstein's patients cut sodium intake and restricted protein, their excretion of urinary calcium dropped 35 per cent.

Some stone-formers — maybe 10–20 per cent — overindulge in sodium, eating more than 5,000mg a day. It's wise to cut that at least in half, say experts. Others prone to stones also have an overreaction to sodium, stimulating calcium excretion.

Dr. Wasserstein advises stone-formers with high urinary calcium not to use salt at the table or in cooking, and to avoid high-sodium processed foods such as bacon and other cured meats, olives, canned soups (unless low-sodium), sauerkraut. smoked fish and frozen and canned "ready meals" (unless low-sodium).

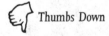 Thumbs Down

BEWARE SPINACH AND RHUBARB

Eating oxalate-rich foods may help boost urinary oxalate, which can combine with calcium to form stones. There's no question that stone-formers often have lots of oxalate in their urine, but some of it gets there through other avenues, say experts. For example, eating too much protein also enriches urine with oxalate. Therefore, it's uncertain how much cutting back on high-oxalate foods helps but it's worth a try. Studies do show high urinary oxalate in stone patients who eat lots of oxalate-rich foods, such as spinach, rhubarb, peanuts, chocolate and tea.

• BOTTOM LINE • *Don't worry about eating up to 180 milligrams of oxalate a day, but more may lead to a "marked increase" in urinary oxalate, says Richard W. Norman,*

STONE-MAKERS: FOODS HIGH IN OXALATES

Food	Serving	Milligrams of Oxalate
Baked beans	12oz (340g)	50
Blackberries	5oz (140g)	66
Chocolate	1oz (30g)	35
Cocoa	1 tablespoon (15ml)	35
Gooseberries	5oz (140g)	132
Leeks	7oz (200g)	89
Peanuts	5oz (140g)	288
Rhubarb	2½oz (75g)	1,092
Spinach, cooked	5oz (140g)	1,350
Squash, mashed	8oz (225g)	40
Swede	6oz (170g)	32
Sweet potato	1 (medium)	63
Swiss chard and beet greens	5oz (140g)	1,000

M.D., director of the Stone Clinic of Camp Hill Medical Centre in Halifax, Nova Scotia. Three foods to particularly avoid: spinach, rhubarb and beet greens.

THE CALCIUM CONUNDRUM

If calcium is the main stuff of kidney stones, why not severely curtail calcium to ward off stones? "For years, when you went to a physician after you had a kidney stone, you were told to stop eating dairy products because calcium is in the stone and the calcium must have come from your diet," notes Dr. Goldfarb. It's actually more complicated, he says, and severely restricting calcium-rich foods may be worthless or actually detrimental. Paradoxically, severe restriction of calcium can actually have the unwanted effect of boosting oxalate in the urine and promoting kidney stones' recurrence. Also, eating calcium does not dump as much calcium in the urine as eating protein does.

Indeed, a large new study has found that men who ate more calcium were less prone to kidney stones than men who restricted calcium! After studying the diets of 45,619 men for four years, Dr. Gary Curhan and colleagues at Harvard's School of Public Health reported that men who ate the most calcium had a 34 per cent lower risk of kidney stones than those who ate the least calcium. Non-stone formers took in about 600 milligrams more daily calcium, the amount in two glasses of milk. In fact, the study also revealed that men who drank two or more 8fl oz (225ml) glasses of skimmed milk a day had a nearly 40 per cent lower risk of kidney stones compared with men who drank only one glass per month. Also, eating 8oz (225g) or more of cottage or ricotta cheese a week reduced risk by 30 per cent compared with eating less than 4oz (115g) per month.

Dr. Curhan thinks calcium ties up food oxalate in the intestines, preventing it from entering the bloodstream and travelling to the kidneys where it forms crystals that become stones. He advises people who have had calcium stones not to restrict high-calcium foods. That means two or three servings of dairy foods or other high-calcium foods (about 800 milligrams of calcium a day) are not only okay, but desirable.

NOTE: *Only calcium in foods, not supplements, seems to deter stones, because to be effective, the calcium must be ingested at the same time as the oxalates in food, says Dr. Curhan. Few people take supplements with every meal.*

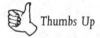 Thumbs Up

THE ANCIENT WATER CURE

Drink more water. Hippocrates' 2,000 year-old advice to thwart kidney stones is still tops among physicians, no matter what the cause or type of stone. One study found that men who drank the most fluids cut their chances of kidney stones 29 per cent. Drinking lots of water blunts the potential damage from calcium, oxalate and every other stone-forming mineral in the urine. The reason is that water dilutes concentrations of minerals that can crystallize into stones. Studies show that people who excrete less than 1¾ pints (1 litre) of urine a day are much more likely to have kidney stones than those who put out twice that much. Fluids are particularly beneficial to the one-third of stone-formers who do not eat excessive protein, sodium, oxalate and calcium, but have an extra sensitivity that promotes high urinary mineral concentrations.

Unfortunately, most people think they drink more fluids than they actually do. The bare minimum should be eight glasses spread throughout the day, and twice that much is sometimes recommended, especially in hot weather when it is sweated off. Dr. Norman says at least half the fluid should be water. Dr. Wasserstein recommends water, dilute apple juice or some diet fizzy drinks, but water is the drug of choice, he says. Fluids to skimp on, especially if you are on a calcium- or oxalate-restricted diet, are tea, hot chocolate, citrus juices and high-sugar soft drinks.

What about alcohol? Stone sufferers should be moderate, says Dr. Norman. There's some suggestion that alcohol boosts levels of urinary calcium and uric acid. And beer, especially draught beer, contains oxalate.

"I prescribe water for recurring kidney stones. I actually take out a prescription pad and write a prescription, saying drink two 8fl oz (225ml) glasses of water every four hours – at 8:00 AM., noon, 4:00 PM., 8:00 PM. and before bedtime. I want them to see it as a medication, not just as a vague by-the-way advice to drink more fluids. And the water prescription is in addition to other fluids they ordinarily drink."
– Dr. Stanley Goldfarb, professor of medicine, University of Pennsylvania School of Medicine

---

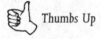 Thumbs Up

UP THE FIBRE

Even when you are eating a high-fluid, low-protein diet, high-fibre foods can further reduce stone-encouraging urinary calcium and oxalate. In one study at Halifax's Stone Clinic at Camp Hill Medical Centre, 21 patients prone to forming stones ate a couple of high-fibre wheat or corn bran muffins or biscuits every day, boosting their fibre intake from 6g per day to 18g. The amount of calcium in their urine dropped sharply. "Fibre may be especially beneficial for people at risk of forming calcium kidney stones," said dietician Janey Hughes.

One fear of a high-fibre diet is that such foods contain oxalate. But rice and corn bran contain only half as much oxalate as wheat bran and these also help prevent kidney stones, Japanese researchers have found. In tests, 182 calcium stone-formers who ate ⅓oz (10g) of rice bran twice a day for an average five years had about a sixfold drop in kidney stone recurrence. Fully 61 per cent did not develop new stones during that time. The greatest benefit was in the most frequent stone formers.

There is a potential for abuse. An excess of fibre could block calcium absorption, resulting in a very low calcium balance, in short, com— parable to a super-low-calcium diet but so far, such problems have not appeared.

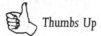 *Thumbs Up*

NO STONES FOR THE PHILADELPHIA BANKER

At age 47 a financial executive in Philadelphia had passed kidney stones for 15 years. In recent years they were coming more frequently – five a year for the last five years compared with a total of five in the first ten years. His distress sent him to the Stone Evaluation Center at the University of Pennsylvania. There some stones were dissolved by shock- wave lithotripsy. Still, X-rays showed more stones were developing.

Physicians took a look at his diet. He was eating lots of protein – about 110g a day, 80g in animal protein (the amount in 12oz (340g) of T-bone steak) and considerable amounts of sodium. With the help of a dietician he changed his diet, dropping his protein intake to no more than 65g a day. He cut down on sodium and avoided high-oxalate foods. He was told to drink an extraordinary amount of water – two 12fl oz (340ml) glasses every two hours while awake.

The last time the physicians checked the Philadelphia banker, he had not developed or passed a stone for three years.

STONE-FIGHTING DIET ADVICE

Try diet first to defeat recurring kidney stones. You can then use drugs if diet fails. Here is general advice from experts:

• Number one: drink more water – at least two glasses every four hours in addition to other fluids you normally drink.

• Restrict sodium to 2,500 milligrams a day, especially if you now eat a lot of sodium.

• Restrict animal protein, namely meat. For most people, that means no more than one 7–8oz (200–225g) serving of meat, poultry or seafood a day. (3oz (85g) of meat, poultry or seafood typically contains around 20 grams of protein.)

• If you eat lots of oxalate-rich foods, such as spinach and rhubarb, avoid them or cut back. Go easy on high-sugar beverages, such as non-diet colas and citrus juices, which are also high in oxalates.

• Eat two or three servings of high-calcium foods, including dairy foods, a day – and do not go on a drastically low calcium diet of less than 650–800 milligrams a day.

• Eat more high-fibre vegetables and grains.

Such a diet can cut your risk of having stones by half or more say many experts. Most likely to benefit are stone-formers who usually eat large amounts of protein and sodium.

CANCER

CANCER

> **Foods That May Help Prevent Cancer:** Vegetables – Notably Garlic, Cabbage, Soya beans, Onions, Carrots, Tomatoes, All Green and Yellow Vegetables • Fruits, Especially, Citrus • Fatty Fish • Tea • Milk
>
> **Foods That May Encourage Cancer:** Meat • High-fat Foods • Vegetable Oils, Such as Corn Oil • Excessive Alcohol
>
> **Foods That May Help Thwart the Spread of Cancer:** Seafood • Garlic • Cruciferous Vegetables, Such as Cabbage, Broccoli, Collard Greens

THE STAKES ARE HIGH

Diet is now considered a major weapon against cancer. The American National Cancer Institute says about one third of all cancers are linked to diet. British expert Richard Doll recently put the figure as high as 60 per cent. Thus, food choices might help prevent some 92,000 to 165,000 new cancer cases and 55,000 to 98,000 cancer deaths in 1993 in the United Kingdom alone – about 450 a day.

HOW FOOD CAN HELP SAVE YOU FROM CANCER

Full-fledged cancer is a long time happening. That means you have years in which to literally starve or feed a potential cancer. Two to three decades are typical and four to five decades not unusual from the time a single cell suffers genetic changes, called mutations, until a tumour appears.

The exciting news is that what you eat may interfere with that cancer process at many stages, from conception to growth and spread of the cancer. For example, some chemicals must be "activated" before they can initiate cancer; food can block that. Food compounds can turn up the body's detoxification system, preventing the genetic rape of cells, a prelude to cancer. Food chemicals in cells can determine whether a cancer-causing virus or natural cancer promoter like oestrogen can turn tissue cancerous. Antioxidant food substances, including vitamins, can snuff out carcinogens, and even repair some of their cellular damage. Even after cells have massed into still-benign tiny structures that can grow into dangerous tumours, food compounds can intervene to *stop further growth or actually shrink the patches of precancerous cells or eruptions!* Diet, though far less powerful at later stages, may still influence the metastasis or spread of cancer. Wandering cancer cells need the right conditions in which to attach and grow. Food agents can foster a hostile or favourable environment. The right foods even after cancer is diagnosed may help prolong your life.

The myriad ways food can influence cancer are indeed complicated, not fully understood and intertwined with many other factors. Even if your genetics and lifestyle are against you, your diet may still make a tremendous difference in your cancer odds. Here is the latest evidence on what to eat to prevent all types of cancer.

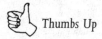 Thumbs Up

READ MY LIPS: MORE FRUITS AND VEGETABLES

It is inarguable. Ever since scientists started probing a cancer-diet connection in the 1970s, the antidote to cancer has been coming up "fruits and vegetables," consistently and relentlessly. It is a striking read-my-lips kind of message. In the words of Dr. Peter Greenwald, Director of the Division of Cancer Prevention and Control at the American National Cancer Institute: "The more fruits and vegetables people eat, the less likely they are to get cancer, from colon and stomach cancer to breast and even lung cancer. For many cancers, persons with high fruit and vegetable intake have about *half the risk of people with low intakes.*"

That fact is substantiated by massive evidence. A recent review of 170 studies from seventeen nations by Gladys Block, Ph.D., of the University of California at Berkeley, came up with the same exciting message: People everywhere who eat the most fruits and vegetables, compared with those who eat the least, slash their expectations of cancer by about 50 per cent. That includes cancers of the lung, colon, breast, cervix, oesophagus, oral cavity, stomach, bladder, pancreas and ovary. Nor are we talking about huge amounts of fruits and vegetables. Some research shows that eating fruit twice a day, instead of less than three times a week, cut the risk of lung cancer 75 per cent, even in smokers. It is almost mind-boggling, says one researcher, that ordinary fruits and vegetables could be so effective against such a potent carcinogen as cigarette smoke.

The evidence is so overwhelming that Dr. Block views fruits and vegetables as a powerful preventive drug that could substantially wipe out the scourge of cancer, just as cleaning up the water supply eliminated past epidemics, such as cholera.

• BOTTOM LINE • *Nobody really knows the best anticancer dose of fruits and vegetables, but at least two fruits and three vegetables a day of various kinds are a goal to aim for. Adding more fruits and vegetables to a typical diet is likely to cut your chances of cancer.*

TOP FRUIT AND VEGETABLE CANCER FIGHTERS

Here are the plant foods the National Cancer Institute has under investigation for their expected anticancer potential:

Garlic, cabbage, liquorice, soya beans, ginger, *Umbelliferae* vegetables (carrots, celery, parsnips), onions, tea, turmeric, citrus fruits (orange, grapefruit, lemon, lime), whole wheat, flax, brown rice, *Solanaceae* vegetables (tomato, aubergine, peppers), cruciferous vegetables (broccoli, cauliflower, Brussels sprouts), oats, mint, oregano, cucumber, rosemary, sage, potato, thyme, chives, cantaloupe melon, basil, tarragon, barley, berries.

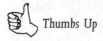 Thumbs Up

THE ANTICANCER TRUTH IS IN YOUR BLOOD

If you had a chemical snapshot of your blood, it would predict your chances of cancer. Your blood reveals the truth about whether you have been getting infusions of anticancer compounds by eating fruits and vegetables. Analyses of blood samples consistently reveal that cancer victims tend to eat lower amounts of fruits and vegetables. For example, a recent 12-year study of about 3,000 men in Switzerland found that those with low blood levels of vitamin A and carotene, reflecting low fruit and vegetable intake, were more likely to die of all types of cancers, especially lung cancer. Low blood levels of vitamin C predicted death from stomach and gastrointestinal cancer.

A recent British study found that cancer rates dropped by 40 per cent in men with the most blood beta carotene, compared to those with the least. Other research has found that those with higher levels of folic acid (found in green vegetables) and lycopene (a tomato compound) are much less vulnerable to all cancers, in particular of the lung, cervix and pancreas.

BEST FRUIT AND VEGETABLE BETS AGAINST VARIOUS CANCERS

Lung cancer: carrots and green leafy vegetables
Colon cancer: cruciferous vegetables and carrots
Oesophageal, oral and pharyngeal cancers: fruit
Laryngeal cancer: fruit and vegetables
Stomach cancer: fruit in general; lettuce, onions, tomatoes, celery,
        squash — especially raw vegetables
Pancreatic cancer: fruits and vegetables
Bladder cancer: vegetables, specifically carrots, and fruit
Thyroid cancer: cruciferous vegetables

                       John Potter, University of Minnesota

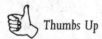 Thumbs Up

GARLIC AND ONIONS: PUNGENT PREVENTIVES

Eat a little of these allium cousins every day. More than 30 different enemies of carcinogens have been identified in garlic and onions. Such compounds include diallyl sulphide, quercetin and ajoene. In animals, they block the most terrifying cancer-causing agents such as nitrosamines and aflatoxin, linked specifically to stomach, lung and liver cancer.

In the county of Georgia where Vidalia onions are grown, the stomach cancer rate is only half that of other Georgia counties, and one-third that of the rest of the United States. — American National Cancer Institute

---

Feeding garlic to animals consistently blocks cancer. Harvard scientists immunized hamsters against certain cancers by putting ground-up onions in their drinking water. A leading researcher on garlic is Michael Wargovich, at Houston's M. D. Anderson Cancer Center. He gave some mice purified diallyl sulphide from garlic, and others plain mice food, followed by powerful carcinogens. Mice eating the garlic substance had 75 per cent fewer colon tumours. More impressive, when given agents that cause oesophageal cancer in mice, not a single one getting the diallyl sulphide came down with cancer!

Similarly, John Milner, head of nutrition at Penn State University, blocked 70 per cent of breast tumours in mice by feeding them fresh garlic. In humans, studies show that those who eat more onions and garlic are less prone to various cancers.

FOODS THAT MAY BLOCK THE SPREAD OF CANCER

Several food substances have been identified that may not only help prevent cancer but also retard its spread (metastasis). They are:

- Fish oil (specifically for breast cancer)

- Cabbage, collard greens and other cruciferous vegetables (for breast cancer)

- Garlic's ajoene and allicin (which may perform as chemo–therapy against cancerous cells in general)

- Beta carotene in deep orange and deep green vegetables and fruits

- Triterpenoids in liquorice (which may stifle quick-growing cancer cells and cause some precancerous cells to return to normal growth)

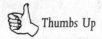 *Thumbs Up*

THE ATTACK OF THE ANTICANCER TOMATOES

Pay attention to the lowly tomato. It may seem too mundane to bother with as an anticancer drug, but new research finds the tomato prominent in the diets of people less prone to cancer. There's no mystery about the tomato's potential anticancer weapon. It's lycopene, a pigment that gives tomatoes their red colour. New research by Dr. Helmut Sies of Germany has found that lycopene is twice as powerful as beta carotene at "quenching singlet oxygen," a rampaging toxic oxygen molecule that can trigger cancer in cells. Tomatoes are the major source of lycopene in the food supply, and that includes all types of tomato products, such as cooked tomatoes, canned tomatoes and sauces, tomato paste and ketchup. Lycopene is also highly concentrated in watermelon, and there is a smidgen in apricots.

STRIVE FOR FIVE

Eat at least five servings of fruits and vegetables every day advises the American National Cancer Institute. One serving means 3½–4oz (100–115g) of cooked or chopped raw fruit or vegetables; 2½–3oz (70–85g) of raw leafy vegetables; one medium piece of fruit, or 6fl oz (170 ml) of fruit juice or vegetable juice. Only 10 per cent of Americans eat that much every day.

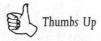 *Thumbs Up*

GO FOR THE GREEN

Make it a point to eat green vegetables, notably green leafy vegetables. They exhibit extraordinarily broad anticancer powers. A recent Italian study showed a "striking" protection from the frequent consumption of green vegetables against the risk of most cancers. The green stuff, such as spinach, kale, dark green lettuce and broccoli, is chockful of many different antioxidants, including beta carotene and folic acid, as well as lutein, a little-known antioxidant that some scientists think may even be as potent as beta carotene in thwarting cancer. Green leafy vegetables are rich in lutein. For example, spinach has a lot of lutein, but kale has twice as much. To get green vegetables with the most carotenoids and other anticancer agents, "Choose the darkest green vegetables," advises Frederick Khachik, Ph.D., a research scientist at the Department of Agriculture. "The darker green they are the more cancer-inhibiting carotenoids they have," he finds. He also says lutein and other carotenoids are not lost during cooking or freezing, although heat does harm more fragile antioxidants, including vitamin C and glutathione.

 Thumbs Up

AMAZING CITRUS POWER

Eat oranges, grapefruit, lemons and limes, urges toxicologist Herbert Pierson, Ph.D., a diet and cancer expert formerly with the American National Cancer Institute. He calls citrus fruits a total anticancer package, because they possess every class of natural substances (carotenoids, flavonoids, terpenes, limonoids and coumarins) that individually have neutralized powerful chemical carcinogens in animals. One analysis found that citrus fruits possess 58 known anticancer chemicals, more than any other food.

Further, Dr. Pierson says: "The beauty of citrus is that several classes of phytochemicals are highly likely to act more powerfully . . . as a natural mixture than when they appear separately." In other words, whole citrus fruits are a marvellous cocktail of anticancer compounds. One is the powerful antioxidant glutathione. Whole oranges contain high concentrations of this tested disease-antagonist. However, when extracted the juice tends to lose glutathione concentrations. Oranges also are the highest of all foods by far in glucarate, another cancer-inhibitor. Some experts greatly credit the wide use of citrus fruits for the dramatic decline of stomach cancer in the United States.

RAW OR COOKED FOR ANTICANCER POWER?

Eat vegetables both raw and cooked. Many studies identify raw vegetables as more anticancer. However, this is not always true with foods high in beta carotene. A little heat changes the form of beta carotene so it is more easily absorbed. Thus, you are likely to absorb more beta carotene from lightly cooked vegetables than raw ones, says researcher John Erdman, Jr., Ph.D., at the University of Illinois in Urbana.

Similarly, you are able to absorb more lycopene, another strong anticancer antioxidant, from cooked tomatoes than raw ones, according to new German studies.

Nor are certain other important anticancer carotenoids: like lutein in green leafy vegetables, harmed by heat.

On the other hand, several fragile anticancer agents, including indoles and vitamin C in vegetables, are destroyed by heat. That's why you should also eat lots of raw green leafy vegetables, such as lettuce, spinach and broccoli and raw cruciferous vegetables, such as cauliflower and cabbage. When you do cook them, do it gently and quickly to preserve the greatest health benefits.

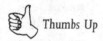 Thumbs Up

SOYA BEANS: CANCER BLOCKERS

Learn to love soya beans; including tofu The soya bean has exciting anticancer potential. It possesses at least five known anticancer agents. Soya beans have anti-oestrogenic activity that may thwart the development of hormone-related cancers, such as breast and prostate cancer. Soya beans are the richest source of so-called protease inhibitors, which in animals totally block or hinder the development of colon, oral, lung, liver, pancreatic and oesophageal cancers.

Two other soya bean constituents – phytosterols and saponins – are strongly anticancer. In animals phytosterols help squelch colon cancer by inhibiting cell division and proliferation. Saponins can stimulate immunity, directly slay certain cancer cells, slow the growth of cancerous cervical and skin cells, and can even reverse the proliferation of cancerous colon cells! Not surprisingly, the Japanese, with low rates of cancer, eat five times more of these cancer-fighters than we do. Our typical Western diet yields 80 milligrams of phytosterols per day; the Japanese typically eat 400 milligrams daily.

Westernized vegetarians eat about 345 milligrams of saponins a day. Ironically, nearly all of the soya beans raised in the United States go into animal feed. Most of the rest is shipped to Japan.

Soya bean compounds also block formation of one of the world's most dreaded carcinogens – nitrosamines; which can lead to liver cancer. In fact, soya substances did the job better than vitamin C, which is put into cured meats explicitly to inhibit nitrosamines.

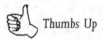 Thumbs Up

TEA: THE ANTICANCER DRINK

Develop an enthusiasm for tea. It has newfound anticancer potential. "It's exciting to discover that black tea, green tea and oolong tea all have anticancer effects," says cancer researcher Dr. John Weisburger, of the American Health Foundation. These three varieties of tea, used worldwide, all come from the plant called *Camellia sinensis*. This is not the same as so-called herbal teas, which are local mixtures of many different herbs and spices, and which may not have the anticancer compounds found in "real tea".

Recent studies in China, Japan and the United States confirm that tea dramatically blocks development of various cancers in animals. Dr. Allan Conney of Rutgers University found that drinking green tea at concentrations normally consumed by humans blocked up to 87 per cent of skin cancers, 58 per cent of stomach cancers and 56 per cent of lung cancers in mice. Other studies show that compounds in oolong and black tea (which is green tea that has been baked and fermented) also inhibit cancer in animals.

You can expect plain old Typhoo and PG tea, as well as other common brands of black tea, to possess these anticancer agents, but for the most potent anticancer effect, drink green tea, usually found in Asian markets and restaurants. It contains the most anticancer substances called catechins. The Japanese have identified one catechin in green tea as especially potent: epigallocatechin gallate (EGCG). Chemist Chi-tang Ho of Rutgers found the highest amounts of EGCG in green tea. Oolong tea has only 40 per cent as much of the anticancer agent as green tea, and black tea has only 10 per cent as much. The reason is that when green tea is processed to make black tea, some of the catechins are destroyed.

ANTICANCER COOKING: OFF THE GRILL AND INTO THE MICROWAVE

What's the best way to cook meat, chicken and fish to ward off cancer? By microwaving, stewing boiling or poaching, says Richard H. Adamson, Ph.D., of the American National Cancer Institute. These lower-temperature cooking methods produce virtually no cancer-causing heterocyclic aromatic amines (HAAs).

In contrast, frying, grilling, broiling and barbecuing meats at searing temperatures produce loads of the cancerous agents. Worst are grilling and barbecuing, in which temperatures reach 176° C. Oven roasting and baking give rise to low to moderate amounts, says Dr. Adamson.

Scientists are increasingly worried about these HAAs. Dr. Adamson estimates that they contribute to about 6,000 new cancer cases a year. In animals, they cause various kinds of cancer, including liver and breast cancer in monkeys, our closest relatives. A recent Swedish study found colon cancer more prevalent in people who eat meat grilled or fried.

Here is Dr. Adamson's anticancer advice for cooking meat: Stew, boil and poach meats more often. Eat beef medium rather than well done. (Longer cooking produces more HAAs.) Microwave meats such as burgers, chops, chicken and fish to cook them partially prior to barbecuing. Drain their juices before putting them on the grill. Resist making gravy from meat drippings. Vary methods of cooking meats.

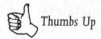 Thumbs Up

CANCER FIGHTER IN MILK?

As you might expect, saturated fat in milk seems to promote certain cancers, but something in milk may also deter cancer. That's the intriguing finding of a study of 1,300 people by researchers at Roswell Park Memorial Institute in Buffalo. They found, not surprisingly, that consumers of semi-skimmed and skimmed milk had lower odds of cancer (oral, stomach, rectal, lung and cervical) than drinkers of higher-fat whole milk. That made sense because high fat is incriminated in promoting some cancers.

Now here's the odd part: Those drinking semi-skimmed milk were also less likely to develop various cancers (oral, stomach, colon, rectal, lung, bladder, breast and cervical) than nonmilk drinkers! Why? Dr. Curtis Mettline, director of the study, suspects milk has unknown anticancer agents that can counteract the procancer milk fat only when there is less fat to neutralize. Some potential anticancer agents in milk are calcium, riboflavin, vitamins A, C and D. "Or the key component may be something we haven't even identified yet," he says.

"Heavy meat eaters are more vulnerable to cancers of the pancreas, colon, lung and breast. The risk jumps even higher if you smoke and do not eat green and yellow vegetables every day." – Takeshi Hirayama, Institute of Preventive Oncology, Tokyo, Japan (based on a seventeen-year study of 265,118 adults in six prefectures in Japan)

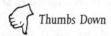 Thumbs Down

BEWARE: SOME FATS FEED CANCER

When you compare diets around the world and within countries, animal fat often pops out as concentrated in the diets of those with higher cancer rates. Additionally, widely used omega-6 polyunsaturated fats, such as corn oil, are a potential cancer danger. For example, feeding animals corn oil sends cancer rates zooming in those exposed to carcinogens.

However, monounsaturated fat, the type predominant in olive oil, has not been designated a cancer culprit, says Dr. Ernst L. Wynder, president of the American Health Foundation. On the contrary, new evidence suggests olive-oil-type fat helps counteract cancer. Seafood's omega-3 fatty acids also help deter certain types of cancer, including breast cancer.

There are several ways fat may foster cancer. Fat acts as a fuel to promote tumour growth. Without the fat, cancer-prone cells might remain relatively quiet. Fat also stimulates bile acids in the colon that can help drive cells toward cancer. Additionally, eating too much fat, both animal and omega-6 vegetable oils, can depress the immune system's tumour surveillance mechanism, according to research at the American Health Foundation and St. Luke's – Roosevelt Hospital Center in New York.

• BOTTOM LINE • *Animal fat and polyunsaturated vegetable oils tend to promote cancer. Olive oil and fish oil tend to deter it.*

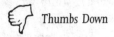 *Thumbs Down*

GO EASY ON ALCOHOL

Alcohol can up your risk of cancers of the upper and lower digestive tract, liver, prostate, breast and in particular, of the colon. If you are a smoker, the combination of heavy smoking and drinking can make you 43 times more likely to develop throat cancer and 135 times more apt to get nasal cancer, according to a large study of European men by the International Agency for Research on Cancer in Lyon, France. Heavy beer drinking is especially linked to rectal cancer. Researchers at the University of Oklahoma found that men who drank five or more beers a day had double the risk of rectal cancer. Usually, the more alcohol consumed, the greater the risk of various cancers.

Moreover, new research suggests that drinking a lot of alcohol at one time can stimulate cancer to spread, by depressing the immune system. According to Gayle Page of the University of California at Los Angeles, even a few episodes of intoxication or one binge appear sufficient to promote tumour progression. In animals, she says, the equivalent of four to five drinks in one hour doubled the number of new lung tumours that had spread from the breast. The clear message is *people who have cancer should be especially wary of excessively consuming alcohol.*

NEW FRONTIER: FOODS THAT MAY SLOW CANCER SPREAD

If certain foods can help prevent cancer, can they also act as chemotherapy after you have cancer? Could food chemicals actually intervene in the course of cancer? It makes scientific sense and there is mounting evidence of foods' chemotherapeutic powers to fight cancer by retarding tumour growth, spread and recurrence, as well as possibly attacking the malignancy itself by destroying cancer cells.

This does not mean, of course, that food should be used *instead* of modern cancer treatments but eating anticancer foods can be a form of adjuvant therapy, helping patients better defeat and survive the cancer.

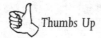 *Thumbs Up*

GARLIC KILLS CANCER KILLS

It's not unreasonable to think that garlic may interfere with cancer progression. A recent German study found that garlic compounds are toxic to malignant cells. Thus, garlic substances might help destroy cancerous cells somewhat the way chemotherapy drugs do. In the German study of human cells, one potent garlic compound, ajoene, was three times as toxic to malignant cells as to normal cells.

Garlic may also antagonize existing cancer by performing as a "biological response modifier," according to long-time garlic researcher Benjamin H. S. Lau, M.D., at Loma Linda University School of Medicine. Some of mainstream medicine's hottest new cancer "cures," such as interleukin, are biological response modifiers that boost immune functions. Dr. Lau found that garlic fits the description. In test tubes, garlic's sulphur compounds boosted the anticancer activity of macrophages and T-lymphocytes, components of the immune system that are summoned to destroy tumour cells. It will take further study to be sure garlic has the same effect in the human body, says Dr. Lau.

Garlic might also discourage colon and stomach cancers by functioning as an antibiotic. New evidence suggests that an infection by *H. pylori* bacteria contributes to these cancers. If so, says Dr. Tim Byers of the Centers for Disease Control and Prevention, garlic might fight cancer by attacking the bacteria.

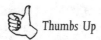 *Thumbs Up*

CAROTENE, A NEW CANCER DRUG

A prime anticancer weapon in fruits and vegetables is beta carotene. Beta carotene seems not only to help prevent cancer, but to help fight it. According to new research, beta carotene can destroy human tumour cells by multiple mechanisms. For example, beta carotene stimulated production of immune products that directly killed tumour cells, resulting in tumours only one-seventh as big as those in animals not fed beta carotene.

Indeed, in remarkable new studies at Harvard, beta carotene proved to have a direct toxic effect on human squamous carcinoma cells taken from solid tumours, thus performing as a chemotherapy agent. The carotene reduced the proliferation of lung cancer cells, reduced pro-cancer free-radical activity in the cancerous cells and bucked up enzyme activity to fight cancer.

Perhaps most exciting of all is new research at Tufts University by Dr. Xiang-dong Wang, showing that beta carotene in the body can actually change into a substance called retinoic acid, now used in the United States and many other countries to treat cancer, notably of the blood and bladder, with considerable success. Amazingly beta carotene is transformed in your intestinal tract, infusing your bloodstream with small amounts of this chemotherapeutic agent. Moreover, beta carotene is stored in lung, liver, kidney and fat tissues, which can also convert it into retinoic acid as needed. It means that when you eat beta carotene you stock your tissues with your own supplies of antitumour medicine to be called forth in case your cells need it. Can there be any more compelling reason to eat beta-carotene-rich fruits and vegetables? (For a list of foods rich in beta carotene, see page 457.)

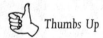 Thumbs Up

FISH OIL PROMISES

In animal experiments, fish oil is a whiz at combating cancer and re–tarding tumour growth. "Numerous studies show that fish oil consistently decreases the size of animal tumours, the number of tumours and their tendency to spread," says Artemis Simopoulos, M.D., president of the Center for Genetics, Nutrition and Health in Washington, D.C.

It seems to hold true for humans too. A new look at a major government study of 6,000 middle-aged men by Therese A. Dolececk, Ph.D., at the MRFIT Coordinating Center in Minneapolis, discovered that deaths from cancer were lower in men whose blood had more fish-oil fatty acids, indicating they were fish eaters. Exciting new studies also show that fish oil suppresses precancer growths leading to colon cancer in humans. George Blackburn, M.D., professor of surgery at Harvard Medical School, believes fish oil can thwart the spread of breast cancer after surgery. He is confident that fish oil can help block new attachments of wandering tumour cells, defeating their attempts to metastasize. He is testing his theory by having breast cancer patients eat more fish and take fish oil after surgery. He says, "I would be dumbstruck after all the data that's been collected so far if we did not find that this diet will help reduce the risk of metastasis from breast cancer."

 Thumbs Up

WHEAT AND CABBAGE CHEMOTHERAPY

Oestrogen is a known promoter of breast cancer; thus, women with breast cancer, especially premenopausal women, should try to lessen the type of oestrogen that may promote the cancer. Cabbage and other cruciferous vegetables, such as broccoli, as well as wheat bran, have accelerated the metabolism of such oestrogen in human studies. Both foods tended to deplete body oestrogen supplies that could otherwise feed cancer. Women with breast cancer may want to try to lower circulating oestrogen by eating raw cruciferous vegetables —cabbage, broccoli, cauliflower, kale and turnips – as well as wheat bran foods, say some researchers.

OTHER POSSIBILITIES

Shiitake mushrooms. Lenitan, found in shiitakes, is a "biological response modifier" that boosts immune activities against cancer.

Yoghurt. Live cultures in yoghurt increase immune functioning by stimulating production of gamma interferon that may slow tumour growth.

Liquorice. Triterpenoids in liquorice may stifle quick growing cancer cells and cause some precancerous cells to return to normal growth.

WHAT PEOPLE EAT WHO DON'T GET CANCER

If you were a newborn infant and could eat right the rest of your life to avoid cancer, you would be a vegetarian or semivegetarian, allowing for some seafood. You would generally shun red meat and high-saturated-fat animal and dairy foods, like cheese and whole milk. You would eat greens and fruits heavily, along with cereal brans, notably wheat bran, and dried beans. You would drink green tea primarily and coffee occasionally when you felt like it. Your milk would be low-fat. You would eat yoghurt, especially that made with the acidophilus culture.

If you drank alcohol, it would be very sparingly. You might eat eel, the highest of all foods in vitamin D, suspected of fighting off breast cancer. You would favour oily fish like mackerel over leaner fish, for the former is brimming with omega-3 type oils thought to help block cancer. You would forgo heavily salted and cured products. If you did touch meat, it would be turkey breast without the skin – never smoked cured meats like bacon and salami. Your bread would be heavy and grainy, and you would eat it without butter or margarine. If you used oil, it would not be traditional vegetable oils such as corn and safflower. You would choose olive oil, rapeseed oil or the more exotic flaxseed oil, the darling of cancer researchers.

You would be a salad freak and always eat your greens. You could never get enough broccoli, carrots, tomatoes, oranges and onions. You would love the taste of garlic – raw or cooked. You would tend toward colourful fruits, like strawberries, raspberries, watermelon, oranges; you would eat red grapes with a passion. You would eat nuts of all kinds for their protective vitamin E and other anticancer agents, namely Brazil nuts for their selenium, walnuts for their ellagic acid, and almonds for their oleic acid – although not so fanatically as to add needless weight. Leaner people who eat fewer calories are less likely to fall prey to cancer.

BREAST CANCER

Foods That May Discourage Breast Cancer: Cabbage • Broccoli • Other Cruciferous Vegetables • High-Vitamin C Fruits and Vegetables • Beans • Soya beans • Oily Fish • Wheat Bran • Olive Oil

Foods That May Promote Breast Cancer: Meat • Saturated Fatty Foods • Omega-6 Vegetable Oils, Such as Corn Oil • Alcohol

What you eat may influence whether you get breast cancer, how fast it grows, whether it spreads to other parts of your body, and even its final outcome. Certainly, many crucial factors are at play in breast cancer destiny, but diet is now considered a major one, and researchers are zooming in on intriguing ways foods can govern cellular events, notably involving oestrogen, that help control expression of breast cancers.

One leading clue has long been evident: To escape breast cancer, eat more like Asian women. For example, Japanese women are only one-fifth as likely to develop breast cancer as American and European women, and such tumours generally grow more slowly in Japanese women. It's not just heredity. When Japanese women move to another area, such as Hawaii, and switch to a Western-style diet, their breast cancer rates creep up and eventually approach those of Western women. Is it any wonder scientists suspect there is some secret in the Asian diet that powerfully prevents breast cancer or something in the Western diet that promotes it – or both?

It's going to take researchers a long time to figure it all out but they have begun to unlock some of the secrets. Right now there is at least enough evidence to tell women who want to escape and defeat breast cancer which foods look like your best and worst bets. In one year 26,990 British women will be diagnosed with breast cancer. Breast cancer in the UK is second to none as a cancer killer. Yet some authorities think that changing the way we eat could make a major dent in breast cancer. British authority Richard Peto, writing in the *Journal of the National Cancer Institute*, declared that changes in the diet might prevent as much as 50 per cent of all breast cancer in the United States.

FOODS UNIQUELY INFLUENCE BREAST CANCER

Breast cancer, as well as uterine and ovarian cancers, is hormone dependent — that is, an excess of the female hormone oestrogen appears to spur growth of the cancers. Thus, foods that can interfere with the metabolism or absorption of oestrogen are thought to be partial antidotes to breast cancer. For example, some drugs, like tamoxifen, are designed to treat and prevent breast cancer by lessening oestrogen's effects. Amazingly, it turns out that several foods can manipulate oestrogen in the body, much the way drugs do. Thus, foods that antagonize oestrogen possess a unique mechanism for discouraging breast cancer. Since oestrogen is a breast cancer risk factor throughout a woman's life, diet is important for both premenopausal and postmenopausal women in defeating the cancer. Premenopausal women have more oestrogen, but even after menopause, when ovaries stop making oestrogen, fat cells produce some oestrogen, so it is still available in the body to promote breast cancer.

Some scientists suspect that excessive oestrogen in early years may set you up for breast cancer in later life, so an anti-oestrogen diet when you are young may act as an important preventive. Also, circulating oestrogen can influence whether breast cancer recurs or moves to another site, including the other breast. Thus, even after breast cancer occurs, it's urgent to pay attention to foods that regulate oestrogen.

Additionally, certain food compounds can have a direct toxic effect on breast cancer cells and still other foods, especially various fats, seem to work in mysterious ways to stimulate or block breast cancer growth.

According to recent scientific discoveries, here are foods most likely to make a difference in the development and survival of breast cancer.

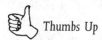 Thumbs Up

THE CABBAGE FACTOR

Put cabbage and its cousins high on your list of foods that may help immunize against breast cancer by managing oestrogen. Certain foods can speed the removal of oestrogen from the body. They speed up the metabolism of oestrogen, burning up the hormone so less is available to feed cancer. That's what compounds in cabbage and other cruciferous vegetables — broccoli, cauliflower, Brussels sprouts — do, according to Dr. Jon Michnovicz and colleagues at the Institute for Hormone Research in New York City. Their research reveals that specific indoles in these cruciferous vegetables accelerate a process in which the body deactivates or disposes of the type of oestrogen that can promote breast cancer.

In tests on women and men, the cabbage compound "turned up" the oestrogen-deactivation process by about 50 per cent, says Dr. Michnovicz. The test dose, as usual, exceeded what people would ordinarily eat: a daily 500 milligrams of indole-3-carbinol, the amount in about 14oz (400g) of raw cabbage but eating less would also burn up oestrogen to a lesser degree. It's known that women with elevated oestrogen metabolism have lower risks of hormone-dependent cancers, such as breast, uterine and endometrial cancer, says Dr. Michnovicz. He suspects Asian women have less breast cancer partly because they eat many cruciferous vegetables, including bok choy.

When mice were fed vegetable indoles, their rates of breast cancer sank dramatically, says Dr. Michnovicz. Researchers at Eppley Cancer Institute at the University of Nebraska also found that feeding animals cruciferous vegetables, particularly cabbage and collard greens, curtailed both the occurrence and the spread or metastasis of breast cancers.

Anticancer indoles are also concentrated in the other cruciferous vegetables, including cauliflower, broccoli, Brussels sprouts, kale, mustard greens and turnips. To get the greatest effect, eat the crucifers raw or lightly cooked, Dr. Michnovicz advises. Heavy cooking tends to destroy indoles, curtailing their anti-oestrogen and anticancer effect.

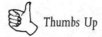 Thumbs Up

WHEAT BRAN MANIPULATOR

Another way to defeat breast cancer by curtailing oestrogen levels in your blood is to eat wheat bran cereals. There's something specifically magical about wheat bran, but not other brans, that can dramatically lower the circulating levels of cancer-promoting oestrogen in the blood. So found a landmark study of 62 premenopausal women, ages 25–50, by David P. Rose, M.D., of the American Health Foundation in New York.

The women ate three to four high-fibre muffins a day made with either oat bran, corn bran or wheat bran. That doubled their fibre intake from about 15g to 30g. After a month, there was little difference in their blood oestrogen levels, but after two months, oestrogen levels had sunk about 17 per cent in the women eating wheat bran. Oestrogen levels did not change in eaters of oat bran or corn bran muffins.

The main difference is that wheat-bran fibre is highly insoluble, giving bacteria in the colon much to chew on. That, through a complex series of biological events, causes less oestrogen to be released back into the bloodstream. How much does it take? You can get the amount of wheat fibre effective in the study by eating an extra 2oz (55g) of Kellogg's All-Bran or Kellogg's Bran Flakes or six tablespoons of raw, unprocessed wheat bran every day. Although the study was done in premenopausal women, Dr. Rose says the wheat bran would curb oestrogen, blocking cancer promotion in older, postmenopausal women also.

In fact, wheat fibre can suppress blood oestrogen even better than a low-fat diet does, according to another study at Tufts University School of Medicine. Investigator Margo Woods reported that both cutting fat and increasing fibre blocked one type of oestrogen – oestrone sulphate – but only fibre decreased levels of oestradiol, thought to be a major villain in breast cancer. In animals, a low-fat, high-wheat fibre diet cuts the incidence of breast tumours in half. Other studies find that women who eat high-fibre diets have lower rates of breast cancer.

"American women should eat more soya beans, especially if they have a family history of breast cancer. This includes plain soya beans, textured soya protein, tofu and soya milk." – Kenneth Setchell, Cincinnati Children's Hospital Medical Center

---

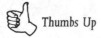 Thumbs Up

BEANS VS. BREAST CANCER

Eating lots of beans may help protect you from breast cancer, possibly because they contain so-called phytoestrogens that help block the activity of cancer-promoting oestrogen. So contends researcher Leonard A. Cohen, Ph.D., at the American Health Foundation in New York. Dr. Cohen says that Hispanic women in the Caribbean and Mexico are known to have less breast cancer than American women. In a new study, Dr. Cohen believes he has found one reason why: Hispanic women eat twice as many beans – mainly pinto beans, chickpeas and black beans – as American women.

Hispanic women average over 4oz (115g) of beans six days a week. That's compared with beans three times a week for African-American women and twice a week for white American women. Beans also possess several anticancer compounds, including protease inhibitors and phytates, says Dr. Cohen.

 Thumbs Up

SOYA BEANS: JAPAN'S WONDER FOOD?

Soya beans, too, contain compounds that can manipulate oestrogen as well as directly inhibit the growth of cancerous cells, theoretically reducing the risk of breast cancer in women of all ages, according to Stephen Barnes, Ph.D., associate professor of pharmacology and biochemistry at the University of Alabama. One soya bean compound, in fact, is quite similar chemically to the drug tamoxifen, given to certain women to help prevent breast cancer and its spread.

The soya bean's phytoestrogens counteract cancer-promoting oestrogen much the same way tamoxifen does, at least in animals, says Dr. Barnes. He put some animals on a high soya bean diet, others on a regular diet, and then subjected all to cancer-causing agents. Rats fed soya beans had from 40 per cent to 65 per cent *fewer* breast cancers. Dr. Barnes and colleagues have isolated what they believe to be the soya bean's most active anticancer agent, genistein. It also prevents breast tumours in animals. Dr. Barnes is now testing whether women who drink prescribed amounts of soya milk show diminished biological risk factors for breast cancer.

Soya beans seem to protect Asian women against breast cancer. A recent study found that premenopausal women in Singapore who ate twice as much soya protein as most people had only half the risk of breast cancer.

Soya beans are regarded as the likely *primary* reason Japanese women have less breast cancer, say Dr. Herman Adlercreutz and colleagues at the University of Helsinki, who studied residents of a rural village near Kyoto who still eat the "traditional" Japanese diet. They found that those who ate the most soya bean foods had the highest urine concentrations of isoflavonoids, which are anticancer agents, particularly against breast cancer and prostate cancer. Typically the women ate 3oz (85g) of soya bean products a day, including tofu (soya bean curd), miso (soya bean paste), fermented soya beans and boiled soya beans.

Eating miso has also decreased both the occurrence and growth of breast tumours in animals. This jibes with the observation that post-menopausal breast cancers grow more slowly in Japanese women than in Caucasian women.

NOTE: *Only soya bean protein appears protective. That includes soya beans, textured soya protein, soya milk, tofu, miso and tempeh, but not soya sauce or soya bean oil.*

THE SOYA BEAN-OESTROGEN PARADOX

Since soya beans are full of plant oestrogens and oestrogen promotes breast cancer, how in the world could soya beans help prevent breast cancer? It's a paradox say scientists. Soya beans seem to mimic the body's oestrogen without having its detrimental effects, says Dr. Barnes. He theorizes that soya beans contain a natural analogue of the drug tamoxifen, which is also, oddly, an oestrogen with antioestrogen activity. Thus, both soya beans and tamoxifen seem to block oestrogen's ability to stimulate malignant changes in breast tissue, while promoting beneficial effects on the skeleton and cardiovascular system, says Dr. Barnes.

One way the active soya bean compound may interfere with cancer is to attach itself to the cell's receptor site for oestrogen, blocking admittance of the dangerous-type cancer-promoting oestrogen. Thus, in effect it starves the cancer; the active oestrogen is unable to attach itself to the cell to perform its dirty work of feeding the cancerous cell. It appears, however, that soya beans also block the growth of cancer cells by another mechanism not related to oestrogen. Studies in cells have found that soya bean agents, for mysterious reasons, can entirely halt the growth of cancerous cells even though they do not have any oestrogen receptors to block, according to Dr. Barnes. That means these soya bean compounds fight cancer in at least two separate ways, he says. Thus, soya may be important in helping prevent cancer in both premenopausal and postmenopausal women, independently of oestrogen supplies.

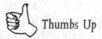 Thumbs Up

EAT FOOD FROM THE SEA

Seafood, especially fatty fish, can also help block breast cancer. So says Dr. Rashida Karmali, associate professor of nutrition at Rutgers University. She has found that supplements of fish oil, equal to the amount Japanese women commonly eat in fish, suppressed biological signs of developing breast cancer in women at highest risk for the disease. Further, a Canadian survey of 32 countries showed that the incidence and death rate from breast cancer is lower in countries, such as Japan, where women eat the most fish.

Most dramatically, fish oil may actually be able to interfere with the progression of cancer, once it occurs. Eating fish oil may help stop the spread (metastasis) of breast cancer, believes Harvard surgeon George Blackburn. He speculates that fish oil strengthens immune activity, thus killing wandering cancer cells before they can start new tumours. He also says fish oil hinders the attachment of travelling cancer cells to new sites; thus they cannot as easily establish new colonies of cells that can build distant tumours. He is conducting a major study of women with breast cancer to test his theory.

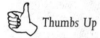 Thumbs Up

VITAMIN D PROTECTION

There's surprising new evidence that older women who skimp on foods rich in vitamin D are more likely to develop breast cancer, according to Frank Garland, Ph.D., of the Department of Community and Family Medicine at the University of California at San Diego. This may also help explain fish's anticancer protection, because fatty fish is packed with vitamin D. Specifically, Dr. Garland finds that dietary vitamin D wards off postmenopausal breast cancer in women over 50 but not in women who get cancer at younger ages.

Unfortunately, most American women eat only one-quarter the recommended dietary allowance (RDA) of vitamin D, which is 200 IU (international units) or 5 micrograms (µg) for women over age 22. Japanese women eat six times that much or 1,200 IU (30µg) a day. When Japanese women move to the United States, their vitamin D intake sinks and their breast cancer rates skyrocket. Further, vitamin D slows the rate of growth of cancer cells in lab studies and cuts the rate of cancer in animals in half. All American women should eat foods with at least 400 IU (10µg) of vitamin D per day, says Dr. Garland. In the U.K. there is no RDA for Vitamin D. It is just recommended you get normal exposure to sunlight and for people for whom this would be impossible the RDA is 400 IU (10µg) per day.

The best sources of vitamin D are fatty fish, such as salmon sardines, mackerel, herring and tuna. The richest source of vitamin D in the world is eel, popular in Japanese sushi bars. 3½oz (100g) of eel contain nearly 5,000 IUs (125µg) of vitamin D. (For a list of foods high in vitamin D, see page 461.)

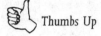 Thumbs Up

VITAMIN C FOODS: YOU CAN'T EAT TOO MANY

Eat fruits and vegetables rich in vitamin C. They can put a big dent in your risk of breast cancer as well as most cancers at all ages. Vitamin C is a formidable antagonist to breast cancer, according to several reviews of the evidence. For example, vitamin C foods came out tops as protective, according to an analysis of 12 major studies on breast cancer and diet by researchers at the National Cancer Institute of Canada. In fact, eating too little vitamin C was more critical than eating too much fat.

On the basis of the finding, researchers predicted that eating enough fruits and vegetables to get 380 milligrams daily of vitamin C would probably reduce the breast-cancer risk by 16 per cent in all women. That's over nine times the RDA (recommended dietary allowance) for vitamin C. Still, it's easy to get that quota of vitamin C by eating lots of fruits and vegetables. (For a list of foods high in vitamin C, see pages 460–1.)

The investigators also found stronger vitamin C protection in post-menopausal women who also cut back on fat in the diet, especially saturated dairy and meat-type fats. Their conclusion was that if you cut saturated fat to 9 per cent of calories, your breast cancer chances drop 10 per cent. However, if postmenopausal women also got 380 milligrams of vitamin C daily, their chances of breast cancer would probably drop a dramatic 24 per cent.

A large Italian study singled out green vegetables, rich in vitamin C, beta carotene and other antioxidant carotenoids, as particularly protective against breast cancer. Women who ate more than one green vegetable every day had only one-third the risk of breast cancer of women who ate less than that.

Drinking coffee or caffeine does not promote breast cancer, though the two may contribute to fibrocystic breast disease. There is no association between coffee and other caffeine-containing beverages, and breast cancer, concluded Dr. F. Lubin, of the University of Toronto, who recently reviewed the subject in Cancer Letter, a medical journal.

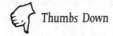 Thumbs Down

TO DRINK OR NOT TO DRINK?

Does alcohol contribute to breast cancer? Yes, according to about two dozen studies that have detected a higher risk in drinkers.

How much alcohol is hazardous is controversial, and how alcohol works to increase breast-cancer risk is unknown.

In 1988 investigator Matthew P. Longnecker, at the Harvard School of Public Health, attempted to sort it all out by doing a "meta-analysis" of all the pertinent studies on alcohol and breast cancer. He found "compelling" evidence of a dose-response relationship between breast cancer odds and alcohol. Drinking roughly a couple of drinks a day boosted the risk of breast cancer by about 50 per cent, he concluded. At one drink a day, there was scant danger. Dr. Longnecker figured that 13 per cent of all breast cancer among American women can be chalked up to alcohol. However, he called the risk so slight for women who imbibe one drink or less a day that he saw no reason for them to give up alcohol totally, especially since heart protection from small amounts of alcohol might outweigh the cancer risk. Other research has given women more leeway, suggesting that two drinks a day may not be dangerous, but that more definitely is.

• BOTTOM LINE: • *One drink a day for women seems safe and beneficial. More alcohol entails some risk of breast cancer, say many experts. Especially if you have a strong family history of breast cancer, you should restrict alcohol to a drink a day.*

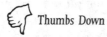 Thumbs Down

BINGE-DRINKING: A SPECIAL THREAT

Women who have breast cancer should not drink heavily and certainly not enough to get intoxicated, cautions Dr. Gayle Page, a researcher at the University of California at Los Angeles. There's evidence that high blood levels of alcohol can help breast cancer spread to other parts of the body, she says.

In studies, she and colleagues gave rats with breast cancer enough alcohol to make them drunk by human standards. The higher their blood alcohol, the more likely their tumours were to spread. Rats with a blood alcohol content of 0.15 per cent (four or five drinks in human terms) later revealed twice as many metastasized lung tumours – offspring of the breast cancers – than rats given no alcohol. Animals with a blood alcohol level of 0.25 per cent had eight times more tumours.

The cancers spread more easily because the alcohol suppressed. the immune system, namely the activity of natural killer cells that otherwise would have destroyed circulating tumour cells. "It's frightening," says Dr. Page, because only a single episode of intoxication incited the cancer to spread.

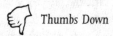 Thumbs Down

HIGH-FAT DANGER?

Does eating too much fat help trigger breast cancer? Some epi–demiological studies find a link with dietary fat. Others do not. One of the strongest bits of evidence came from a study of 750 Italian women, showing that those eating the most saturated fats and animal protein had triple the odds of breast cancer compared with those eating the least. Other major studies, including a recent one at Harvard that tracked nearly 90,000 women, turned up no link between breast cancer occurrence and fat intake.

Regardless, compelling evidence indicates that eating too much fat can influence the spread and virulence of an existing breast cancer, its recurrence and your survival chances. Some research shows that the more saturated animal fat in your diet, the greater the odds of axillary lymph node involvement or spread of the cancer, and the more total fat in your diet, the greater your chances of dying from breast cancer. A low-fat diet may be one reason the five-year survival rate for Japanese women with breast cancer is 15 per cent greater than that for Western women.

The hazard also appears to depend on the type of fat. The worst fats appear to be saturated animal fat and omega-6-type vegetable oils, such as corn oil. Animals eating high amounts of those fats have breast tumours that grow faster and bigger and metastasize more readily. In contrast, omega-3 fish oil and olive oil appear to discourage growth of breast cancer. Additionally, Mediterranean women who eat lots of olive oil have low rates of breast cancer, as do Japanese women who eat lots of fish oils but little animal fat. In countries where animal fat consumption is high, so are breast cancer rates.

Theoretically, there are solid reasons to suspect fat's role in breast cancer. For one thing, saturated animal fat promotes high blood levels of the hormone oestradiol considered a marker for high susceptibility to breast cancer. An American National Cancer Institute study, of 73 healthy women past menopause, found that cutting fat intake from 38 to 20 per cent of calories reduced oestradiol by 17 per cent. A high-fat diet also depresses immunity, possibly curtailing the body's ability to fight off cancer.

"There is evidence that dietary fat may be a stronger risk factor for postmenopausal breast cancer than for premenopausal breast cancer." – Lawrence H. Kushi, School of Public Health, University of Minnesota, Minneapolis

---

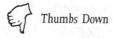 Thumbs Down

BEWARE FAT IF YOU HAVE BREAST CANCER

If you have breast cancer, you should be very wary of eating fat, especially animal fats, including cheese, butter and meat fat. Such fat may spur a recurrence of the cancer after it is surgically removed, according to a recent Swedish study of 220 women. Specifically, investigators found that dietary fat prodded the growth of new tumours that were oestrogen dependent – that is, tumours with lots of receptors for oestrogen. (Fat did not influence growth of tumours with few or no oestrogen receptors.) The theory is that high-fat diets boost blood concentrations of oestrogen that becomes fuel to feed the growth of further tumours.

In the Swedish study of 220 women, those who commonly ate the most animal fat were 20 per cent more likely to suffer another bout with breast cancer in the next four years after their initial breast cancer surgery.

Thus, even if it's debatable whether too much fat actually causes breast cancer, it can prod the growth of an existing tumour, says Norman F. Boyd of the Ontario Cancer Institute in Toronto. He says switching to a low-fat diet after detection and removal of a breast cancer may be lifesaving by preventing a recurrence.

DIET PRESCRIPTION *AGAINST BREAST CANCER*

- Whether you are premenopausal or postmenopausal, eat fatty fish and beans, including soya beans – foods that may prevent both occurrence of breast cancer and its growth.

- Eat foods that interfere with the pro-cancer activities of oestrogen. This includes soya beans, cruciferous vegetables and wheat bran cereals.

- Additionally, eat a variety of green vegetables, which generaly seem to deter breast cancer.

- Confine alcohol intake to a drink a day. Never binge.

- To prevent breast cancer or suppress its growth if you have it,eat omega-3 fatty acids in oily fish and omega-9 fatty acids of the monounsaturated type found in olive oil. Restrict saturated animal fats as well as omega-6 fatty acids predominant in corn, safflower, and sunflower seed oils, and shortenings and margarines made from such oils.

- Eat more like Japanese women do, or used to before World War II. Here's the daily diet of a traditional Japanese woman: about 8oz (225g) of fruit, 9oz (255g) of vegetables, 3oz (85g) of soya bean products (mostly tofu), 3½oz (100g) of fish and very little meat, milk or alcohol.

COLON CANCER

> **Foods That May Help Control Colon Cancer:** Wheat • Bran
> • Vegetables, Especially Cabbage, Broccoli, Cauliflower and Other
> Crucifers • Milk • Yoghurt • Seafood • Foods Rich in Fibre,
> Calcium and Vitamin D.
>
> **Foods That May Promote Colon Cancer:** High-Fat Foods • Red
> Meat • Alcohol

HOW FOOD CAN BLOCK COLON CANCER

Even if there is a history of colon cancer in your family, and even if
you are well into middle age, you may still be able to defeat this
potentially fatal malignancy with diet. Astounding research on humans
shows that food can intercede in colon cancer by squashing the rate
of proliferation of cancer-prone cells in the intestines and even stifling
or shrinking small, precancerous eruptions in the colon, called polyps,
that can grow into full-blown malignant tumours! The theory goes that
if such rapid and uncontrolled cell growth is curbed or the later-stage
polyps are prevented from appearing and flourishing, colon cancer
does not materialize.

In short, food may help prevent small benign events from
becoming large catastrophic ones – even blocking recurrence of
new growth after colon cancer surgery. Thus, food acts as a powerful
and safe chemopreventive and even chemotherapeutic drug against
a cancer that strikes about 18,000 Britains every year and kills
some 12,800. Indeed, as much as 90 per cent of the colon cancer toll
might be influenced by diet, says British cancer authority Dr. Richard
Peto of Oxford.

IT'S NEVER TOO LATE

So you are already in middle age? Don't despair. It can still be an excellent time to start an anti-colon-cancer diet. It's exciting to realize, says Peter Greenwald, M.D., of the American National Cancer Institute, that it may never be too late to try to interrupt the colon-cancer process with diet. He explains that scientists now better understand how cancer can be stopped by "hits" at various stages of the progressive chain of events leading to tumours. Researchers can judge a food's effect on colon cancer by measuring "markers," such as cell proliferation and the small precancerous masses called polyps. For example, doctors can tell rather quickly whether a specific food has spurred or curbed precancerous polyps simply by counting and measuring them during an internal examination of the colon. If the polyps grow, you're in trouble; if they don't or if they regress, you are doing something very right.

"That's important," says Dr. Greenwald, "because most of these changes in early polyp formation actually happen in people late in life – who are in their forties, fifties and sixties." Thus, he says, these are critical ages during which to intervene and break the chain. "We ought to be able to modify diet even at that late point in life and have a major impact on risk of colorectal cancer."

The trick is to discover which foods encourage or discourage these potentially cataclysmic changes in the colon. Here are your best bets for curtailing colon cancer.

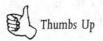 Thumbs Up

THE MIRACLE FOOD TO SAVE 9,000 BRITAINS

What if someone discovered a new drug that could slash your odds of colon cancer by one-third to one-half, preventing 6,000–9,000 colon cancers a year? Furthermore, suppose that the drug was utterly safe and incredibly cheap? Wouldn't it be acclaimed one of the miracle drugs of the century? Well, the fibre in food has the astonishing potential to prevent colon cancer on such a grand scale, according to a group of cancer experts, writing in the *Journal of the National Cancer Institute.* The dose of fibre needed to accomplish this massive lifesaving feat is very slight.

According to senior author Geoffrey R. Howe, Ph.D., of the University of Toronto, if Americans ate an additional 13 grams of food fibre a day (about the amount in a bowl of extra-high-fibre wheat bran cereal), colon cancer rates in the United States would drop 31 per cent, and that would mean 50,000 fewer diagnosed cases of colorectal cancer a year perhaps nearly 9,000 cases in the U.K. He and colleagues based the prediction on a new analysis of 13 recent studies of colon cancer and diet.

To slash the toll by 50,000 cases yearly, most Americans would have to up their fibre intake by about 70 per cent, the experts figured. You get fibre in cereal, fruits, vegetables, legumes and nuts. All such foods also contain a plethora of natural anticancer chemicals, in addition to fibre per se.

Although studies consistently show that fibre-rich foods in general ward off colon cancer, some specific foods have shown out–standing powers. Wheat bran has the best documented reputation as a formidable colon cancer fighter.

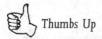 Thumbs Up

THE AMAZING POWER IN ALL-BRAN

If you do nothing else to protect yourself against colon cancer, eat wheat bran cereal. That breakthrough advice first came from a study by Jerome J. DeCosse, M.D., a surgeon at Memorial Sloan-Kettering Cancer Center in New York. Dr. DeCosse chose 58 patients who had an inherited "familial" tendency to develop polyps and thus were at high risk for colon cancer. He found that two ordinary bowls (1oz (30g) each) of Kellogg's high-fibre All-Bran cereal caused the premalignant polyps to shrink, thus halting their inevitable march toward cancer.

For four years the patients ate either All-Bran or a look-alike low-fibre cereal. No one, including doctors, knew who was eating what. The All-Bran group ate a total of 22g of fibre a day; the others, 12g, typical for Americans. Periodically, the patients' colons were examined by endoscopy to measure changes in the growth of the polyps.

After the code was broken, Dr. DeCosse discovered that the polyps in the All-Bran eaters had begun to decrease distinctly in size and number within six months! The polyps continued to shrink for the next three years. Most remarkable is that such a small amount of food could have such an impact within such a short time on such a major killer – thus illustrating that dietary intervention can work at fairly late stages after precancerous warning signs have appeared. If the findings apply across the board to others with polyps, it means anyone diagnosed with colon polyps should run for the cereal box. There may still be much time to head off malignancy. Usually, it takes about ten years for polyps to grow into malignant tumours.

"Only wheat bran, not oat bran or other brans, has been found to have some protective effect in cancer." – Bandaru S. Reddy, American Health Foundation

---

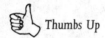 Thumbs Up

REACH FOR THE CEREAL AFTER CANCER SURGERY

Suppose colon cancer develops and the tumour is then excised. Astonishing as it seems, eating wheat bran can even act as a drug following cancer surgery to block the return of the cancer, suggests research by David S. Alberts, M.D., at the Arizona Cancer Center in Tucson. He documented that after malignant tumours were surgically removed, All-Bran cereal curbed cell changes that would stimulate a recurrence of colon and rectal tumours.

For two months 17 men and women who had undergone surgery for colon or rectal cancer each ate about 1½oz (40g) of All-Bran (13.5g of fibre) per day. Researchers then measured the rate of proliferation of rectal surface cells, which they say is a good sign of whether cancer is likely to recur or even to develop in the first place. In those most in danger, those with a baseline rapid rate of cell proliferation, All-Bran dramatically suppressed the cell-growth rates in half of the patients. Once again, researchers noted how quickly – in a mere 60 days – high-fibre wheat cereal acted to curtail whatever stimulates cancer in the colon," as Dr. Alberts puts it.

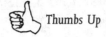 *Thumbs Up*

ONLY WHEAT BRAN WORKS

Don't accept substitutes. Nobody really knows why wheat bran works but they do know that the magic ingredient does not seem to be present in other cereals. In a study by American Health Foundation researchers, 75 women ate two or three muffins a day made from wheat, oats or corn for a total of 30g daily of fibre for eight weeks. Only the wheat bran squelched cancer-promoting changes in the colon. Presumably, wheat contains a type of biologically active fibre and/or other constituents that specifically engage and conquer colon cancer promoters. One clue is that wheat bran, but not oat bran or corn bran, reduces the concentration of bile acids and bacterial enzymes in the stool that are believed to promote colon cancer. Some think wheat's main anticancer agent is phytate, which does block colon cancer in animals. Dr. DeCosse thinks perhaps pentose, a sugar in wheat, is an active polyp inhibitor.

• BOTTOM LINE • *Eating too little fibre triples your prospects of polyps. In a large Harvard study, men who ate the most fibre—more than 28g a day — had only one-third the rate of polyps of men who ate the least fibre or 17g a day. The protective dose is the amount of fibre in 3oz (85g) of high-fibre All-Bran or 100% Bran cereals. Check the label to be sure.*

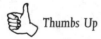 *Thumbs Up*

EAT SEAFOOD, STOP POLYPS

One of the quickest ways to stop the growth of polyps, and thus curtail cancer, is to eat lots of fatty fish. So suggest the remarkable results of an Italian study from the Catholic University of Rome. Researchers discovered that patients with polyps who ate fish oil exhibited a suppression of precancerous colonic cell growth in just two weeks! "It's exciting new evidence of fish oil's ability to interfere with the cancer process in an incredibly short time," said Harvard's George Blackburn.

In the study men with polyps ate either daily doses of fish oil or a dummy capsule for three months. In 90 per cent of the fish oil group, cell proliferation, a sign of colon cancer activity, dropped an average 62 per cent. The abnormal cell growth came to a complete halt in one patient. Further, the researchers detected the slowdown in cell growth within only two weeks.

The fish oil doses were fairly high – equal to eating about 8oz (225g) of mackerel a day. However, Dr. Blackburn says that such "fish oil loading" is necessary at first to correct a longtime deficit in the oils. After that, lower amounts are probably enough to keep the cells from going haywire. That's why some authorities think regularly eating small amounts of fish over many years prevents polyps and colon cancer from ever erupting.

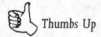 Thumbs Up

BRING ON THE VEGETABLES

Follow the example of medicinal plant expert Dr. Jim Duke at the U.S. Department of Agriculture, who has a family history of colon cancer. He eats lots of vegetables. Dr. Duke says his colon polyps diminished dramatically after he deliberately ate raw cabbage every other day. It appears that other high-fibre vegetables can also put a dent in colon cancer, according to Dr. Greenwald. His analysis of 37 studies done in the last 20 years showed that eating either high-fibre foods and/or vegetables cut the chances of colon cancer by 40 per cent. Dr. Greenwald says it was impossible to tell which offered more protection – fibre per se or vegetables that have fibre plus other known anticancer compounds.

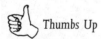 Thumbs Up

CABBAGE VS. COLON CANCER

Among vegetables, your best bets to prevent colon cancer are cabbage and its cruciferous cousins. There is something peculiar about these vegetables – perhaps their high concentrations of indoles – that empowers them to intervene in colon cancer. In Dr. Greenwald's survey, eight out of nine "case-control" studies declared crucifers, including cabbage, broccoli, Brussels sprouts and cauliflower, to be enemies of colon cancer.

The evidence is striking and consistent. The first study to put cabbage on the colon cancer scene was done among men in Buffalo, New York. It found that those who ate more vegetables – notably cabbage, including coleslaw and sauerkraut – were less likely to get colon cancer. Men who ate cabbage more than once a week were only one-third as likely to develop colon cancer as those who ate it only once a month or never. Even eating cabbage once every two or three weeks cut the risk of colon cancer nearly in half. A more recent, larger study of 600 persons at the University of Utah School of Medicine again revealed that men who ate the most cruciferous vegetables had a 70 per cent lower risk of colon cancer than those who ate the least of such vegetables. Eaters of cabbage and other crucifers are also less likely to have premalignant polyps.

The main anticancer agents in cruciferous vegetables are probably indoles, which consistently save animals from colon cancer after they have been dosed with potent cancer-causing agents. The cabbage compounds apparently act as an antidote to carcinogens.

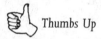 Thumbs Up

THE CALCIUM CONNECTION

Don't skimp on calcium foods; the mineral seems to be an antagonist to cancer. Decidedly, calcium appears to suppress disastrous physiological events leading to colon cancer, according to an impressive array of studies. Dr. Cedric Garland, director of the Cancer Center at the University of California at San Diego has noted that men who drank a couple of glasses of milk daily over a 20 year period were only one-third as prone to developing colon cancer as nonmilk drinkers. Dr. Garland estimates that 1,200–1,400mg of calcium per day might prevent an astonishing 65–75 per cent of colon cancers. Currently, middle-aged men average 700mg daily and middle-aged women average 450mg he says. That means even an extra two or three glasses a day of skimmed milk – each with 316mg calcium – might determine whether misbehaving cells progress to full-blown malignant tumours, especially in people who are at high risk, for example, those who have polyps.

One reason is that calcium can suppress the proliferation of surface cells on the inner lining of the colon, thus preventing the rapid cell growth that is a sign of developing cancer. When researchers at Ichilov Hospital in Israel gave 35 men and women 1,250–1,500mg of calcium for three months, abnormal cell pro–liferation dropped 36 per cent after one month, as determined by examinations of the colon. Further, when the patients stopped taking the calcium, abnormally high rates of proliferation returned. Scientists at Henry Ford Hospital in Detroit found that giving 1,250mg of calcium every day to men with polyps for just *one week* reduced by about half the activity of enzymes in the colon that promote tumour growth in some patients! The calcium was not effective in some individuals.

A CUP OF MILK, A BOWL OF CEREAL AND . . .

As a dietary antidote to colon cancer, a hard-to-beat combination seems to be a bowl of cereal (make it wheat bran) doused with low-fat milk. That's what Swedish researchers found when they compared the diets of colon-cancer-surgery patients and normal men and women over a 15 year period. Two foods stood out in the diets of cancer-free individuals: high-fibre cereal and calcium. Additionally, they ate less fat.

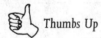 Thumbs Up

ANTICANCER VITAMIN IN MILK

Drink milk for its vitamin D, another potential cancer suppressor, according to Dr. Garland. He says vitamin D blood levels can predict colon cancer risk. He examined 25,620 blood samples collected in Maryland in 1974 for vitamin D content; then he compared colon cancer rates over the next eight years. His conclusion was that those with high blood levels of vitamin D were 70 per cent less likely to develop colon cancer than those with low levels. A fascinating fact revealed by this study was how little vitamin D it took to protect against the cancer. To get anticancer blood concentrations, you need to eat daily only 200 IU (5 micrograms) of vitamin D. Seafood is especially rich in vitamin D.

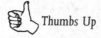 *Thumbs Up*

ACIDOPHILUS – THRICE A CANCER FIGHTER

Give your colon some yoghurt made with the acidophilus culture. This adds another potential colon cancer antagonist to the calcium and vitamin D duo already present in dairy foods. Research shows that *Lactobacillus acidophilus* helps suppress enzyme activity needed to convert otherwise harmless substances into cancer-causing chemicals in the colon. Proof comes from studies done by leading researchers Barry R. Goldin and Sherwood L Gorbach at the New England Medical Center. For a month, volunteers drank two glasses of plain milk every day. Then they switched to acidophilus milk (available in the United States). Researchers measured the enzyme activity in the subjects' colons. Drinking acidophilus milk caused dangerous enzyme activity to drop by 40–80 per cent. This means certain carcinogenic activity in the colon was dramatically suppressed. Some yoghurts available in Britain contain acidophilus bacteria. Check the label to be sure.

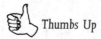 *Thumbs Up*

HOW ABOUT MARMALADE?

Pectin, the fibre in apples as well as many other fruits and vegetables promises to keep colon cancer away, according to Dr. Ivan Cameron, professor of biology at the University of Texas Health Science Center in San Antonio. When he fed rats pectin, which is a soluble fibre their rates of colon cancer dipped 50 per cent. (As a bonus, their cholesterol also went down about 30 per cent.) Dr. Cameron calls pectin "unique" among soluble fibres in inhibiting colon cancer. Typically, insoluble fibre, the type found in wheat, has been shown to block colon cancer. Look for pectin in apples, bananas, pears, prunes, apricots, carrots, dried beans and the white membranes of citrus fruits. "Marmalade is a surprisingly good source," advises Dr. Cameron.

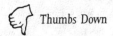 Thumbs Down

ANIMAL FAT – BIG DANGER

If you have colon polyps, colon cancer, a family history of colon cancer, or any concern about colon cancer, severely restrict meat and animal fat; they are energetic promoters of colon cancer, according to strong evidence.

Around the world, people who eat more fat, namely animal fat, have much more colon cancer, study after study shows. Eating lots of saturated animal fat also doubles your chances of precancerous polyps, according to Edward Giovannucci and colleagues at Harvard. In their study of 7,248 men, those who ate the least saturated fat (7 per cent of calories in animal fat) had half the rate of precancerous polyps compared with men who ate twice that much (14 per cent of calories in saturated fat). Skimping on fibre also boosted polyp formation, leading researchers to conclude that fat interacts with other food substances, including fibre in determining whether colon cancer occurs.

HOW FAT PROMOTES CANCER

Eating lots of fat, one theory goes, prompts microorganisms in the colon to make more bile acid, a cancer promoter. According to cancer researcher Dr. Michael J. Wargovich, "We think these products of dietary fat digestion wound the colon." Cells then start proliferating in attempts to heal the colon wall, but if you eat too much fat, the process gets out of hand and "may go on continuously in the colon," he explains. Such rapid, excessive cell proliferation may eventually stimulate growth of colon polyps and possibly malignant tumours. Dr. Wargovich also theorizes that one way calcium, fibre and perhaps other food constituents neutralize carcinogenic fat is by binding to the bile acids so they cannot injure the colon, setting the cancer process in motion.

"If you step back and look at the data [on colon cancer], the optimum amount of red meat you eat should be zero!" – Dr. Walter Willett, M.D., Harvard researcher

---

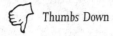 Thumbs Down

THE LESS RED MEAT, THE BETTER

Be wary of red meat, regardless of the fat. There's something in red meat that makes it even more hazardous than its fat alone, studies suggest. For example, Norwegian men who ate the most processed meat had the highest rates of colon cancer. In a 14-year follow-up study of Swedish men, meat (beef and lamb) was the only food linked to higher rates of colon cancer.

The most disturbing evidence comes from a six-year Harvard study of 90,000 women, directed by Walter Willett, M.D., of the Harvard School of Public Health. The study declared no amount of red meat safe when it comes to colon cancer. Dr. Willett and colleagues found that women who ate a main dish of meat daily – about 5oz (140g) of beef, pork, or lamb – were 250 per cent more likely to develop colon cancer than those eating meat less than once a month. The more they ate, the greater the risk. Further, even women who ate red meat infrequently – once a week or once a month – were still 40 per cent more likely to get colon cancer than those who ate red meat less than once a month. In fact, no amount of red meat was safe, that is, unable to promote colon cancer, according to the data.

In contrast, fish and chicken seemed to stave off colon cancer. Eating fish two to four times a week reduced colon cancer chances 25 per cent. Eating skinless chicken every day pushed down the risk 50 per cent. A possible explanation, says Dr Willett is that the type of fat in chicken and fish tips the balance away from colon cancer. Eating more fibre also reduced colon cancer odds.

Dr. Willett, who does not eat meat, said the results would apply equally to men and women.

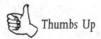 Thumbs Up

FOOD-ASPIRIN ANTIDOTES?

Don't neglect fruit. Fruit may contribute more than its fibre in staving off colon cancer, so goes an intriguing new theory. There's a new kid on the block in colon cancer prevention," as Tim Byers of the Centers for Disease Control and Prevention (CDC) puts it. It's aspirin. A major study has found that taking aspirin daily cut the risk of colon cancer dramatically. That brings up the question: What about natural aspirin in foods, so-called salicylates? Many foods contain them. Might eating high-salicylate foods also help curb colon cancer? Dr. Byers thinks it's a possibility. "At least it s a whole new line of inquiry, to be pursued," he says. Foods highest in natural salicylates are fruits such as apples, dates, berries. (For a list of such foods, see page 440.)

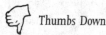 Thumbs Down

THE DRINKER'S COLON CANCER

Beware of excessive drinking. The sobering news is that heavy drinking may double or triple your chances of colorectal cancer, and generally, the more alcohol you consume, the more likely the malignancy. So concluded Australian researchers who reviewed 52 human studies on the subject. They identified beer as by far the principal villain. Alcoholic spirits were much less dangerous and least hazardous was wine. They also blamed drinking for promoting colon polyps. How alcohol promotes colon cancer is unclear. The researchers speculated that a steady intake of alcoholic beverages may chronically suppress immune functioning, making the body less able to combat the cancer process. Some beverages, notably beer, may contain carcinogens such as nitrosamines.

Alcohol poses a particularly formidable threat in cancer of the sigmoid colon, the S-shaped part of the colon that lies in the pelvis. According to a 17-year study of 26,118 Japanese over age 40, drinkers were four times more likely to have sigmoid colon cancer than nondrinkers. Again most incriminated was beer. Daily beer drinkers racked up nearly 13 times the odds of this cancer as nondrinkers. Consumers of sake and shochu, Japanese rice wine, were four to six times more likely to develop colon cancer. Consuming too much meat also looked bad.

DIET ADVICE TO CURTAIL COLON CANCER

• The research all points in the same direction, suggesting that two mighty important things you can do to prevent colon cancer are to eat high-fibre wheat bran cereal regularly and stay away from red meat and meat fat. If you do eat meat, roast it or microwave it instead of grilling or barbecuing it.

• Make it a point to eat more vegetables, especially the cru-ciferous vegetables, such as cabbage, broccoli, cauliflower and Brussels sprouts. Cruciferous vegetables two or three times a week seem to go a long way in preventing colon cancer. Daily doses of cabbage are not necessary and could be detrimental to some. These vegetables provide fibre as well as other compounds, such as indoles, that act as antidotes to colon cancer in animals.

• Eat chicken and fish, which both appear to counteract a propensity to colon cancer. If you already have polyps, eating lots of fatty fish could cause them to regress.

• Skimmed milk and very-low-fat yoghurt, especially containing acidophilus cultures, can also be part of an anti-colon-cancer regimen. If you cannot tolerate milk, eat yoghurt.

• Restrict your drinking to no more than two drinks a day, and be particularly wary of beer.

• Such dietary changes are all the more critical if you have had colon cancer surgery or have colon polyps that could become cancerous. In such cases, think of a daily bowl or two of All-Bran (or equally high-fibre wheat cereal) and milk as a natural medi-cation that could help save you as surely as prescription drugs might.

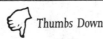 Thumbs Down

BEER DANGER IN RECTAL CANCER

Beer is a special villain in rectal cancer. A study at the State University of New York at Buffalo determined that men who drink two to three beers a day over a lifetime boost their chances of getting rectal cancer. The same was not true of wine and spirit drinkers. It took more – at least four – daily alcoholic drinks of other types to boost the odds. The scientists speculate that alcohol itself stimulates rectal cancer, but that beer has an added hazard of being contaminated with other cancer-causing chemicals.

Swedish researchers also agree, after tracking 6,230 male brewery workers for 19 years. Compared with the average Swede these workers had a slightly higher rate of almost all types of cancer, but rectal cancer in particular. The brewery workers also drank about seven times as much beer as their compatriots.

LUNG CANCER

Foods Most Likely to Prevent Lung Cancer: Any Dark Green Leafy
Vegetable, the Darker Green the Better • Any Yellow-Orange
Vegetable or Fruit, the Deeper Orange the Better • Carrots •
Broccoli • Spinach • Kale • Dark Green Lettuces • Collard Greens
• Brussels Sprouts • Pumpkin • Sweet Potatoes • Green Tea •
Beans • Low-Fat Milk

Foods That May Prolong Survival Time: All Vegetables,
Especially Broccoli and Tomatoes

ATTENTION SMOKERS AND EX-SMOKERS: HERE'S WHAT TO EAT

The evidence is compelling: If you are a smoker or former smoker, or
if you live around smokers or have any other reason to believe you are
vulnerable to lung cancer, make it a point to eat fruits and vegetables
every day, especially carrots and broccoli and other green leafy veg–
etables. Amazingly, research suggests that eating only an extra single
carrot, 3oz (85g) of dark yellow-orange or dark green vegetables, a
piece of fruit or a glass of juice daily, or even more than once a week,
could mean the difference between getting and not getting lung cancer.
In fact, such a tiny amount appears to cut your odds of developing lung
cancer by half or even more! Eating vegetables even seems to fight lung
cancer after it occurs by slowing its pace and prolonging survival time.

It may seem faintly preposterous – a piece of carrot, broccoli floret or
spinach leaf fending off dreaded lung cancer. Yet it is a prospect taken
very seriously by knowledgeable scientists around the world. The medical literature bulges with support. In a sweeping review of the evidence,
Gladys Block, Ph.D., formerly at the American National Cancer Institute
and now at the University of California at Berkeley, found that a
whopping 30 of 32 studies on the impact of diet on lung cancer odds
identified fruits and vegetables as potent food antidotes.

"It is striking," says Tim Byers, an epidemiologist at the CDC "Of all cancers, the smoking cancers, notably cancers of the lung and oral cavity, are most consistently related to dietary prevention. Study after study on all continents show that people who have diets deficient in fruits and vegetables are at increased risk of such smok– ing cancers." He suggests that tobacco has a "synergistic effect – that is, it becomes a far more potent carcinogen in people with "poor diet"

"Smokers should switch from cancer sticks to carrot sticks and soya beans." – James Duke, Ph.D., U.S. Department of Agriculture

---

If you smoke or once smoked, you can ill afford a vegetable deficiency". It's a new twist in perspective, seeing the tragedy of lung cancer not only as a curse of smoking and 20th-century pollution, but also as a dietary lack that may be partly countered by "edible plant chemoprevention" – infusions of natural drugs to help shield lung cells from anticipated carcinogenic damage. John Potter, M.D., an epidemiologist at the University of Minnesota, calls fruits and vegetables "essential nutrients" for combating cancer, especially lung cancer.

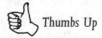 Thumbs Up

ALL HAIL THE CARROT CHEMICAL

Learn to love the orangest and greenest. All kinds of vegetables and fruits may rescue your lungs from the ravages of cancer. Premier are those rich in beta carotene, an orange pigment isolated from carrots 150 years ago. Beta carotene is concentrated in deep orange and green vegetables (green chlorophyll covers up the orange) and the deeper the colour the more beta carotene. Beta carotene acts as an antidote to lung cancer; it has been described as "a morning-after pill," because it nullifies cancer in animals fed powerful cancer-causing chemicals.

In humans, the most dedicated beta-carotene eaters are only 40–70 per cent as likely to get lung cancer, according to virtually all epidemiological studies done in the last ten years. Typical is a recent study at the State University of New York at Buffalo. It showed that eating beta-carotene-rich vegetables more than once a week drama—tically depressed lung cancer odds when compared with non-eaters of the vegetables. Munching down a single raw carrot at least twice a week reduced lung cancer odds 60 per cent; a more-than-weekly 5oz (140g) of raw broccoli depressed odds 70 per cent, raw spinach by 40 per cent.

A TIME BOMB IN YOUR BLOODSTREAM

Don't let your blood levels of beta carotene drop. If you skimp on vegetables, carotene levels in your bloodstream sink; such low levels are a time bomb – a grim predictor of death from cancer, specifically lung cancer. In a landmark study, Marilyn Menkes, Ph.D., of Johns Hopkins University, tracked down donors who in 1974 had given blood samples that had been analyzed for beta carotene content. She discovered that by 1983, some 99 of the donors had developed lung cancer. She compared the beta carotene blood levels of the lung cancer victims with those of similar donors free of the cancer.

The message was startling. Those with the least beta carotene in their blood had twice the lung cancer rates of those with the most blood beta carotene. More striking, the lack of blood beta carotene correctly forecast the appearance nearly a decade later of the most deadly type of lung cancer among smokers – squamous cell carcinoma – a sort of skin cancer of the lung lining. The seemingly small matter of skimping on beta carotene foods had massive consequences. Those with the lowest blood beta carotene had quadruple the chances of developing this dreaded "smoker's" cancer as those with the highest blood beta carotene.

The American National Cancer Institute is testing the carrot compound in capsule form on thousands of people in 14 large-scale studies worldwide to see if it helps fend off cancer. Five studies are specifically geared toward lung cancer.

"Eating one extra carrot a day might help prevent from 15,000 to 20,000 lung cancer deaths a year." – Marilyn Menkes, Ph.D., cancer researcher, Johns Hopkins

---

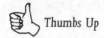 Thumbs Up

A BITE OF CAROTENE A DAY

Eat some carrots, sweet potatoes, spinach and other leafy veg–
etables every day; even one bite a day is better than none.
3–6oz (85–170g) is better yet. How much carotene you must eat
to deflect lung cancer depends on such factors as heredity, the
amount of damage your lungs have suffered from cigarette smoke
and how well you absorb beta carotene. The difference in intake is
generally staggeringly small between those most likely and least likely
to get lung cancer. Regina Ziegler, Ph.D., of the American National
Cancer Institute, figured the daily carotene gap separating the high
and low lung cancer risks among ex-smoking men to be a mere
3oz (85g) daily of a deep yellow-orange or deep green vegetable.
Similarly, researchers at the State University of New York at
Buffalo calculated that a cancer-protective dose is found in just one
carrot a day!

British researchers at the Imperial Cancer Research Fund in
Oxford recently narrowed that lifesaving gap to an extra bite of carrot
a day! In a study of 193 men, investigators calculated that those who
ate a mere 2.7mg of beta carotene a day were only 45 per cent as
likely to develop lung cancer as those who ate 1.7mg. The anti–
cancer difference was a mere 1mg. An average carrot contains
about 6mg of beta carotene. The study also found a dose response;
eating more beta carotene further reduced the lung cancer odds.

Beta carotene's anticancer power theoretically comes from both
its antioxidant capabilities and its ability to enhance immunological
defences important in preventing and fighting cancer.

Note: Such studies do not reveal an optimum anticancer dose be–
cause even those who eat the most beta-carotene-rich foods still eat
fairly low amounts. The anticancer impact of eating two or three carrots
a day or comparable beta-carotene doses is untested and unknown.
Who knows? A shift to heavy vegetable eating – five or more servings
a day – might make a much bigger dent in cancer than is currently
anticipated.

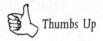 Thumbs Up

GREENS' AND BEANS' SECRET WEAPON

Give your lungs some chemical ammunition that bucks up cell resistance, namely folic acid or folate, a B vitamin. It's another potent protector concentrated in green leafy vegetables. University of Alabama researcher Douglas Heimburger discovered how critical folic acid is in warding off lung cancer. By measuring folic acid levels in the lung tissue of men with and without the cancer, he discovered that cancer victims were more likely to have a localized deficiency of this B vitamin in their lung tissue. This lack, he says, led to more chromosome breakage in cells, making them more vulnerable to formation of tumours.

Smokers, also, not surprisingly, had much lower levels of folic acid in their blood, once again indicating that a predisposition to lung cancer may be partly due to a "vegetable deficiency". Folic acid is concentrated in spinach, collards, turnip and beet greens, broccoli and Brussels sprouts. It is also high in all kinds of dried beans, including soya beans. Folic acid may be another secret weapon that explains why lovers of green leafy vegetables are more immune to lung cancer.

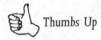 Thumbs Up

EAT TOMATOES AND CABBAGE, TOO

Spread your bets widely. Eating all kinds of other vegetables may also save you from lung cancer. Beta carotene and folic acid are not the only potential lung-cancer fighters in vegetables. A major study from the Cancer Research Center at the University of Hawaii showed that all vegetables, including dark green vegetables, cruciferous vegetables and tomatoes, cut the risk of lung cancer dramatically – even more than did beta carotene alone. Eating these various vegetables pushed down the lung cancer rate sevenfold in women and threefold in men, whereas beta carotene alone depressed odds threefold in women and twofold in men. This suggests that other carotenoids besides beta carotene, such as lutein, lycopene, indoles and others, found generally in vegetables, can also be strong protectors against lung cancer.

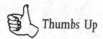 *Thumbs Up*

TEA-DRINKING ANIMALS DON'T GET LUNG CANCER

To protect your lungs, you may want to drink more tea. Even among smokers in Japan, the lung-cancer rate is not as high as among American smokers. One possible reason is that the Japanese drink so much green tea, suggests Dr. Fung-lung Chung, a researcher with the American Health Foundation in New York. His tests on mice show that a potent cancer-causing agent in tobacco, known to help induce lung cancer in smokers, is partly neutralized by a compound in green tea. Mice drinking green tea or the concentrated tea compound in water had 30–45 per cent fewer lung cancers than mice drinking plain water. Other studies in the United States and Japan show essentially the same thing. Dr. Hirota Fujiki an official with Japan's National Cancer Center Research Institute calls the green tea protection "dramatic," saying "drinking green tea could be one of the most practical methods of cancer prevention available to the general population at present". Ordinary black tea contains smaller amounts of the compound that prevented mouse lung cancer. Asian markets, as well as food speciality shops and some supermarkets, carry green tea, which is noted on the label.

WHAT CAN SMOKERS EXPECT FROM FOOD ANTIDOTES?

The truth is that smokers, past and present, as well as nonsmokers, reap varying degrees of protection against lung cancer from eating more anti-cancer vegetables and other foods. Still, many researchers dislike mentioning that, lest it take some of the fear out of smoking. In fact, some studies suggest that the greatest vegetable-eating beneficiaries are those who still smoke or have recently quit. One Hawaiian study found veg-etables were most likely to cut the cancer odds in men who were current heavy smokers or recent ex-smokers and in women who were light smokers or quitters who had smoked for a long time. Other studies note that fruits and vegetables exert more anticancer clout among ex-smokers, but that even current smokers get considerable protection.

Obviously this does not mean by any stretch that you can eat lots of vegetables and continue to smoke with impunity in the futile hope that nature's medicines will erase lung cancer from your future. Quitting is always the first and most potent action. There is no way the powers of diet can totally offset the carcinogenic catastrophe of filling your lungs with smoke. Even fervent eaters of anticancer vegetables who continue to smoke are at least ten times more susceptible to lung cancer than are nonsmokers, says one expert.

Still, if you must continue smoking, it makes eminent sense to load up on vegetables and fruits to try to cut your odds as much as possible. Quitters can know that such foods may hasten the healing of their lungs, more rapidly cleansing lung tissue of the cancer threat. The constant infusion of antioxidant, anticancer agents may help interrupt the long, slow progression toward lung cancer that characteristically proceeds for years after a person has stopped smoking.

Pioneering research by Richard Shekelle, Ph.D., of the University of Texas at Houston, discovered that even long-time male smokers – some who had smoked for thirty years – could find some salvation in veg–etables. Those who ate the least beta-carotene foods were seven times more likely to develop lung cancer than those who ate the most.

"A diet relatively high in beta carotene may reduce the risk of lung cancer even among persons who have smoked cigarettes for many years." – Richard Shekelle, Ph.D., University of Texas, Houston

---

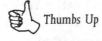 Thumbs Up

VEGETABLES AGAINST PASSIVE SMOKING

If you have never smoked, eating "right" may also save you from lung cancer. A group of nonsmoking New Jersey women – who were "passive smokers," exposed to others' cigarette smoke – cut their risk of lung cancer nearly in half by eating an extra 3oz (85g) of dark-yellow and orange vegetables every day. In another study, researchers looked at a group of 88 women in Hong Kong, including many who had never smoked and yet had lung cancer. Certain foods were highly protective against the lung tumours – primarily, fresh leafy green vegetables, carrots, tofu or other soya bean products, fresh fruit and fresh fish. Once again, vegetables had a profound impact. Women eating the most carrots, fresh green leafy vegetables, and fresh fruit cut their chances of lung cancer by 90, 70 and 40 percent respectively.

WHAT TO EAT IF YOU HAVE LUNG CANCER

If you have been diagnosed with lung cancer, it's still good to eat more vegetables and fruits. The time has come when food may serve not just to ward off cancer but help actively treat it. Alternative medicine practitioners have long prescribed a vegetarian or macrobiotic diet for those with cancer, including lung cancer. Now, growing mainstream evidence reveals that eating more fruits and vegetables may pay off for people who have lung cancer. New research shows that food substances, such as beta carotene, can attack and destroy tumour cells and retard the growth and spread of tumours. A recent report from the University of Hawaii's Cancer Research Center in Honolulu indicated that vegetables'

VEGETABLE CRAZE: THE BEST DIET PRESCRIPTION

• The best dietary bet for escaping lung cancer, whether or not you ever smoked, is to eat plenty of vegetables, especially those rich in carotenoids, including beta carotene – namely carrots, broccoli, spinach, dark green lettuce, pumpkin, sweet potatoes. (For a list of high-beta-carotene foods, see page 453.)

• If you were or are a smoker, that advice is magnified. It is critical after you quit smoking to eat at least 3oz (85g) of dark green or dark orange vegetables every day. They may intercede in the long, slow march toward lung cancer that continues for ten years or more after you quit. Vegetable chemicals may retard promotion of the cancer and formation of tumours.

• It also seems smart to drink tea, particularly green tea, and eat more legumes, although the evidence is less solid.

• If you have been diagnosed with lung cancer, adding anti-cancer chemicals to your diet by eating more vegetables, specifically tomatoes, broccoli and those rich in carotenoids such as beta carotene, lycopene and lutein, may help fight the cancer, prolonging life.

---

chemotherapeutic powers stifled cancer progression and virulence, and prolonged survival time.

In that study of 463 male and 212 female lung cancer patients, researchers discovered that eating lots of vegetables of all types nearly doubled survival time in women. Females who ate the most vegetables, especially broccoli, were likely to survive 33 months compared with 18 months for those eating the least vegetables. Fruit, and tomatoes specifically, also prolonged life. Among men with lung cancer, eating more tomatoes and oranges appeared to extend survival time. The researchers credit anticancer compounds in the fruits and vegetables.

The most likely candidates were lycopene in tomatoes and carotenoids in other vegetables, including beta carotene, which in test-tube experiments has destroyed human tumour cells by multiple mechanisms.

PANCREATIC CANCER

> **Foods That May Help Prevent Pancreatic Cancer:** Fruit, Especially Citrus • Tomatoes • Legumes
>
> **Foods That May Promote Pancreatic Cancer:** Cured Pork Products (Bacon, Ham, Cold Cuts) • Red Meat

Eating to prevent pancreatic cancer can be critical because this cancer is especially resistant to treatment. There is some persuasive evidence that the right diet can help keep this virulent cancer from ever developing.

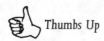 *Thumbs Up*

FRUIT POWER

The most urgent advice for escaping pancreatic cancer has to be: Eat more fruit. Study after study strikingly confirms that heavy fruit eaters have lower rates of this cancer. Examples include a Swedish study which found that eating a citrus fruit a day cut the risk of pancreatic cancer by *one-half to two-thirds* compared with eating a citrus fruit less than once a week. A Seventh-Day Adventist study revealed that even dried fruit protected against pancreatic cancer. In that study, tomatoes and fresh citrus fruit were also protective.

Now here's the most fascinating bit of fruit-power evidence. A study among a Cajun population in Louisiana, with one of the highest pancreatic cancer rates in the country, revealed that fruit might even be an antidote to a meat diet that encourages pancreatic cancer. In other words, fruit may blunt meat's propensity to promote cancer of the pancreas. An American National Cancer Institute research team found that a group of Cajuns in Louisiana, who ate the most pork (mainly bacon, ham, sausage, cold cuts and unprocessed fresh pork, usually eaten with rice) had tremendously high rates of pancreatic cancer. A once-a-day pork eater was 70 per cent more likely to have the cancer than a person eating pork less than twice a week. Those consuming pork more than once a day tripled their risk for pancreatic cancer. At the same time, twice-a-day fruit eaters (bananas, oranges, strawberries, canned fruits, orange juice and apples) were only 40 per cent as likely to get the cancer as those eating fruits less than once a day. There was a dose response: the more fruit, the lower the risk. No real surprises there.

Most startling was the fact that heavy pork eaters could get away with it if they also ate a lot of fruit. Prodigious pork eaters who also loaded up on fruit were *no more likely to have pancreatic cancer than skimpy pork eaters!* There was a wipe-out effect, which researchers generally credited to vitamin C in the fruit, but it's well known that there are dozens of other cancer-counteracting chemicals in fruits that might also be influential.

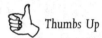 Thumbs Up

EAT TOMATOES FOR SURE

Lycopene is a seemingly formidable deterrent to pancreatic cancer Lycopene means tomatoes. The tomato is the major source of lycopene in the diet. Having low levels of lycopene in your blood is predictive of pancreatic cancer, according to a Johns Hopkins University study. The investigators examined blood samples of 26,000 people, collected ten years ago, in a search for clues that might identify those most likely to develop pancreatic cancer.

Indeed, the cancer victims' blood showed one outstanding dietary difference: low levels of lycopene. Those with the least blood lycopene had over five times the risk of pancreatic cancer as healthy people with the most blood lycopene. Primarily, low lycopene denotes low consumption of tomatoes. Watermelon also is extremely rich in lycopene, a pigment that gives these foods their red colour. (Red berries are not a good source of lycopene; they get their colour from a different chemical.)

• BOTTOM LINE • *An orange – or grapefruit – a day may cut your chances of developing pancreatic cancer in half People who don't eat tomatoes or watermelon are five times more likely to have pancreatic cancer.*

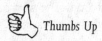 Thumbs Up

THE BEAN DEFENCE

Eat dried beans at least once a week. One large-scale study showed that those who ate legumes weekly, including soya beans, were 40 per cent less likely to die of pancreatic cancer than those who ate legumes less than once a week. Study director Paul K. Mills of the Department of Preventive Medicine at Loma Linda University School of Medicine believes compounds in beans, called protease inhibitors, may be the saviour. However, legumes also have other proven anticancer agents.

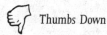 Thumbs Down

THE CASE AGAINST MEAT AND FAT

Cut down on meat. Pancreatic cancer is greatest among populations that consume the most fat. That may be due more to meat itself than to the fat. Numerous studies show that too much fried or barb–ecued meat, as well as smoked and cured pork products, boost chances of pancreatic cancer. As noted previously, in the Louisiana study of Cajun populations, cured bacon, ham, sausage, cold cuts and unprocessed fresh pork dramatically elevated the odds of pancreatic cancer.

In Japan, eating meat at least once a day boosted the pancreatic cancer risk by 50 per cent. A Swedish study found that eating fried and barbecued meats – but not meats cooked in other ways – boosted pancreatic cancer odds. In Los Angeles, those who ate beef at least five times a week had twice the rate of pancreatic cancer. Animals fed lots of fats often show damaged cells in the pancreas.

If it is not entirely the fat in meat that encourages pancreatic cancer, what could it be? Nobody knows for sure, but likely culprits are cancer-causing nitrosamines that can form from sodium nitrite used as a preservative in cured meats. Vitamin C helps counteract the nitrosamines, which perhaps explains why vitamin-C-laden fruits seem to be such a potent preventive.

WHAT ABOUT COFFEE, TEA AND ALCOHOL?

In the early 1980s, a couple of studies suggested that coffee promoted pancreatic cancer and, in fact, that a mere one or two cups of coffee a day could nearly double the risk. Since then, a dozen or so well-conducted studies have shown no danger from either regular or decaffeinated coffee, leading the overwhelming majority of researchers to dismiss coffee as a culprit in pancreatic cancer.

Nor does tea seem a threat. At least ten studies examining the impact of tea on pancreatic cancer have been done, and the preponderance of evidence showed nothing. One British analysis did report that drinking three or more cups of tea a day doubled the risk of pancreatic cancer. On the other hand, Italian scientists found that tea-drinking actually cut the risk in half! The remaining 80 per cent of the reports found no relationship at all. It seems likely that tea is neutral in pancreatic cancer.

Despite several reports in the 1960s, as well as a few recent ones declaring alcohol, notably beer, a culprit in pancreatic cancer, most researchers do not find a connection, says Pelayo Correa, M.D., professor of pathology at Louisiana State University Medical Center; If alcohol is related to pancreatic cancer, its effect appears to be slight.

STOMACH CANCER

Foods That May Prevent Stomach Cancer: Cabbage • Tea • Garlic • Onions • Soya beans • Fruits and Vegetables Rich in Vitamin C

Foods That May Promote Stomach Cancer: Salt • Cured, Smoked Meats

Stomach cancer is no longer the villain in the United States that it was at the turn of the century, but it still ranks as a major killer in other parts of the world, namely Japan. Many authorities credit diet for the dramatic decline in stomach cancer among Americans, mainly because fruits and vegetables are available year round due to refrigeration. The magic ingredient? Maybe vitamin C. Vitamin C has undisputed ability to neutralize such powerful stomach carcinogens as nitrosamines, and in fact, is added to cured meats specifically for that purpose. Additionally, fruits and vegetables contain an array of other compounds, such as carotenoids, indoles and sulphurous chemicals that have demonstrated anticancer potential.

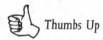 *Thumbs Up*

ANTICANCER SALAD BAR

Munch on raw vegetables. You're two to three times more susceptible to stomach cancer if you skip fruits and raw vegetables. So many studies have found an array of fruits and raw vegetables protective that anyone worried about stomach cancer should step up to the salad bar. If you don't consume fruit daily, your risk of stomach cancer doubles or even triples, according to studies in Japan, England and Poland. Raw vegetables of various types are formidable opponents of stomach cancer, according to much research. Especially protective are raw celery, cucumbers, carrots, green peppers, tomatoes, onions and lettuce.

In fact, veggies seem to beat out fruit in discouraging stomach cancer, according to a large-scale Hawaiian study of nearly 70,000 men of Japanese descent. The men were first interviewed in 1965 about their dietary habits. After 18 years of follow-up, 111 had developed stomach cancer. When their diets were compared with those of cancer-free men, vegetables of all types popped out as the strongest factor in suppressing stomach cancer. The men who ate at least 3oz (85g) of vegetables a day were only 60 per cent as likely to have stomach cancer. Especially good guards against stomach cancer were cruciferous vegetables and green vegetables. Cabbage was the most popular vegetable among the men.

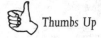 Thumbs Up

A COUPLE OF TABLESPOONS OF CABBAGE A DAY

Indeed, cabbage may have super powers against stomach cancer. A remarkable study done in Heilongjiang Province in northeast China, where stomach cancer is the worst cancer killer, singled out cabbage as the leader among vegetables in fighting the malignancy. Various vegetables, including Chinese cabbage, spinach, squash, aubergine, green beans, were all linked to lower rates of the cancer. But outstanding was Chinese cabbage. Those who ate only one ¾oz (25g) of raw cabbage every day or a mere two tablespoons of cooked cabbage had less stomach cancer.

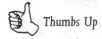 Thumbs Up

SPRING ONION SURPRISE

Eat an onion a day. One of the most convincing studies on the power of diet over stomach cancer comes from Shandong Province in China, where stomach cancer rates are also high. The study was sponsored by the American National Cancer Institute. When researchers delved into the diets of 564 stomach cancer patients compared with 1,131 healthy individuals, they found that those who ate 3oz (85g) of garlic and onions daily were only 40 per cent as likely to develop stomach cancer as neighbours who ate only 1oz (30g) daily of garlic and onions. That included garlic, garlic stalks, spring onions, chives and onions.

Most potent were spring onions followed by garlic and chives. There was a dose-response relationship – the more garlic and onions consumed, the lower the chances of cancer. Considering the magnitude of protection, the quantities were fairly low. You get the 3oz (85g) protective dose in one medium-size onion. Such a finding makes sense, say researchers, because the allium vegetables possess known anticancer compounds, and have saved many a laboratory animal from death by cancer. Onions and garlic, for example, contain sulphrous compounds that have been tested in labs and found to block cancer.

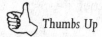 Thumbs Up

TEA-TOTALLING JAPANESE

Try drinking tea. In one Japanese study of 4,729 adults, heavy tea-drinkers were designated least likely to get stomach cancer. Drinking at least ten cups (small Japanese size) of green tea a day was protective. That amount of tea would provide 40–50mg of vitamin C, the researchers estimated. Furthermore, it has been shown that green tea (as well as black tea) does neutralize the formation of nitrosamines – potent carcinogens – in both test tubes and in the stomachs of humans.

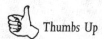 Thumbs Up

MAKE YOURS MISO SOUP

Soya beans may help fight off stomach cancer. Looking for clues to which foods help prevent cancer, Japanese scientists hit on miso (soya bean paste) as a possibility. Specifically, they found that men and women who ate a bowl of miso soup a day were only one-third as likely to develop stomach cancer as those who never ate it. Even eating it occasionally cut the odds of stomach cancer by 17 per cent in men and 19 per cent in women. At the time – about a decade ago – this finding was a surprise. Analyses of soya beans have now shown them to be full of various anticancer compounds. Apparently, the soya bean constituents overcame any cancer-promoting effects of high sodium in miso.

Surprising fact: A bowl of miso (soya bean paste) Japanese soup a day cut the risk of stomach cancer by two-thirds!

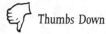 Thumbs Down

SODIUM, MEAT AND FAT – TRIPLE THREAT

Avoid excessive salt. Sodium has long been hailed as a cancer threat to the stomach, especially in collusion with other carcinogens, such as residues and smoke from barbecuing and grilling meat. Cured meats, such as hot dogs, ham, salami's and bacon are also high in sodium. Salt is bad stuff in fostering cancer. It is an irritant to the stomach that induces gastritis, increases precancerous cell replication and boosts the potency of chemical carcinogens. Salt appears particularly virulent when the diet is also low in fruits and vegetables that may counteract the cancer process.

OTHER CANCERS

AN ANTI-SKIN CANCER DIET

If you're worried about melanoma (skin cancer), which has doubled in the United States since 1980, the best <u>diet</u> advice is to cut back on oils high in omega-6 fatty acids. That includes corn oil, safflower oil and sunflower oil. Eat more of the omega-3 type fat in fish. The reason being that when your cells have too much omega-6 fat and not enough omega-3, the production of prostaglandins goes into overdrive, encouraging the onset and growth of skin tumours. A proper balance of fish oil helps block that disastrous biochemical cascade of events.

In mice, safflower and sunflower oils, high in omega-6, definitely spur the growth of melanoma. Also, a recent study showed that patients with melanoma ate about twice as much omega-6 type polyunsaturated oil as a similar group without the cancer.

Keep the ratio of omega-3 to omega-6 fatty acids high, says Dr. James Duke. "Eat fish at least twice a week, and avoid high linoleic acid vegetable oils," such as corn oil. Olive oil is okay. An international conference on melanoma in 1989 concluded that eating butter, with a higher ratio of omega-3 to omega-6, was safer than eating high omega-6 vegetable oils. Also, eating antioxidants, concentrated in fruits and vegetables, combats the ability of omega-6 fats to promote melanoma. For example, putting antioxidant vitamin C in the drinking water of mice with melanoma inhibited tumour growth, size, in–vasiveness, and increased survival time.

As further protection against melanoma, diet-and-cancer authority Dr. Herbert Pierson advises eating garlic, flaxseed, quercetin (onions) and walnut oil.

VEGGIES VS. ENDOMETRIAL CANCER

Diet may "play an important role in the etiology [cause] of endome–trial cancer," according to researchers at the University of Alabama School of Public Health in Birmingham. A comparison of the diets of women who did and did not have endometrial cancer showed that those who ate carrots, spinach, broccoli, cantaloupe melon or lettuce (foods high in carotene) at least once a day were only 27 per cent as likely to have the cancer as women who ate those foods less than once a week. Eating yoghurt, cheese and other calcium-rich foods also reduced the risk significantly.

BROCCOLI AND TOMATOES BLOCK CERVICAL CANCER

It's astonishing but true. Eating the right stuff – foods such as greens and dried beans, high in folic acid, a B vitamin – can stop the virus that can lead to cervical cancer. About 80 per cent of all cases of cervical cancer occur in women infected with the virus. Yet women who have high levels of folic acid in their red blood cells are much less likely to develop the cancer, according to new research by Charles Butterworth, Jr., M.D., of the University of Alabama at Birmingham. His study of 464 women infected with the virus found that those with lower levels of folic acid were five times more likely than those with higher folic acid levels to develop cell changes leading to cervical cancer.

A lack of folic acid provokes a kind of "double whammy," says Dr. Butterworth. Chromosomes are more likely to break at "fragile" points. This allows the virus to slip into the healthy cell's genetic material, promoting initial changes that foreshadow cancer. Eating a diet rich in folic acid is preventive, he says. "A couple of spears of broccoli a day" give you about half the recommended dietary allowance of folic acid, which is 400 micrograms a day. Once cancer occurs, loading up on the vitamin does no good, he says. (For a list of foods high in anticancer folic acid, see page 458–9.)

Eating tomatoes also appears to prevent precancerous signs of cervical cancer, namely an inflammation called CIN (cervical intraepithelial neoplasia). Researchers at the University of Illinois at Chicago found that women with the highest blood levels of lycopene (tomatoes are the primary source of lycopene) had a five times lower risk of developing the precancerous condition than those who had the lowest blood levels of lycopene.

CARROTS FOR THE LARYNX

Because cancer of the larynx typically strikes smokers and former smokers, the same dietary prescriptions that help avert other smoking-related cancers, such as lung cancer, may also work against cancer of the larynx.

Eating foods high in carotene (carrots, sweet potatoes, green leafy vegetables, pumpkin) seems to be a boon notably to ex-smokers in the early years after they stop smoking, from two to ten years after they lay down that last cigarette. So finds a major study done at the University of Texas Health Science Center by Dr. Dorothy Mackerras and colleagues.

Comparing the diets of those who got laryngeal cancer with those who did not, Dr. Mackerras found that among those who had quit smoking two to ten years ago, the consumers of the least carotene in the diet were five and a half times more likely to develop laryngeal cancer than those with the highest intake of carotene. "Once you stop smoking, it would seem that carotene can help the larynx heal, so you're less likely to get laryngeal cancer," she said.

Caution: eating lots of high-carotene foods did not protect current smokers from laryngeal cancer — only ex-smokers.

PROSTATE CANCER AND DAIRY DANGER

Concerned about prostate cancer? Danger may lurk in a fatty diet, particularly from dairy foods, according to recent research. For example, Seventh Day Adventists who drank two glasses of milk a day had nearly double the risk of prostate cancer as those drinking one glass. Three daily glasses of milk hiked the odds about two and a half times. Prodigious eaters of cheese, eggs and meat were also more likely to develop prostate cancer.

The main culprit in milk appears to be fat. Researchers at Buffalo's Roswell Park Memorial Institute who examined the diets of those with and without prostate cancer found a link to whole milk, but not skimmed milk. Drinking more than three glasses a day of high-fat milk boosted the cancer risk two and a half times.

FEEL BETTER AND BRIGHTER

STAY AWAKE, BE ALERT

Downers: Sugar • Honey • Other Carbohydrates, Including Pasta, Bread and Alcohol

Uppers: Caffeine • Protein

If food can have such an enormous impact on cancer, heart disease, arthritis and digestive problems – the so-called chronic diseases of Western civilization – why can't it influence how your brain works? It can and does. Pioneering new research reveals that what you eat can help determine how alert and energetic you are, how good your memory and concentration are, whether you are depressed or anxious, how aggressive you are, whether your brain waves are abnormal and perhaps whether you have a vulnerability to certain mental illnesses and degenerative neurological diseases. Big things – such as carbohydrate, protein and fat, as well as caffeine – may have a profound and almost immediate impact on your mood and mental energy.

Even subtle deficiencies of certain nutrients over time can throw your brain waves and functioning out of whack, according to new studies. This comes as a surprise to investigators in the field, who did not previously think the brain was susceptible to such consequential permutations from such mild events. Fortunately, you can easily eat your way back to brain-wave normality.

"A child who comes home, has potato crisps and Coke in the afternoon, pizza with little or no cheese on it for dinner and ice cream for dessert has been priming himself with carbohydrates for several hours. When it comes time to do homework, that child will [have difficulty] because of sleepiness and lethargy." – Judith Wurtman, researcher at MIT

DR. WURTMAN'S BRAIN-FOOD THEORY

Much of the credit for discovering how food can manipulate brain activity goes to a neuroendocrinologist, Richard Wurtman and colleagues at the Massachusetts Institute of Technology (MIT) in Cambridge.

According to their pioneering research, the secret is in neurotransmitters, chemicals that pass information among cells in the brain. These neurotransmitters are manufactured by nerve cells using specific food components, called precursors, as raw material. Foods help create various neurotransmitters with different functions, depending on the type of raw material supplied by specific foods. For example, tryptophan, an amino acid in protein foods, is made into serotonin, the calming chemical that usually makes you more relaxed, drowsy and fuzzy-headed. From tyrosine, also an amino acid, are born dopamine and norepinephrine, neurotransmitters that enliven the brain, making you more alert; you think and react more quickly, are more attentive, motivated and mentally energetic.

Since brain chemistry is extremely complex, this does not necessarily mean that eating a food high in certain amino acids sends them directly to the brain. Amino acids, because of their varying size and concentration in the blood, compete for entry into the brain. Thus, paradoxically, when you drink milk that contains tryptophan, levels of tryptophan do not increase in the brain, but actually decrease because tryptophan molecules are crowded out of the brain by other more plentiful amino acids in milk. On the other hand, eating high-carbohydrate meals without tryptophan, actually raises brain tryptophan that creates serotonin, calming most people down, say Dr. Wurtman.

Not all scientists agree with Dr. Wurtman's intricate explanations of brain chemistry. Still, there's fairly wide scientific agreement that in normal persons, eating very-high-carbohydrate foods tends to subdue brain activity, and protein foods can counteract carbo-induced mental sluggishness. Some exceptions are people with PMS (premenstrual syndrome), the winter depression known as Seasonal Affective Disorder (SAD) and smokers going through nicotine withdrawal. For unknown reasons eating carbohydrates seems to perk up the brains of such individuals.

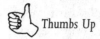 Thumbs Up

FIRST ALERT! EAT PROTEIN

One of the first rules of the brain for most people is that carbohydrates, notably sugar, are downers. Protein-containing foods are relatively uppers. When you want to stay mentally sharp, do not load up on sweets, cake, doughnuts, ice cream, sorbet or sugary cereals, rice or pasta (without meat, milk or other protein-containing foods). Instead, to maximize your mental alertness, eat protein-rich foods either alone or along with sweet and starchy foods. Good bets are low-fat seafood, turkey breast, skimmed milk, low-fat yoghurt and lean beef. Fat is also a downer, making brain functioning sluggish, because it takes so long to digest. Other foods, like green leafy vegetables, appear to be fairly neutral, neither stimulating nor muddling the brain.

It is not that such protein-rich foods energize the brain or make you cleverer than you basically are, says Bonnie Spring, a professor of psychology of the University of Health Sciences at the Chicago Medical College and a food-mood researcher. She explains that the protein simply keeps the carbos from making you fuzzy-headed. That's why including a little protein in a meal can block the brain-dulling effects of carbohydrates, she says. Nor do you have to eat much protein to blunt carbo effects. Studies show, says Dr. Spring, that including five to ten per cent protein in a meal helps block the build-up of serotonin in the brain, the sleep-inducing neurotransmitter that many think is the reason carbohydrates can make you drowsy and fuzzy-headed. That means a little, meat or cheese with your pasta, milk with your cookies or tuna fish on your roll will do the trick, say experts. It also means that when you want to be extra alert, particularly avoid pure carbos, such as boiled sweets, caramels, gum drops, plain chocolate bars, fudge, marshmallows, honey or sugar in your tea or coffee. All have no or very little protein.

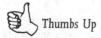 Thumbs Up

COFFEE: AN EXTRAORDINARY ENERGIZER

Since the 1600s when coffee was introduced first into the pharmacies and then the coffeehouses of Europe, users have marvelled at its ability to stimulate the brain. Initially, it was considered so powerful and hazardous to mental sensibilities that only physicians could dispense it and some wanted it banned for common folk. Today millions of people use coffee to pep up and feel better, and its druglike effects on the brain are undisputed.

New scientific probes of caffeine activity in the brain find that it is an odd type stimulant. It suppresses "down" brain chemicals instead of releasing "up" chemicals. According to researchers, caffeine works because of its fluky chemical resemblance to a brain substance called adenosine, secreted by nerve endings to put the brakes on brain cell activity. Caffeine, masquerading as adenosine, ensconces itself on the cell's receptor sites, displacing adenosine and keeping it from dampening brain cell activity. Thus brain cells remain in a state of excitability. Further, only a little caffeine has an effect. The caffeine in a couple of cups of coffee can knock out half of the brain's adenosine receptors for a couple of hours, say experts. This means it takes only a little caffeine to put your brain on alert, so numerous refills are needless.

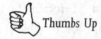 Thumbs Up

HIGH ALERT ON A CUP OR TWO

Consistent findings show that exceedingly low doses of caffeine can improve mental performance, according to Harris R. Lieberman, a psychologist with the U.S. Army Research Institute in Natick, Massachusetts and a leading expert on caffeine and behaviour. In one experiment, Dr. Lieberman had men take various doses of caffeine in the morning, ranging from the amount found in a carbonated cola (32mg) to that in a ½ pint (285ml) mug of brewed coffee (256mg). Then he administered a series of subtle mental tests that measured reaction time, attention span, concentration and accuracy with numbers.

Amazingly, all the caffeine doses, even the smallest, boosted the subjects' performance on the tests, stimulating their brains into quicker thinking, faster reactions and increased concentration.

Much other research confirms that caffeine increases alertness, improves performance on mental tasks and reduces fatigue. What's the best dose? Around 100–200mg of caffeine, the amount in a ¼–½ pint (140–285ml) mug of coffee downed in the morning and later in the afternoon when the caffeine wears off and energy sags. Interestingly, researchers do not find that taking in more caffeine boosts mental performance further. So it's futile to try to juice up brain power by load-ing up on numerous cups of coffee during the day. When you need to stay alert, researchers say, the caffeine in a cup or two of coffee can give your mental powers a beneficial edge.

 Thumbs Up

NO AFTER-MEAL SLUMP

That shot of caffeine can even counteract the mental slump you ordinarily get after eating. Many Europeans and Americans have instinc-tively followed meals with a cup of coffee. Now there's new proof that it's a self-prescribed natural antidote to the letdown of eating, according to psychologists at the University of Wales College of Cardiff. First, the investigators demonstrated that feeling let down after lunch is a common phenomenon, even if you keep your lunch small. In a test, 32 men and women felt drowsy, less alert, less clear-headed and less energetic after lunch, regardless of the size of the lunch. Furthermore, they were likely to make mistakes in tasks requiring sustained attention.

What researchers wanted to know was whether caffeinated coffee could counteract this post-lunch dip in performance by boosting alertness and attention. The answer was yes. Decaf coffee did not combat the after-lunch letdown, but regular coffee virtually wiped it out. Those who drank coffee after lunch had much longer attention spans, allowing them to perform tasks with greater speed and accuracy.

THE CAFFEINE FIX

If you use caffeine – in coffee, tea, soft drinks and chocolate – as a brain pick-me-up, you should know you are quite likely to become addicted to it. Although an addiction can be mild and harmless – a small price to pay for the benefits – it can, in some, be destructive, leading to an overconsumption of caffeine with severe ill effects on mind, mood and body. New research finds that caffeine provokes the classic physical signs of addiction. In short, it makes you feel good when you get it and awful when you don't.

Caffeine definitely is "reinforcing" says Roland Griffiths, M.D., professor of psychiatry and neuroscience at Johns Hopkins University.

Also, abruptly deprived of caffeine, you are likely to suffer pangs of withdrawal – lethargy, headaches, depression – for a few days to a week. This means caffeine is clearly addictive, he says. Nor does it take much to hook a person on caffeine. Experts once thought it took more than five cups of coffee a day to produce signs of dependence. Dr. Griffiths documents that a single ¼ pint (140ml) of coffee – a mere 100mg of caffeine – a day can do it.

Telling whether you are addicted to caffeine is simple, says Dr. Griffiths. Just give up your caffeine sources – coffee, tea, soft drinks – for a couple of days and see if you feel tired, headachy, unmotivated, grumpy and depressed. Headaches and fatigue are the classic signs of caffeine deprivation. For advice on kicking the caffeine habit, see page 295.

• BOTTOM LINE • *It usually takes only a cup of coffee in the morning and one in mid- to late afternoon to give your brain all the energy it can use. Heavy caffeine doses, usually more than five or six cups a day, in misguided attempts to juice up energy, concentration or attention, can produce anxiety, restlessness, excitement, even tremors, indicating "caffeinism". Such symptoms can be caused by lower doses in those who are very sensitive to caffeine. Since individuals vary greatly in their tolerance of caffeine, one person's ecstasy is another's poison.*

COFFEE SEDATES SOME? HARVARD SAYS YES

At Harvard they have discovered the most extraordinary thing – that coffee – or caffeine – actually gives some people the snoozes instead of waking them up! When a group of such people quit caffeine, all of them woke up, according to the *Harvard Medical School Health Letter*.

Dr. Quentin Regestein, a psychiatrist at Brigham and Womens Hospital in Boston, suggested that these odd individuals suffered from the rare and paradoxical condition in which caffeine kept them in a state of sleepiness instead of stimulation. In fact, the more they drank coffee to overcome their sleepiness, the more groggy they got during the day. One 35-year-old woman said she slept 12 hours a night, stayed in bed all day Sunday and yet drank ten cups of coffee and 3½ pints (2 litres) of cola a day.

It's a mystery, but Dr. Regestein speculates that some individuals just have an idiosyncratic reaction (the opposite of that expected) to caffeine. *The Health Letter's* advice: If you drink caffeine and still fall asleep, stop it for two to four weeks and see if matters improve.

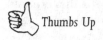 Thumbs Up

MORE BRAINPOWER FROM FRUITS AND NUTS

Fruits and nuts are brain food? Yes, according to recent experiments by research psychologist James Penland, Ph.D., at the U.S. Department of Agriculture's Grand Forks Human Nutrition Research Center. That's because fruits and nuts are high in boron, a trace mineral that appears to affect the electrical activity of the brain. Skimping on boron can subdue your mental alertness, says Dr. Penland, meaning you could have difficulty performing certain tasks.

He put 15 people over age 45 alternately on a low-boron or high-boron diet for about four months. When the subjects ate little boron, the electrical activity in their brains was more sluggish, indicating a slowdown in mental activity. "Their brains produced more theta waves and fewer alpha waves, which happens when you become drowsy," he says. The lack of boron seemed to "downshift their brains". When their diets were very deficient in boron, their performance on the simplest tasks slowed down. They could not tap their fingers as fast, track a target as accurately with a computer joystick, or as rapidly pick out specific letters of the alphabet. They were just much slower. When they went on a high-boron regimen (3mg a day) their brain wave activity picked up, as detected by electroencephalograms.

Dr. Penland was surprised to find the brain subject to such fine-tuning by minute amounts of a food constituent. "It's somewhat amazing to think that the brain is so sensitive to such mild differences in nutritional status. It's a whole new discovery," he says.

Where, specifically, is boron? In nuts, legumes, leafy vegetables such as broccoli and fruits, especially apples, pears, peaches and grapes. You would get your entire test dose of 3mg of brain-stimulating boron if you ate only a couple of apples (1mg of boron) and 3½oz (100g) of peanuts (2mg of boron) in a day.

POTION FOR AGEING BRAINS

Get your daily quota of thiamin, riboflavin, carotene and iron. Even slight deficits of these may also slow down thinking and memory in older people, according to Dr. Penland's research. Specifically, when he and colleagues compared the nutritional status with the brain functioning of 28 healthy people over age 60 here is what they found:

•   Low thiamin levels were linked to some impairment in brain activity. Thiamin, known as the "nerve vitamin," is concentrated in wheat germ and bran, nuts, meat and fortified cereals.

•   People who got enough riboflavin did better on memory tests. Best sources: liver, milk, almonds, fortified cereals.

•   Those getting adequate carotene did best on thinking (cognitive) tests. Carotene comes from deep green leafy vegetables and deep orange fruits and vegetables.

•   Especially fascinating: Older people with high iron status showed the same type of EEG (electroencephalogram) brain-wave activity as found in young adults. Iron comes from such foods as greens, liver, shellfish, red meat and soya beans.

•   The amounts of vitamins that restored top mental functioning in the study were so small – just the recommended dietary allowances (RDA) – that you need not take supplements to get them. You can get enough to protect your brain through food, says Dr. Penland.

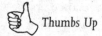 Thumbs Up

HOW COULD YOU FORGET? – SEAFOOD IS BRAIN FOOD

If your memory is sagging and your attention lagging, you may not be getting quite enough zinc. In startling new discoveries, scientists are finding that even marginal lacks of zinc can mildly impair mental functioning, including memory. "It's surprising," says Dr. Harold Sandstead, an expert on zinc at the University of Texas Medical Branch in Galveston. He and colleagues found that normal healthy men and women, marginally deprived of zinc, did poorly on memory and concentration tests. When their zinc was replenished their mental faculties improved. For example, women's recall of words and visual designs jumped 12 per cent and 17 per cent respectively when they ate adequate zinc.

In another study, men on a very low intake of 1–4mg of zinc made more errors and had slower responses to 10 out of 15 mental and sensory-motor tests in a seven-month live-in study at the U.S. Department of Agriculture's labs in Grand Forks, North Dakota. Decidedly, mental functions that suffered most from deficits of zinc were short-term memory and attention.

This does not mean you need to load up on zinc supplements to maintain proper memory. You can get the memory-boosting amount in the diet by eating seafood, such as oysters and fish, legumes, cereals, whole grains and dark-meat turkey. A mere 1 oz (30g) of raw oysters supplies 20mg of zinc, more than the recommended dietary allowance (RDA) of 15mg. Even better 3oz (85g) of smoked oysters contain 103mg of zinc, according to Agriculture Department figures.

"There's a theory. . . that man evolved in areas bordering seas and lakes because fish provided material for brain development which other species lacked. So the folklore that said fish is food for the brain may be vindicated." — A. E. Bender, professor emeritus, University of London

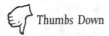 Thumbs Down

LARD AND FADING MAZE MEMORIES

Too much animal fat may dim your mental faculties. Rats fed lard cannot find their way through mazes as easily as rats fed soya bean oil. The spatial memories of the lard eaters are simply not as good, dooming them to make more mistakes. Whether this applies to people who down Big Macs instead of tofu is quite unknown, say researchers. Scientists have, however, begun fascinating inquiries into the possibility that the type of fat in a diet over a period of time can affect brain functioning, including memory. The biggest culprit in experimental animals is saturated-type animal fat.

Theoretically, fat's brain effects make sense. Brain cells, like other cells, are held together by membranes, and there is plenty of evidence that the type of fatty acid eaten changes the fatty composition of cell membranes, which influences the production of a great many bodily messengers, including neurotransmitters.

That fat can affect memory and learning was first documented in young rats in 1986 by researchers at the Clark Institute of Psychiatry in Toronto, Ontario. When rats were fed either lard (saturated animal fat) or soya bean or mixed fats for 21 days, soya bean fed rats were best able to manoeuvre their escape from a particular maze.

In follow-up studies, Carol E. Greenwood, Ph.D., and colleagues at the University of Toronto fed rats lard or soya beans for longer periods (three months) and put them through their paces on several sophisticated maze tests of memory. The chronic consumers of lard turned in the worst performances. The lard-eaters were deficient in learning certain maze configurations, and their temporal memory over short and long intervals was "severely impaired".

So far, researchers do not know precisely the mechanism by which fat alters brain functioning, affecting memory, but speculate that fats cause "widespread and diffuse alteration in the brain".

"The brain of a 30-year-old alcoholic looks like the brain of a 50-year-old." – Gene-Jack Wang, M.D.. Brookhaven National Laboratory

---

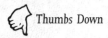 Thumbs Down

CURB YOUR DRINKING – *SAVE YOUR BRAIN*

Too much alcohol is not good for your brain. Alcohol abuse causes decided brain damage, and is especially hard on memory, says Gene-Jack Wang, M.D., Brookhaven National Laboratory in Upton, New York. Using sophisticated PET scanning and MRI (magnetic resonance imaging) to study the brains of young alcoholics, he documented brain damage, including shrinkage of the cortex, impaired cerebral structures and decreased metabolic activity. "They have decreased metabolic activity throughout their whole brain, but especially in the frontal cortex and in the parts of the brain having to do with memory," he says.

• BOTTOM LINE • *Most experts suggest restricting alcoholic intake to two drinks a day. Some favour only one daily drink.*

 Thumbs Up

HIGHER IQ FROM MOTHER'S MILK

There's "very strong evidence" that an unknown substance in mother's milk spurs mental development, giving breast-fed children higher IQs. So says Alan Lucas, head of Infant and Child Nutrition at the Medical

Research Council's Dunn Nutrition Unit in Cambridge, England. In a study of 300 children born prematurely, he found that the babies fed breast milk showed higher intelligence as youngsters than those fed infant formula. Specifically, premature babies fed either breast milk alone or breast milk plus formula scored 8.3 points higher on IQ tests at ages seven and a half and eight. Further, the more mother's milk the babies got, the higher their IQ scores. Formula-fed babies averaged IQ scores of 93.1. Babies fed mother's milk averaged 103.7 points.

The intelligence edge from mother's milk cannot be due to factors

---

EATING TIPS FOR MAXIMUM ALERTNESS AND BRAINPOWER

Just before an examination, a speech, an important business meeting or any task that demands mental alertness, eat low-carbohydrate high-protein, low-fat foods, urges Judith Wurtman, Ph.D., a nutrition researcher at MIT. Here are some of her suggestions, as detailed in her book, *Managing Your Mind and Mood Through Food*.

Breakfast. Yes: Skimmed milk, non-fat yoghurt, fruit, hard boiled egg, coffee, tea, juice or fruit

No: Bacon and eggs, fried potatoes, toast and jam, croissants, pancakes, waffles, bagel

Lunch. Yes: Plain tuna, green salad (go easy on dressing), steamed or boiled shrimp, fruit salad, low-fat cottage cheese, 3–4oz (85–115g) turkey, chicken, lean roast beef

No: Spaghetti or pizza, chips, peanut-butter-and-jelly sandwich, biscuits, regular soft drink (not diet)

Dinner. Yes: Grilled salmon or other fish, green vegetables, tomatoes, soft fruits (strawberries etc)

No: Roast beef; baked potato with soured cream, corn on the cob, fruit pie

• When starting a meal, to stay alert, don't eat a carbohydrate, such as bread, before a protein, such as fish. Doing so cancels out the maximum brain-energizing power of protein. Always eat the protein first, and carbohydrates later only after you've started to digest protein, which must get to the brain first. The sequence of courses is important.

> • Don't eat carbohydrates on an empty stomach or without a protein food. (For example, high-carbo cereal with high-protein milk is okay.) Eating bread, rolls, pasta, crackers alone on an empty stomach makes you as sleepy and relaxed as taking a drink of alcohol on an empty stomach, says Dr. Wurtman.
>
> • Don't eat a large, high-fat meal if you want to be mentally sharp afterward. Too much food brings on lethargy. Fat stays in the digestive tract longer, prolonging tiredness. The fattier and heavier the meal, the longer it takes you to recover mental alertness and energy.

such as bonding during breast-feeding. This study eliminated that prejudice by giving the breast milk and formula by tube because the infants were too premature to suckle.

Some experts insist that omega-3 fatty acid, the type found in fish, may be the magic intelligence-boosting ingredient in mother's milk. Omega-3s have been found critical in foetal and infant brain development. Thus, experts advise pregnant and lactating women to eat seafood to ensure that their children's developing brains are supplied with omega-3 oils. (Caution: Fish contaminated with PCBs or methylmercury could harm a foetus or infant. To be extra safe, pregnant and lactating women can restrict swordfish, shark and fresh tuna to once a month; limit canned tuna to 7oz (200g) a week, avoid fish caught in rivers, lakes, ocean bays and harbours near industrial sources of pollution; avoid eating fish skin or internal organs such as roe; eat a variety of sources of fish. Small, young fish, such as sardines, are safest.)

LIFT YOUR MOOD

> **Food That May Help:** Folic-Acid-Rich Foods, Such as Spinach • Selenium-Rich Foods, Such as Seafood • Carbohydrates (Including Sugar) • Caffeine • Garlic

There is no scientific dispute anymore that what you eat can affect your mood – whether you feel up or down. Although your food choices may seem based on taste or other conscious criteria, there's evidence that people often make unconscious food choices that change brain chemistry and put them in a better mood. They unwittingly "self-medicate" with food antidepressants. Additionally, chronic depression has been linked to a long-term subtle deficiency of certain nutrients that presumably can go unnoticed and uncorrected by the body for long periods.

Except for caffeine and sugar, few food substances have been meticulously studied to determine how they manipulate mood. However, it seems clear that food substances affect neurotransmitters, the brain's cell-communicators. One such neurotransmitter that has been tied to depression, as well as violence, is serotonin. It is known to lift the mood generally, and dramatically, in some people prone to depression. Depression expert Simon N. Young of the Department of Psychiatry at McGill University in Montreal, says that low brain serotonin equals psychiatric symptoms. For example, depressed persons who commit or attempt suicide as well as criminals who commit impetuous, violent acts commonly have low levels of brain serotonin. Getting more serotonin into the brain, or stimulating serotonin activity, sometimes relieves depression. That's why those with the winter blues often turn to sugar.

FOOD REMEDY FOR THE WINTER BLUES

With the dark days of winter, about one million Britains fall into a depression known as SAD (seasonal affective disorder) and another one million have 'sub' SAD. The theory is that light deprivation alters brain chemistry in biologically susceptible persons. Such depressed individuals often crave sweets and starches. No wonder. "Carbohydrates are a self-administered, much-needed dose of brain medication to fight off the winter blues," says Norman Rosenthal, M.D., a leading SAD researcher at the American National Institute of Mental Health. He explains that normal people after eating carbos, like sugar, are less alert and less energetic, regardless of the seasons, but people with SAD get the opposite effect. To them, carbohydrates are an antidepressant. "Carbohydrates energize them, and put them in a better mood," says Dr. Rosenthal.

In a series of experiments at the NIMH labs, he tested the effects of carbohydrates on both patients with SAD and normal nondepressed patients. He fed both of them sugary cookies. Within two hours after eating six cookies, containing a hefty 105g of carbohydrates, the depressed patients were more frisky and energetic and less tense, depressed and fatigued. The normals who ate the cookies were zonked out. One possible explanation is that such depressed persons have abnormal brain chemistry, involving metabolism of the antidepressant serotonin. Eating carbohydrates, some believe, helps overcome this problem by boosting serotonin levels and/or serotonin activity.

"Some people who eat lots of pasta and pastry may be using carbohydrates as an edible antidepressant." – Judith Wurtman, Ph.D., Massachusetts Institute of Technology

---

Regardless of the reason, if you have the "winter blues," don't deprive your brain of the carbo medicine it craves, says Dr. Rosenthal. Doing so only puts you in a deeper, more serious funk, because the cravings for sweets and starches have a biological intensity. "Some of our patients call it an addiction, like craving cocaine," he says. Skimping on carbohydrates when your body cries out for them is also probably doomed to failure. Dr. Rosenthal advises people with this type depression, for example, not to go on high-protein, low-carbohydrate diets, notably in the dark winter months.

To relieve SAD you can eat sweets, but it's more healthy to eat complex carbohydrates like dried beans, pasta, vegetables, cereal, bread and crackers. They work, too – just a little more slowly. Also, Dr.

Rosenthal warns against using excessive alcohol or caffeine (more than a couple of cups of coffee a day) to fight the winter blues. Too much of both substances can increase anxiety, adding to mood problems.

 Thumbs Up

THE MIGHTY CAFFEINE LIFT

As if anyone who uses it needs to be told, caffeine, the most widely used psychoactive drug in the world, has mood-lifting powers. Caffeine's recently discovered mood benefits tend to explain why humans have been self-medicating with caffeine for centuries to fight off the morning blahs, get an afternoon and evening lift and perhaps even alleviate chronic bad moods or depression, say experts. When people claim that a morning cup of coffee brings a smile to their faces, it's often true.

According to Roland Griffiths, M.D., professor of psychiatry and neuroscience at Johns Hopkins University, who has studied the effects of caffeine extensively, it "produces elevations of feelings and well-being, sometimes even euphoria," which is what makes people want to self-administer it. Those hooked on caffeine automatically seek the proper caffeine fix to give them a feeling of "contentedness" and reduce their anxiety and cravings for caffeine, his studies show.

Without being told, regular caffeine users can sense through body wisdom whether coffee has caffeine. In blind tests of unlabelled coffee, with and without caffeine, regular coffee drinkers consistently seek out and drink more of the coffee with the caffeine.

Fortunately, coffee is unique in that you don't constantly have to take more to get the same kick, says Dr. Andrew Baum, professor of medical psychology at the Uniformed Services University of the Health Sciences in Bethesda, Maryland. You get the same lift from a cup of coffee every morning – day after day – no matter how addicted you are, he concluded after blind tests of 48 heavy coffee drinkers.

On the mornings the subjects unknowingly got a cup of decaffeinated coffee or caffeine-free tea, they were grumpy, irritable, lethargic, complained of headaches and performed poorly on mental tasks. On days they secretly were given a cup of coffee with caffeine, they had a surge in mood, were less stressed and performed much better mentally. The good news, says Dr. Baum, is that it takes but a single cup of coffee to provide that morning "jump start," day after day even for normally heavy caffeine consumers.

"It seems not only possible, but likely, that some of the millions of heavy coffee drinkers are, in fact, using caffeine – consciously or not – to medicate themselves for depression, our most widespread psychiatric condition." – Melvin Konner, M.D., Emory University

Melvin Konner, M.D., of Emory University notes that new studies on brain physiology support caffeine's use as a mild antidepressant, and he sees nothing wrong with that if the depression is mild and does not need medical attention. He cites caffeine's long history of safety. "Unlike antidepressant drugs or prescription stimulants, caffeine has been taken billions of times over a period of centuries. There are no prescription drugs for which we have comparable experience, and the absence of clear disaster speaks volumes about its safety, at least in the area of two, three or four cups of coffee a day."

However, excessive caffeine can wreck your mood, disturb your sleep and trigger anxiety, depending on your individual tolerance for the drug.

• BOTTOM LINE • *Small doses of caffeine may improve your mood and performance; heavy doses can be detrimental to your psyche and well-being.*

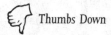 Thumbs Down

I-MISS-MY-CAFFEINE DEPRESSION

Take away caffeine and see what happens. "In addition to causing headache, abrupt withdrawal from the habitual use of caffeine may induce depression," says Seymour Solomon, M.D., of the Montefiore Medical Center in New York. Usually you suffer a day or two of mild depression, but depending on individual reactions, it may last a week or so, according to Dr. Griffiths' research. It's a normal consequence of going off caffeine cold-turkey. You can lessen the depression of withdrawal by giving up caffeine gradually. For advice on how to do that, see page 295.

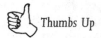 Thumbs Up

SPINACH FOR DEPRESSION?

Has anyone ever told you that greens are good for your mood? Or that you may be depressed because you are not eating enough broad beans or spinach? It's hardly likely. Yet, the medical literature is astonishing in its agreement that a folic acid (folate) deficiency, which is widespread in the United States, especially among women, fosters psychiatric disorders, notably depression, but also dementia and schizophrenia. Folic acid is a B vitamin first isolated from green leafy vegetables. It is also heavily concentrated in legumes. That folic acid can act as an anti-depressant is no secret among scientists.

McGill University's Dr. Young finds "accumulating evidence that folic acid deficiency can contribute to depressed mood," and that eliminating the deficiency often cures the depression.

The evidence on how extensively folic acid affects the brain is indeed sobering. Dr. Young notes that patients with various psychiatric disorders, particularly depression, have much higher rates of folic acid deficiency than the general public. Also, psychiatric patients with low folic acid are more severely disturbed. There are good reasons why a lack of the vitamin can cause depression, he says. For one thing, folic acid deficiency causes serotonin levels in the brain to sink.

People deliberately deprived of folic acid in tests have lapsed into sleeplessness, forgetfulness and irritability after five months; restoring the vitamin caused symptoms to mostly disappear in two days.

How little folic acid may be needed to fight depression was shown strikingly in a double-blind study of 75 patients with depression who were on the drug lithium. Researchers gave only 200mg of folic acid a day – that's the amount in about 5oz (140g) of cooked spinach – to half the group for a year. The others got a placebo. Decidedly, those getting the folic acid had a dramatic relief of depression.

Dr. Young suggests that 200–500 micrograms of folic acid a day may help fight depression in certain susceptible people. That much is easily attainable in food. High folic acid doses can be toxic, he cautions.

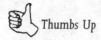 Thumbs Up

GOOD-MOOD SEAFOOD MINERAL

You've probably heard that fish is brain food. Now there's fascinating new evidence that eating seafood could improve your mood. The reason is that seafood is extra high in the trace mineral selenium, and several bits of evidence suggest that people who skimp on selenium are more likely to suffer the blues. Psychologists David Benton and Richard Cook, at University College in Swansea, recently documented that people eating the least selenium were the most anxious, depressed and tired, and generally felt much better when they got adequate selenium.

In a controlled study, 50 healthy men and women, aged 14 to 74, took either 100 micrograms of selenium a day or a placebo for five weeks. After six months, they switched to the opposite pill. The selenium in their diet was also measured. Throughout, they were given tests to judge their moods – whether they were more composed or anxious, agreeable or hostile, elated or depressed, confident or unsure, energetic or tired and clearheaded or confused.

The surprising results were that mood improved markedly when the subjects got enough selenium. Further, the greater their previous selenium lack, the greater their lift in mood. The researchers figure that a subtle selenium deficiency, not enough to cause overt disease symptoms, puts a damper on mood. Thus, correcting that slight deficiency normalizes mood, but getting more of the mineral does not boost mood further.

Bad moods tied to selenium deficiency may be pervasive. Researchers noted that the study subjects who felt better after increased selenium were eating about 72 micrograms a day prior to the test. The average Briton eats much less, a mere 43 micrograms daily. Americans' diets too are commonly selenium-deficient.

How selenium influences mood is unknown, but its antioxidant powers may be involved. In other research, elderly people given selenium plus vitamin E or other antioxidants had significant improvements in mood and mental functioning, as well as increased blood flow to the brain. In a study of patients with early Alzheimer's disease, antioxidants, including selenium, boosted mood and mental performance. However, the Welsh researchers speculate that selenium may have some unknown neural function.

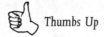 *Thumbs Up*

A NUT A DAY KEEPS THE BLUES AWAY

Most selenium in the diet comes from grains, seafood, cereals, seafood and meat but for a real selenium booster, try Brazil nuts. They are richest of all foods in selenium, and eating a single nut a day will guarantee you are never deficient, says Donald J. Lisk, director of Cornell University's Toxic Chemical laboratory. He found Brazil nuts, because they are grown in selenium-rich soil, to be super high in the mineral – about 2,500 times as selenium-rich as any other nut. Eating half a dozen nuts rapidly boosts blood selenium levels by 100–350 per cent, Dr. Lisk found. Don't eat more than that in a day, he cautions. because selenium can be toxic.

GOOD-MOOD SELENIUM "FOOD PILLS"

You don't need to take selenium pills to get enough of the good-mood compound. Each of the following foods contains the same amount of selenium as the 100 microgram pill that boosted mood in the above-noted British study. Getting a little here and there can easily add up to a good-mood dose.
- 1 Brazil nut
- 4½oz (125g) canned light tuna
- 7oz (200g) swordfish or clams
- 5oz (140g) cooked oysters
- 4½oz (125g) sunflower seeds
- 12 slices of white bread
- 8oz (225g) dry oat bran
- 8oz (225g) puffed wheat cereal
- 5oz (140g) chicken livers

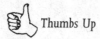 Thumbs Up

GARLIC – A MOOD ELEVATOR?

Strange as it seems, many investigators testing garlic for its positive effects on blood and cholesterol noticed that garlic eaters also experienced a decided lift in mood – "had a greater feeling of well-being". Indeed, several researchers have commented on this as a welcome and surprising side effect.

Garlic's effect as a mood elevator was especially striking to German researchers at the University of Hanover who recently tested a special garlic preparation on people with high cholesterol. The garlic takers, according to questionnaires, felt much better after the garlic therapy. They experienced measurably less fatigue, anxiety, sensitivity, agitation and irritability. This mood-lifting bonus of "garlic medication" is important and in sharp contrast to the adverse side effects of many pharmaceutical drugs, the researchers commented, speculating that "The widespread popularity of garlic preparations might possibly have its origin in their positive effect on people's feeling of well-being." Garlic supplements are the largest-selling over-the-counter drug in Germany.

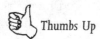 Thumbs Up

THE CHILLI PEPPER HIGH

Eating hot chilli peppers may give you a thrill that is more than purely sensory. The capsaicin, the hot stuff, in chilli peppers can actually induce in the brain a rush of endorphins that give you a temporary high, says Paul Rozin, a psychologist at the University of Pennsylvania, who has done extensive research on reactions to hot peppers. Dr Rozin explains that for unknown reasons, when you eat hot chillies, the capsaicin "burns" the nerve endings of the tongue and mouth, causing them to send false pain signals to the brain. In response, attempting to protect the body from perceived injury, the brain secretes natural painkillers or endorphins that, like a shot of morphine, cause a high. Another bite of pepper incites further release of endorphins, and so on, building up into a pleasurable rush, according to Dr. Rozin. He maintains that some people get addicted to peppers because of this high, eating hotter and hotter peppers. You can get hooked on peppers because they make you feel so good, he says.

ANXIETY AND STRESS

> **Foods That May Help Relieve Anxiety:** Sugar • Starches
>
> **Foods That May Produce Anxiety:** Caffeine • Alcohol

Feeling tense, edgy, stressed out, and anxious is natural and happens to everybody at times. For some people however, anxiety can be chronic and severe, triggering not only feelings of fear, apprehension and uncertainty, but also sudden attacks of tachycardia (rapid heartbeat), sweating and shakiness. Intense and persistent anxiety can even lead to frightening panic attacks and incapacitating phobias.

Decidedly, you can help relieve these stressful and anxious states of mind by what you eat. Certain food and drink act as tranquillizers or anxiety generators, charging up or cooling down your nervous system.

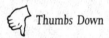 Thumbs Down

CAFFEINE CATASTROPHE

You probably won't be surprised to learn that one of the prime purveyors of high anxiety is caffeine – the psychotropic (active) drug in coffee, tea and colas. For most people caffeine in doses ordinarily consumed is a safe drug that can improve mood and performance but not for all. For a sizable group of people whose brain cells are particularly sensitive to caffeine, drinking five or six cups a day can trigger well-recognized signs of psychiatric illness. Upping the caffeine dose further can overwhelm the anxiety centres of larger numbers of ordinarily mentally sound persons depending on their individual sensitivities to caffeine. Indeed, the American Psychiatric Association classifies "caffeine intoxication" as a mental disorder; symptoms include nervousness, excitement, restlessness, tachycardia, insomnia, psycho-motor agitation and rambling thought and speech.

As John F. Greden, M.D., former director of psychiatric research at

Walter Reed Army Medical Center in Washington, D.C., has pointed out, the symptoms of such "caffeinism" are "essentially indistinguishable from those of anxiety neurosis". The medical literature is, full of cases of futile medical tests, prescriptions of heavy tranquillizers and psychiatric care, all in search of a nonexistent underlying physical illness when the actual culprit was an overload of caffeine.

"Some people may really need drugs to alleviate anxiety, but for an undetermined number of others, subtracting one drug — caffeine — may be of greater benefit than adding another." – John F. Greden. M.D., formerly Walter Reed Army Medical Center

THE SKEPTICAL COLONEL'S CAFFEINISM

You may recognize yourself, family members or friends in the ordeal of one 37-year-old army lieutenant colonel who ended up in a psychiatric clinic after suffering two years of chronic anxiety characterized by almost daily attacks of dizziness, tremulousness, apprehension about job performance, butterflies in the stomach, restlessness, frequent episodes of diarrhoea and persistent problems in falling asleep and remaining asleep. His scores on a standard anxiety test were high.

Three complete medical checkups had found nothing. Daily doses of Valium and other tranquillizers did no good and interfered with his job performance. When he finally saw Walter Reed's Dr. Greden, who informed him caffeine toxicity might be the cause of his anxiety, the colonel was incredulous. To him 8–14 daily cups of coffee were routine and necessary. Eventually, when the anxiety became unbearable, he cut back on caffeine. Within a month his symptoms began to subside and three months later his long-standing anxiety had disappeared.

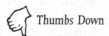 Thumbs Down

CAFFEINE TRIGGERS PANIC ATTACKS

Caffeine's danger is escalated for about three million Americans who have an overvigilant alarm system that predisposes them to panic disorder – frequent attacks of disabling fear that can lead to terrifying phobias. For genetic reasons, such people's brains are wired differently, making them more sensitive to stress and other stimuli including caffeine. Their reaction to anxiety goes beyond the expected norm and is a physiologically distinct condition.

That caffeine can provoke excessive anxiety and panic attacks in people with panic disorder – and, more surprisingly, also in ordinary individuals – has been documented by Thomas Uhde, M.D., chief of the anxiety and affective disorders branch at the American National Institute of Mental Health. He tested the effects of caffeine on patients with panic disorder and normal healthy individuals. Those with the disorder developed panic attacks after fairly moderate doses of 480mg of caffeine, or four to five cups of coffee.

Amazingly, Dr. Uhde was able to induce panic attacks in two out of eight normal subjects by upping the dose of caffeine to 750mg (about seven to eight cups of coffee). That such frightening and incapacitating reactions can be inflicted by caffeine is proof positive of its enormous pharmacological hold over the brain.

Obviously, some brains are more sensitive to the drug, and as Dr. Uhde notes, people who suffer with panic disorder tend to drink less caffeine perhaps out of a sense of self-preservation.

The possibility exists, however, that caffeine, depending on the dose, can stir up fear and anxiety in many unsuspecting individuals, including children who may be prone to panic disorder. Caffeine, of course, is but one of several factors that can trigger anxiety and panic attacks in susceptible nervous systems (stressful life events are certainly critical), but caffeine is unique in that it can be easily eliminated.

THE INSTANT NO-CAFFEINE ANXIETY CURE

How common are caffeine-induced anxiety and panic disorders? Malcolm Bruce, M.D., at London's Institute of Psychiatry, calls caffeine "a seriously underrated cause of severe anxiety disorders". In a recent study, he discovered that about 25 per cent of his patients with anxiety disorder dramatically recovered after giving up caffeine.

Typical, says Dr. Bruce, is a woman patient, age 33 who came to him with severe and long-standing anxiety disorder She had suffered two to three panic attacks every week for about ten years. Neither medication nor extensive psychotherapy had done much good. Every day she drank about nine cups of strong tea containing about 540mg of caffeine – equal to five or six cups of coffee.

As a test, Dr. Bruce asked her to give up caffeine for a week. She felt better immediately. Shortly afterward, he took her off medication. Her panic attacks disappeared, never to return – that is, except on the rare occasions when she drank more than her customary half cup of tea a week. With more caffeine, the panic attacks came rushing back.

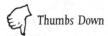 Thumbs Down

BOOZE IS NO SOLUTION

Alcohol and anxiety often go together but do people drink to cure their anxiety? Could it be that certain vulnerable people who drink excessively end up with pathological anxiety as the alcohol wears off? That's a matter of controversy but Dr. Uhde notes that some patients do have panic attacks or more frequent panic attacks within 6 to 12 hours after drinking even a small amount of alcohol. Dr. Uhde describes it as a kind of "mini-withdrawal syndrome," as the alcohol wears off. Some authorities also theorize that panic patients can tolerate less alcohol, and get the same brain neurotransmitter activity from drinking small amounts that normal people get from drinking larger amounts.

Regardless, Dr. Uhde advises anyone with panic disorder to cut out alcohol or take no more than one or two drinks a day as a test to see whether alcohol is involved in promoting panic attacks. If, he says, you find that even a little alcohol provokes increased anxiety or more frequent panic attacks, you should stay away from alcohol entirely.

"The right food at the right time in the right amount is as effective as a tranquillizer . . . 1½–2oz (40–55g) of carbohydrates (about two and a half teaspoons of white sugar) will trigger production of a mood-altering chemical, serotonin, which eases anxiety within about 20 minutes." – Judith J. Wurtman, Ph.D., Massachussets Institute of Technology

---

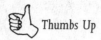 Thumbs Up

THE SWEETEST ANXIETY CURES

Nature's way of calming down the brain and relieving stress and anxiety may be surprising, although the remedy has been used for centuries. A taste of honey before going to bed was commonly recommended by our forefathers to bring on sleep. "In times of stress, sweeten the tea," advises an ancient Chinese proverb. Yet the notion that sweets quiet the brain runs counter to popular belief. Ask almost anyone, and they will say sugar is a quick fix for energy; it revs you up, gives you a "jump start". Recent research on brain biology suggests that all carbohydrates, including sugar and starches, have the opposite effect on most ordinary, normal people. They typically are sedatives, inducing relaxation and drowsiness. A string of experiments shows carbohydrates to be a downer, not an upper.

Typical is a classic test in which Dr. Bonnie Spring, a professor of psychology at the Chicago Medical School, had a group of healthy men and women eat either carbohydrate-rich sorbet or high-protein slices of turkey breast. Two hours later the subjects took standardized tests to measure alertness and moods. Compared with those eating the turkey, the women who ate the sugary sorbet were drowsy and the sorbet-eating men were relaxed. Dr. Spring says certain individuals, including women and people over age 40 appear more sensitive to the sedation of sugar. In some people, eating carbos makes them exhausted, inducing what some call the "sugar blues".

Why carbos act as tranquillizers, experts say, could be due to several complex biochemical reactions in the brain. The most publicized theory is that eating carbohydrates makes way for more tryptophan, an amino acid, to enter the brain, where it is converted into serotonin, the neurotransmitter well known as the "calming chemical".

Incidentally, carbohydrates do not make people sleepy by causing a sharp rise and then a dip in blood sugar (so-called hypoglycemia). Tests often find high blood-sugar levels in drowsy people. Alertness and fatigue in the vast majority of people are due to brain chemistry, not blood sugar.

• BOTTOM LINE • *When you want to calm down, one of the best medicines is carbohydrates, and that includes complex carbos like potatoes, pasta, bread, beans and cereal. For the fastest acting tranquillity fix, eat nature's sweet stuff — honey or sugar. Artificial sweetners, such as aspartame and saccharin, do not tranquillize the brain.*

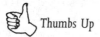 Thumbs Up

DR. WURTMAN'S FAST-ACTING ANTI-STRESS, ANTI-ANXIETY RECIPE

When you want to wind down and feel more calm, eat sugar or starches, says Judith Wurtrnan, Ph.D., a researcher at the Massachusetts Institute of Technology. Her husband, neuroendocrinologist Richard Wurtman, has mapped some of the puzzling and seemingly contradictory mechanisms by which carbohydrates affect brain chemistry. Judith Wurtman has translated those findings into practical advice for using carbohydrates as a calming drug to allay stress and anxiety, as detailed in her 1986 book *Managing Your Mind and Mood Through Food*. Here are her observations and tips:

• Both sugar and starches are tranquillizers, but sugar works faster. A sugary drink can work in as little as five minutes. It can take from half an hour to 45 minutes for starches like cereals and bread to work.
• The best calming dose for most people is 1½–2oz (40–55g) of pure carbohydrate, as found in 2oz (55g) of gumdrops or breakfast cereal (without milk and sugar), such as Cheerios, or 9fl oz (255ml) of a nondiet cola. There is no need to overdo it. The brain chemical changes inducing the calm feeling begin with the first few bites of sweet, biscuit, cereal or soft drink.
• Don't mix protein with your carbohydrate. Eat the carbo alone. That means don't put milk, high in protein, on your high-carbo cereal. Even a little protein can blunt the carbohydrate's calming effect.
• Eat low-fat carbohydrate foods. It takes longer for fat-laden sweets and desserts to work. Nearly pure sugar gumdrops, caramels, mints, and lollipops give faster relief than a higher-fat chocolate bar.
• For fastest stress relief, drink your carbos, because liquids pass more quickly through the stomach. "Sip a cup of herb tea with two full tablespoons of sugar mixed in or a cup of instant cocoa with water, not milk, or very slowly drink 8fl oz (225ml) of caffeine-free regular [nondiet] soft drink," suggests Dr. Wurtman. Slowly sip the liquid through a straw until you feel more mellow.

• If you anticipate a long stress-filled period of time – such as 12–14 hours – nibble on low-fat, high-carbohydrate foods such as air-popped popcorn, rice cakes, miniature marshmallows, and Cheerios and other dry breakfast cereals. Also, sucking on sugary foods like lollipops and gobstoppers helps keep stress under control.

ANTI-ANXIETY DIET PRESCRIPTION

• If you have anxiety, give up or severely restrict caffeine for at least a week, and see if the anxiety begins to dissipate. That includes less or no caffeinated coffee or tea, cocoa, chocolate or cola drinks. Be prepared for caffeine withdrawal symptoms, such as headache, which ordinarily occurs within 19 hours, gets worse in the first day or two and then tapers off. If you want to be sure caffeine is what triggers your anxiety, do a test later by drinking some and watching to see if the anxiety returns.

• If you have panic attacks or panic disorder, cut out caffeine or cut back on it. "Probably a couple of cups of coffee a day won't bring on panic attacks," says Dr. Uhde "but more may." Notice whether the onset of panic attacks is linked to caffeine. Consult a professional for proper treatment.

• If you are more anxious or panicky after drinking alcohol, cut down or abstain entirely.

• To allay general stress and anxiety, eat more complex carbohydrates, such as pasta and potatoes. For a faster calming effect, eat something containing sugar or honey, long recognized as mild tranquillizers.

TAKE AN ONION

The ancient Egyptians used onions to induce relaxation and sleep. There may be something to it. Yellow and red onions are the richest source of a compound, quercetin. It's an antioxidant, anti-inflammatory agent and also a mild sedative. At least it seemed to make mice drowsy by acting on their central nervous systems, according to recent French studies.

ANTISOCIAL BEHAVIOUR

> **Foods That May Help Curb Aggression:** Carbohydrates, Including Sugar and Starch

Does eating sugary foods promote criminal, antisocial or disruptive hyperactive behaviour? The theory received much acclaim in the 1970s and 1980s, leading some correctional facilities to ban snacks and sweets from their premises in hope of subduing the criminal psyche. A crowning example of sugar phobia was the now-famous "Twinkie Defence". In 1978, Dan White gunned down San Francisco's mayor, George Moscone, and City Supervisor Harvey Milk, and then blamed his criminal activity and mixed-up mind on his chronic overconsumption of Hostess Twinkies (a sweet snack of a sponge finger with a sugar-laden creamy filling).

NO SUGAR HYPERACTIVITY AT NIMH

The belief that eating sweets promotes hyperactivity and aggression is extremely popular. Thus it comes as a shock to discover that when the theory is tested in tightly controlled and monitored laboratory situations, few facts emerge to support it. Studies at the American National Institute of Mental Health repeatedly contradict parents who contend their kids react badly to sugar. Typical was a test of 18 preschool boys aged two to six years, who were called "sugar responsive" by parents and 12 boys who reportedly had no aggressive reaction to eating sugar.

All of the boys were fed either sugar or the artificial sweetener aspartame and saccharin in a carbonated lemon drink at separate times, and then left to play together. Nobody knew who was getting what when. All of the boys wore a special device to measure their physical activity.

No one could detect from their play which boys had secretly drunk the sugar. Neither parents, teachers nor trained observers accurately spotted aggressive changes that could be tied to eating sugar. The sugar-fed boys did not display more physical activity as determined by the measuring devices either. Researchers concluded that "acute sugar loading did not increase aggression or activity in preschool children". Virtually every study ever done in this double-blind fashion lets sugar off the hook as a behavioural villain.

"I'm aware of maybe 50 or 60 different research projects that have looked at children and behaviour. And if you look at the studies, you'll find that sugar has nothing to do with hyperactivity in children." – Dian Gans, assistant professor of nutrition at the University of Hawaii at Manoa.

After reviewing all the objective scientific evidence on the subject in 1991, Dian A. Gans, Ph.D., of the University of Hawaii, concluded that sugar does not foster antisocial behaviour or hyperactivity in children who are either normal or hyperactive. However, she left open the possibility that it could happen in rare instances. Indeed, Dr. Gans cautions parents that restricting sugar and other carbohydrates to curb behavioural problems could backfire and be harmful. The reason being that research shows carbohydrates, including sugar, are more likely to calm than arouse the brain, and thus, ironically, tend to reduce hyperactive and aggressive behaviour.

Psychologist Bonnie Spring, at Chicago Medical School, a pioneering researcher in the area, even suggests that highly active children may overindulge in carbohydrates precisely because the foods do exert a calming effect. Parents may then mistakenly conclude that sugar is "causing" the problem, when it may be alleviating it, she says.

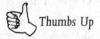 Thumbs Up

SURPRISE! SUGAR MELLOWS OUT DELINQUENTS

The astounding truth is that eating sugar actually seems to improve behaviour in some delinquents, according to a study by researchers at the University of Wisconsin in Madison. In a blind test, the researchers fed 115 imprisoned teenage male delinquents and 39 nondelinquent male high school students breakfasts that included cereal sweetened with either plain table sugar or the artificial sweetener aspartame. The total sugar intake was about 1½oz (40g). Then they gave the subjects a battery of neuropsychological tests, measuring such factors as concentration, hyperactivity, mood and behavioural disturbances. Each male took all the tests twice – after eating both the sugary and nonsugary breakfasts.

"There was absolutely no evidence that sugar had any bad effects on any of the groups," concluded study author Joseph P. Newman, associate professor of psychology at the university.

In fact, he says sugar may help curb hyperactive and destructive behaviour, especially in kids with the worst problems. Such individuals "demonstrated better performance after sucrose [table sugar] than after the no-sucrose breakfast". Also, nondelinquents, after eating the sugary breakfast, were rated better in behaviour and mood. However, Dr. Newman notes that non-hyperactive delinquents had slightly impaired performance on mental tasks, like finger tapping and short-term memory, after eating the sugar. That was not unexpected because it is known that sugar and other carbohydrates tend to induce drowsiness and slow down mental activity in normal people.

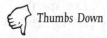 Thumbs Down

POW! BANG! – MY CHOLESTEROL'S TOO LOW

Is it possible that having low cholesterol could make you more aggressive and moody than having high cholesterol? As farfetched and zany as that might seem, it is a legitimate talked-about theory in scientific circles and is supported by some evidence. The first clues came from the results of a large-scale 1981 National Institutes of Health study of men, showing that reducing cholesterol cut the risk of heart attacks. To the surprise of the authors, lower cholesterol did not prolong life. Instead, the men in the study somehow offset their fewer fatal heart attacks by dying from accidents, homicide and suicide. Studies in Finland also discovered a link between lower cholesterol and violent, aggressive behaviour.

STRAIGHT TALK ABOUT SUGAR

There's little cause to worry that eating sugary foods will spark aggressive, violent or hyperactive behaviour. On the contrary, the evidence indicates that in most children and adults, eating carbohydrates, including sugar, tends to calm and tranquilize, reducing aggressive behaviour. Thus eating carbohydrates may be an act of self-medication rather than self-destruction. Totally depriving youngsters of carbohydrates may, in fact, exacerbate poor behaviour.

This does not mean, however, that you or your family should routinely overdose on sugar to modify brain chemistry and behaviour. Too much sugar on a regular basis can foster obesity and undesirably high blood levels of insulin and glucose. It is usually better to eat complex carbohydrates, such as pasta, cereals and bread, which also have a calming effect on the brain, although it takes longer for the effect to occur.

Sometimes scientists have to think the unthinkable. That's what Jay Kaplan, a behavioural scientist at Bowman Gray School of Medicine, and Stephen Manuck, a psychologist at the University of Pittsburgh, did. They decided to find out how our closest biological cousins, monkeys, behave when fed low-fat diets that lower their cholesterol. They studied 30 monkeys for two years. Half the monkeys ate low-fat diets – less than 30 per cent of calories from fat; consequently, their cholesterol was low. The other monkeys ate a high-fat diet that tripled their cholesterol.

Remarkably, the monkeys with low cholesterol were 50 per cent more likely to display violent behaviour – grabbing, biting, shoving and tormenting their neighbours. "We have no idea what the mechanism might be," says Dr. Manuck. "We don't know if high cholesterol mellows the monkeys or if low cholesterol makes them mean." He speculates, however, that fatty cholesterol could influence how brain cells release neurotransmitters, such as serotonin, that can affect mood.

New research also finds that some elderly men with low cholesterol (under 4.16) are more depressed than men with higher cholesterol.

HEADACHES

Foods That Often Trigger Headaches: Chocolate • Red Wine •
Caffeine • MSG • Aspartame • Cured Meats • Mature Cheese •
Nuts • Alcohol • Ice Cream

Foods That May Relieve or Prevent Headaches: Fish and Fish Oil
• Ginger

Believe it – all your headaches, whether they are so-called sinus
headaches, tension and stress headaches or the dreaded migraine, could
be triggered by food compounds you eat every day, according to
revolutionary new findings. Many people endure nearly constant
headaches, never dreaming the cause could be something in their
diet. Diet-induced headaches in children are tragically common and
unrecognized. If you have the severe type of headache known as
migraine, food triggers are a particular worry. It's now recognized,
however, that the same foods that trigger migraines can also trigger
ordinary less severe vascular headaches, according to leading headache authorities.

The reason is that all these common headaches, now known as
tension, stress and sinus headaches, are actually milder versions
of migraines, stemming from the same brain biology, and are
more accurately called "vascular" headaches. Thus, diet must now
be considered a possible culprit in all such benign headaches that
regularly torture more than 50 million Americans.

NEW HEADACHE THEORIES

Whether you have frequent and severe headaches depends a great deal
on your genetic susceptibility. The more genetically prone you are, the
more likely certain factors are to trigger headaches. Some triggers you
just can't control, such as weather changes, bright lights, strong odours

and menstrual cycles. The single easiest headache-provoking factor you can control is your diet; thus, avoiding food culprits can be critical in preventing headaches, says David W. Buchholz, M.D., director of the Neurological Consultation Clinic at Johns Hopkins University Hospital.

It's complicated because food rarely acts alone in precipitating a headache. Usually two or more factors are needed to overwhelm the brain's regulatory mechanisms, generating a headache. It's akin to creating a short-circuit by too much electrical input. That's why drinking red wine might trigger a migraine one time but not another. Your chances go up if, for example, you drink red wine and eat a chunk of blue cheese at a time when you are under stress. How much of a triggering food you eat also counts. One piece of chocolate may not bring on a headache, but eating a whole box of chocolate might, says Seymour Solomon, M.D., director of the headache unit at Montefiore Medical Center in New York City and author of *The Headache Book*.

Further, the headache may not appear until a day or so later, making detection of the food trigger even more tricky, especially if it is a food you eat frequently, says Dr. Buchholz.

"You either do or do not have a headache tendency; it is built-in and it's genetic. What you eat can then influence that susceptibility, triggering headaches." – Joel Saper, M.D., clinical professor of medicine, Michigan State University

---

MAJOR WAYS FOOD CAN AFFECT HEADACHES

Many common foods contain chemicals, particularly tyramines and nitrite, that have a direct effect on the brains of genetically prone individuals, triggering neural and blood vessel changes culminating in headaches. How often headache strikes and how severe it is depends on the degree of vulnerability and the cumulative impact of food and other triggers on the brain. In some cases, the food factor stimulates constriction of blood vessels leading to bloodflow dysfunctions and transient neurological symptoms, such as vision disturbance. In other cases, the blood vessels outside the brain dilate and become inflamed, triggering pain.

Under this theory, all foods containing certain known chemical headache triggers are suspect. Examples: chocolate, mature cheese, bacon and red wine.

On the other hand, some researchers fervently believe many headaches in adults and children result from widespread and generally unrecognized food allergies or intolerances. Thus the body's immune system may perceive a certain food as an antigen (foreign substance), setting off events leading to vascular changes and headache. Such a theory supposes that a wide variety of foods, apparently having no chemical in common, could bring on headaches depending on an individual's peculiar sensitivity.

Further, foods may have an indirect effect on pain and inflammation by working through the complex prostaglandin system. Because headaches are related to blood vessel changes and inflammatory processes, certain foods that affect these processes also have the potential to alleviate headaches. Two examples are fish oil and ginger.

HOW COMMON IS FOOD HEADACHE?

How many headaches owe their origin to food triggers is debatable. Some experts say very few, 5–20 per cent. Others say the majority. Dr. James Breneman, former chairman of the food allergy committee of the American College of Allergy, said "I am convinced three-quarters of migraines are food related." Although certain foods are more likely to cause headaches, the list is growing longer and some experts believe almost any food could be a trigger. One woman, for example, found her migraines triggered by cinnamon, which is not on doctors' lists of common migraine provocateurs. Joel Saper, M.D., clinical professor of medicine at Michigan State University and director of the Michigan Head Pain Neurological Institute in Ann Arbor, now lists milk as a common food trigger of headaches, although the mechanism is unknown. Dr. Buchholz thinks the number-one headache danger for most people is caffeine.

Cutting down on or avoiding headache-triggering foods may well stop the headaches. In a recent review of research, Cynthia L. Radnitz, Ph.D., assistant professor of psychology at Fairleigh Dickinson University, noted studies finding that 70–85 per cent of migraine sufferers who restricted trigger-foods had fewer and less severe headaches.

Here are foods with the worst reputations for triggering headaches. Most of the research has been done specifically on people with extreme vascular headaches known as migraines, but experts say the same foods are expected to trigger the run-of-the-mill type headaches typically suffered by most people.

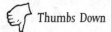 Thumbs Down

BEWARE THE AWFUL AMINES

Food constituents called amines may simply strike your brain all wrong. The ancient Greek philosopher Plinius proclaimed fresh dates a cause of headaches. We now know dates contain proteins with an amine in their chemical structure. Such amines are well-recognized headache-activating agents. For example, chocolate, a legendary reputed trigger of migraines, contains phenylethylamine. Citrus fruit, another common headache trigger, contains octopamine but the most notorious amine implicated in migraine is tyramine. It's widespread in the food supply, found in varying amounts in alcoholic beverages (particularly red wine), dairy products (mature and hard cheeses, yoghurt, soured cream), certain meats and fish (cured or processed meats, herring), yeast products (certain breads and fresh cake), fruits (figs, dates, raisins), nuts and sauerkraut. Interest– ingly, feeding test subjects pure tyramine alone does not always bring on headaches, confirming that additional triggers must combine with food to precipitate pain.

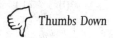 Thumbs Down

RED WINE HEADACHE

Suspect red wine. If you think it triggers your headache, it probably does. Red wine has the worst reputation among alcoholic beverages as an instigator of headaches. The probable reason is that red wine is rich in many grape substances, called congeners, including tyramine. Proof that red wine can trigger headaches comes from several studies, including a recent controlled British test of 19 migraine patients.

CHEESES THAT GIVE THE MOST PAIN (CHEESES WITH THE MOST
TYRAMINE)

Cheese	Milligrams of tyramine per ½oz (15g) cheese
English Stilton	17.3
Blue cheese	15.0
Mature cheddar	7.5
Danish blue	5.5
Mozzarella	2.4
Swiss Gruyère	1.9
Feta	1.1
Parmesan, grated	1.1
Gorgonzola	0.8

Investigator Julia T. Littlewood, of the Princess Margaret Migraine
Clinic at Charing Cross Hospital in London, had subjects drink
from small brown bottles, chilled to obscure the taste of the contents.
Some contained a little over 8fl oz (225ml) of Spanish red wine.
Others held vodka mixed with lemonade. Both had the same
alcohol content, and subjects drank the concoctions from a straw to
disguise identity. Some thought it was cough medicine, others the
dregs of boiled sweets. After they sucked up the mixtures, they were
watched closely for reactions.

Sure enough, within three hours, 9 of 11 migraine patients who got
the red wine developed a full-blown migraine headache with unilateral
throbbing, nausea and light sensitivity. Those who secretly got the
vodka showed no signs of headache. Nor did any of a nonmigraine
group who drank the red wine.

The main point, contends Dr. Littlewood, is that red wine indeed
provokes migraine, and obviously not because of the alcohol. Dr.
Littlewood also says the red wine she used was deliberately low in
tyramines, the often-blamed culprit in red wine. She thinks the active
agent is a natural phenolic compound – not present in white wine – that
some migraine victims cannot metabolize properly because of an
enzyme deficiency.

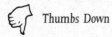 *Thumbs Down*

THE CHOCOLATE HEADACHE

Chocolate is an infamous trigger of migraine headaches. In a recent survey of 490 migraine sufferers, 19 per cent named chocolate their greatest dietary threat, next to alcohol.

That the threat is very real was shown by a double-blind British study of 20 patients with classical migraine. All were sure that chocolate triggered their headaches. As a test, the researchers gave 12 patients a 1.4oz (40g) chocolate bar. The other eight got a placebo or "phony chocolate" bar. Within an average 22 hours, five of the patients (40 per cent) who got the real chocolate felt the oncoming signs of a migraine. None of the patients who got the phony chocolate bar had a migraine.

Note: White chocolate, which contains cocoa butter but not chocolate liquor (a source of tyramine), does not stimulate headaches.

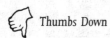 *Thumbs Down*

HOT-DOG HEADACHE: THE NITRITE NEMESIS

If you're headache-prone, beware of hot dogs, bacon, salami, ham, and other meats cured with sodium nitrite or nitrate, well-known headache triggers. Neurologists William R. Henderson and Neil H. Raskin, of the University of California at San Francisco, pinned it down with the help of a "hot-dog headache" sufferer. He was 58 years old and complained of headache attacks, and sometimes facial flushing, about 30 minutes after eating hot dogs, bacon or other nitrite-cured meats. The head pain lasted several hours.

As a test, he agreed to drink odourless, tasteless solutions containing 10mg or less of sodium nitrite or a look-alike solution lacking the nitrite. He did not know which he was drinking. Yet, eight out of 13 times when he drank the nitrite solution, he developed a headache. He never got a headache from drinking the look-alike placebo drink. After the man gave up eating nitrite-cured meats, his headaches disappeared

FOODS MOST LIKELY TO TRIGGER HEADACHES

- Caffeine (coffee, tea, iced tea, cola)
- Chocolate
- Cheese (except cream cheese, cottage cheese and processed cheese)
- Yoghurt and soured cream
- Nuts (including peanut butter)
- Processed cured and aged meats (including hot dogs, sausage, bacon, salami and bologna)
- Alcoholic drinks (especially red wine, champagne and dark or heavy drinks; vodka is least likely to provoke headaches)
- MSG (monosodium glutamate)
- Citrus fruits (oranges, grapefruit, lemons, limes) and pineapples and their juices
- Other fruits (bananas, raisins, red plums, canned figs, avocados)
- Certain vegetables (broad, butter and navy beans, pea pods, sauerkraut and onions)
- Certain bread products (homemade yeast breads, sourdough breads and other yeast-risen baked goods)
- Aspartame (NutraSweet)

Source: David Buchholz, M.D., Johns Hopkins University

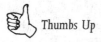 Thumbs Up

THE ASPARTAME HEADACHE

Can aspartame (NutraSweet) trigger headaches? Its makers say the artificial sweetener is blameless but enough complaints received by the federal government and by headache experts make many conclude that aspartame can cause headaches in susceptible persons. "Aspartame may be an important dietary trigger in a significant proportion of headache sufferers, particularly migraineurs," insists Dr. R. B. Lipton, a neurologist with the Headache Unit of Montefiore Medical Center in New York City, who studied aspartame's impact on headaches in 117 patients.

Another study, by Shirley M. Koehler, at the University of Florida, showed that aspartame boosted migraine frequency in more than half of a group of subjects. In fact, their overall number of migraines more than doubled (from an average 1.55 to 3.55) after they took four doses daily of 300mg of aspartame for four weeks compared to taking a placebo. Also, their headaches lasted longer, and some subjects experienced an increase in "unusual symptoms" during aspartame-inspired headache, such as dizziness, shakiness and diminished vision. Why aspartame triggers migraines is unknown but, like other headache food triggers, it apparently strikes those with an inborn vulnerability.

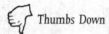 Thumbs Down

MSG HEADACHE

Some say there is no such thing as MSG (monosodium glutamate)-inspired headache, which may also be accompanied by other signs of so-called "Chinese restaurant syndrome," such as a burning and tingling in the face and chest, perspiration, excessive abdominal cramps and dizziness. Yet many headache experts include MSG among the most common food triggers of vascular headaches. Dr. Saper says some people don't metabolize MSG well, so it may build up in the blood-stream, resulting in a chemical overreaction and headache.

The use of MSG as a flavour enhancer is widespread in processed foods. MSG does not have to be listed separately on labels if it is part of a compound item making up less than 25 per cent of the total product. So if you are MSG-sensitive, beware of such ingredients as hydrolyzed vegetable protein (HVP), hydrolyzed plant protein (HPP), and Kombu extract, all of which contain MSG, warns Alfred L. Scopp, M.D., of the Northern California Headache Clinic. It is also often listed just as 621.

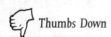 Thumbs Down

CAFFEINE: GOOD GUY, BAD GUY

Don't be innocent about caffeine. It is a paradox, able to relieve or cause headaches. A single cup of strong coffee may zap a mild headache, and caffeine alone is a painkiller equal to acetaminophen, according to tests by Nicholas Ward, M.D., a psychiatrist at the University of Washington.

But there is a dark side to caffeine that makes it a widespread headache threat, says Dr. Buchholz. He finds that caffeine feeds headaches in many unsuspecting persons, and, in fact, is probably the nation's number-one headache instigator. "If you have headaches, one of the first things to do is eliminate caffeine," he urges. He contends that while it is true that caffeine can temporarily relieve headaches by constricting dilated and swollen blood vessels, the cure backfires in the long run. "When the caffeine wears off, the once-constricted blood vessels swell up with a vengeance and dilate in a rebound action, causing even worse headaches." Thus, in the long run, regular use of caffeine promotes headaches in many people even though they think they are getting a quick fix, he says. He cautions against using caffeine to cure headaches.

How much caffeine is a headache hazard? It depends, because tolerance to caffeine varies enormously. A single cup of coffee promotes headaches in susceptible individuals, whereas others can down many cups without getting a headache, says Dr. Buchholz. "I'm not saying everyone needs to give up caffeine," he adds, "but for those who are headache prone and susceptible to caffeine, eliminating it is probably the most important thing they can do to stop headaches." Caution: To avoid caffeine-withdrawal headaches, be sure to taper off caffeine over a couple of weeks, instead of quitting suddenly.

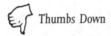 Thumbs Down

CAFFEINE-WITHDRAWAL HEADACHE

If you are used to caffeine and don't get it, you can feel awful. In fact, millions of Americans suffer debilitating caffeine-withdrawal headaches and other symptoms, never suspecting the cause, say experts. They used to think caffeine-withdrawal headache was fairly rare and trivial, striking only heavy caffeine indulgers (more than five cups of coffee a day) who were abruptly severed from their usual caffeine. Not true. Although heavy-caffeine consumers do suffer the most when they abstain, withdrawal headaches commonly strike those who average only one or two cups of coffee a day.

Most people who kick caffeine, or who otherwise don't get their daily dose, experience headaches, often severe ones. Subjects deprived of caffeine in research projects often term their headaches "as severe as any" they have ever had. Some cannot function normally and are temporarily incapacitated. So disturbing and severe is caffeine withdrawal for many people that experts, recently writing in the *American Journal of Psychiatry*, said it should officially be declared a form of mental disorder.

Tests at Johns Hopkins University School of Medicine by Roland R. Griffiths, M.D., show that caffeine withdrawal can strike people who drink a single cup of strongly brewed coffee or three caffeinated soft drinks a day. Further, Dr. Griffiths discovered that caffeine-withdrawal symptoms include not only headache, but also fatigue, mild depression, muscle pain and stiffness, flu-like feelings, nausea and vomiting. In a major study, Dr. Griffiths and colleagues had 62 coffee drinkers go "cold turkey" for two separate two-day periods, during which they got either a caffeine pill (equal to a little over two cups of coffee) or a dummy pill. When deprived of caffeine an astounding 52 per cent complained of headaches; 11 per cent were depressed; 11 per cent felt fatigued; some exhibited severe flu-like symptoms and 13 per cent were in such pain they broke the rules of the study by taking aspirin or other such painkillers.

Symptoms, including headache, typically start about 12–24 hours after you stop caffeine, peak at 20–48 hours and usually last about a week.

ONE MAN'S CAFFEINE-BINGE HEADACHES CURED

At 34 he was suffering severe throbbing headaches that lasted several hours at a time, and frequently came on weekends. After determining there was nothing physically wrong with him, his doctor recommended a psychiatric evaluation. Nothing showed up there either except that he scored rather high on an anxiety test. One major clue was that the only thing that relieved his headaches were over-the-counter analgesic drugs containing caffeine; he regularly took eight to ten such tablets a day; ordinary aspirin had no effect.

He bragged about his coffee capacity. "I can easily put away 10–15 cups a day. I drink more coffee than anyone in my office." His average intake was about 1,500mg of caffeine on a workday. Not surprisingly, he usually cut back on weekends when he was home and away from job stress.

His doctor surmised the cause – caffeine withdrawal headaches that left him a miserable mess when his blood levels of caffeine sank. Within several weeks after the man was persuaded to give up his caffeine binges, his headaches had almost totally disappeared. His anxiety scores also returned to normal.

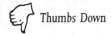 *Thumbs Down*

IF YOU HAVE MORNING HEADACHES, CHECK OUT CAFFFEINE

Amazingly, you can have caffeine-withdrawal headache without ever knowing it, and without deliberately giving up caffeine. In fact, this headache can be an almost constant and unacknowledged companion to some frequent caffeine consumers. If you commonly wake up in the morning with a headache, it could be due to caffeine withdrawal during the night. That morning cup of coffee then provides the caffeine fix that obliterates the headache but it is a vicious circle, requiring more fixes.

If you suffer from headaches on weekends and holidays, they may well be due to a cut back in your regular workaday dose of caffeine. A new study even shows that postoperative headaches, long thought to be sparked by the anesthesia, in many people are simply caused by the absence of their customary caffeine while under the knife and in the hours preceding their surgery!

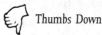 *Thumbs Down*

HOW TO KICK CAFFEINE WITHOUT THE HEADACHES

To keep your body from expressing its displeasure at suddenly being deprived of caffeine, cut down gradually. Here is advice from experts at Tufts University: Try cutting back by one cup every few days until you feel comfortable. Mix regular and decaf coffee to dilute the amount of caffeine, gradually increasing the amount of decaf over the caffeinated coffee. Of course, cut back on other sources of caffeine, such as colas, opting for "caffeine-free" soft drinks, noted on labels. The biggest jolts are found in colas and Mountain Dew.

If you're a smoker, you need more caffeine to get a caffeine "buzz," the Tufts authorities point out, because smokers metabolize or use up caffeine in the blood more quickly than nonsmokers. This means that if you quit smoking, you should cut back on caffeine, too. Otherwise, you may get caffeine jitters from having so much more caffeine in your bloodstream.

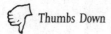 Thumbs Down

ICE CREAM HEADACHE: SURPRISINGLY COMMON

Drink something ice-cold or bite off a chunk of ice cream or frozen yoghurt, and zowee – the shock of cold in the mouth suddenly turns into a sharp pain in the forehead! It's a phenomenon known as ice cream headache. It usually doesn't last long, 20–30 seconds, and sometimes strikes deep in the nose, in the temples or behind the cheeks. What happens, says Dr. Saper, is that the cold contacts the roof of the mouth, stimulating a reaction in the fifth cranial nerve via a branch stretching from the mouth's surface to the head. This cranial nerve is the main carrier of headache pain.

Why some people experience "ice cream headache" and others do not is unknown. However, it is extremely common. A recent British study found that applying ice cream to the palates of 50 student volunteers produced headaches in 46 per cent of them.

The solution, says Dr. Saper, is to eat and drink cold things slowly. Keep them momentarily in the front of the mouth, giving the mouth's roof a chance to cool gradually. That lessens the cold shock that triggers the pain.

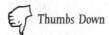 Thumbs Down

THE HANGOVER HEADACHE

Watch not only how much you drink, but what you drink. It's not only the alcohol that can give you a hangover headache, says Dr. Solomon, but also the other constituents, ingredients or flawings called congeners that help distinguish different tastes among varying alcoholic beverages. Some congeners are natural to the source, such as phenols in grapes or aldehydes from the distilling or ageing process. Others are additives, such as sulphites.

Drinks with a lot of congeners are red wine, champagne and bourbon, which may account for why they are commonly mentioned as headache triggers. Vodka has the lowest concentrations of congeners, and is less likely to cause hangover symptoms. That doesn't mean you can get away with swilling vodka with no expectation of consequences. Drink enough alcohol and, of course, you can get a headache.

Exactly how the hangover headache happens is unclear, but it appears to result from metabolic disturbances in the brain as a result of too much alcohol and may cause a type of "brain hypoglycemia," or low sugar. Thus, some experts advise eating a snack before going to bed that is high in fructose sugar, such as fruit juice. "Fructose may help metabolize the chemical products of alcohol that tend to cause headaches and other hangover symptoms," says Dr. Solomon. It's also important to drink lots of fluids, since alcohol causes dehydration. As with other types of headaches, your susceptibility to a hangover headache also is inherited.

FOOD MIGRAINES IN CHILDREN: THE FAMOUS EGGER STUDY

Your child may suffer from migraines brought on by food without your ever suspecting it, according to recent revelations by British paediatric neurologist Joseph Egger, of the Hospital for Sick Children in London. Dr. Egger studied the effects of food intolerances on 88 children with severe migraines. The landmark findings of this first carefully controlled double-blind study of its type were a shocker, jolting the medical community into a new realization of the vast potential of foods in provoking childhood migraines.

To his surprise, Dr. Egger found that an astounding 93 per cent of the boys and girls, aged 3–16, became headache-free when they stopped eating certain foods. Some recovered almost immediately when the offending foods were stricken from their diets; in others, their headaches lingered for three weeks after they stopped eating the "allergic" foods.

Particularly surprising was that 55 different foods produced the headaches, as well as other symptoms such as abdominal pain, diarrhoea, asthma, eczema and hyperactivity. The number one villain was cow's milk; it triggered migraines in 30 per cent of the children. Next in order were eggs (27 per cent), chocolate (25 per cent), oranges (24 per cent), wheat (24 per cent), cheese (15 per cent); and tomatoes (15 per cent). Farther down the list were pork, beef, corn, soya, tea, oats, coffee, peanuts, bacon, potatoes, apples, peaches, grapes, chicken, bananas, strawberries, melon and carrots.

Most children reacted to several foods, although about 20 per cent reacted to only one. Some of the migraines struck within minutes of eating an offending food; in other cases there was an interval of more than a week before the onset of pain. The average was two to three days. Another eerie note: The children were usually very fond of the foods that brought on their pain, "sometimes craving them, and often ate them in very large amounts," reported Dr. Egger. He speculates that unlike typical food allergies that strike instantly and require only minute amounts to do harm, food allergies that spark migraines develop slowly over time from chronic exposure to antigens in foods, and require larger amounts of food to provoke reactions.

NO MORE "HEADACHE EPILEPSY"

In another groundbreaking study, Dr. Egger discovered that children who had migraines often had epileptic seizures, and that the seizures, too, could be controlled by avoiding certain foods. Dr. Egger studied 63 children, 18 with epilepsy alone and 45 who regularly had epileptic seizures as well as migraine headaches. For four weeks the youngsters ate a so-called "oligoantigenic diet," consisting of foods not known to provoke an allergic reaction.

The diet worked wonders in the youngsters with both epilepsy and migraine: 55 per cent ceased to have any seizures at all, and 25 per cent had fewer seizures. The diet had no effect on children with epilepsy alone.

As additional proof, Dr. Egger did a double-blind, placebo-controlled study, in which suspected foods were secretly slipped back into the diet one by one. In 32 youngsters – 89 per cent – the seizures came back! Here are the foods that most often triggered seizures: cow's milk (37 per cent of youngsters), cow's cheese (36 per cent), citrus fruits and wheat (29 per cent), eggs (19 per cent), tomatoes (15 per cent), pork (13 per cent), chocolate (11 per cent) and corn (10 per cent). All the children reacted to at least two foods.

After seven months to three years of avoiding such foods, more than half the youngsters had their seizures under complete control; others had fewer than half as many seizures. In most, their migraines were gone or diminished. Diet can be a powerful treatment for epilepsy-migraine syndrome, insists Dr. Egger.

The connection between epilepsy and migraine has long puzzled neurologists, says Dr. Egger. He speculates that both are somehow linked to brain chemistry changes in neurotransmitters that in turn are influenced by food components. For example, opioid peptides have been implicated in epileptic seizures and immunological changes, he says, and a number of foods, especially milk and wheat, contain opiate-like peptides. Perhaps there is a connection, he theorizes.

Note: Dr. Egger and other researchers do not find that such diets work in children with epilepsy alone, only in those who also have migraines.

 Thumbs Up

CURE MIGRAINE WITH GINGER

Try ginger. The old fashioned spice may be just as effective at aborting and preventing migraines as powerful prescription drugs with potentially serious adverse effects. Used for centuries in some cultures to treat headaches, nausea and nervous disorders, ginger makes physiological sense, according to Dr. Krishna C. Srivastava, at Odense University in Denmark. Ginger, like aspirin and some other sophisticated antimigraine drugs, affects prostaglandins, the body's hormonelike substances that help control inflammatory responses, involving histamine, and pain, he says. Ginger, indeed, operates much like aspirin in blocking prostaglandin synthesis, leading to reduction in inflammation and pain.

As a test, Dr. Srivastava and colleagues suggested to a 42-year-old patient that she take ginger at the first sign of visual disturbances (the aura) that often signal an oncoming migraine. She did so, downing 500–600mg (about one-third of a teaspoon) of powdered ginger mixed with plain water. It was a dramatic success, according to Dr. Srivastava. Within 30 minutes, the "abortive effect on the headache was perceivable," he notes. For the next three to four days the woman also took another one-third of a teaspoon of powdered ginger four times a day.

The experiment was so successful the woman took to eating uncooked fresh ginger root regularly as part of her diet, and both the frequency and intensity of her migraines decreased markedly. Prior to the ginger regimen, she used to have two or three severe headaches a month. During 13 months of using ginger, she suffered only a fairly mild headache every other month.

The doctors speculate that ginger aborts or prevents migraines through one mechanism or a combination of various mechanisms, much the same way modern drugs do. Since no side effects of ginger have been documented, Dr. Srivastava suggests adults and children could safely try ginger to thwart migraines.

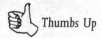 *Thumbs Up*

FISH OIL VS. MIGRAINES

Eat fish as a headache preventive. Experiments at the University of Cincinnati College of Medicine by Dr. Timothy McCarren have shown that taking fish oil capsules for six weeks blocked migraines in about 60 per cent of subjects with severe migraines, cutting the number of attacks in half — from two a week to two every two weeks. The pain and severity of the headaches also lessened. Men were more apt than women to get relief from fish oil, for unknown reasons. Dr. McCarren also suggests that eating less saturated animal fat can sometimes prevent migraines because saturated fat stimulates formation of a particular hormone-like substance, triggering events that can lead to migraines.

This does not mean you can take a bite of fish like a pill when you feel a headache coming on. The research, however, suggests that regularly eating fish, especially fatty fish such as salmon, tuna, mackerel and sardines may have long-term effects on brain chemistry, helping lessen migraine attacks over a period of time.

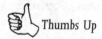 *Thumbs Up*

ODD FOOD PAINKILLERS

Oysters, lobster, liver, nuts, seeds, green olives and wheat bran as painkillers? Maybe, according to new studies at the U.S. Department of Agriculture. All these foods are rich in copper, a mineral that seems to help ward off common aches and pains ordinarily relieved by over-the-counter painkillers. That is a surprising finding by James G. Penland, Ph.D., a psychologist at the U.S. Department of Agriculture.

Dr. Penland made the discovery by analyzing several studies of both men and women who were on low-mineral diets in a special hospital unit. He noted that when the subjects were on low-copper diets, they asked for painkillers twice as often as when they were on copper-adequate diets. They requested over-the-counter analgesics like aspirin for run-of-the-mill pain, including headaches.

Dr. Penland theorizes that a deficiency of copper, which is quite common among Americans, might affect brain chemicals and/or constriction of blood vessel walls, precipitating more general pain and headaches.

DIET PRESCRIPTION TO COMBAT HEADACHES

First, try to prevent headaches by identifying and avoiding food triggers. Here's advice Dr. David Buchholz of Johns Hopkins gives his patients.

• For one month avoid all foods on the "Foods Most Likely to Trigger Headaches" list (page 291). Also avoid caffeine-containing medications such as over-the-counter painkillers like Phensic and others such as Actifed. Check the labels.

• If you regularly drink caffeine, be sure to taper off over a two-week period. You can drink decaf coffee and tea and carbon–ated soft drinks that do not contain caffeine.

• If your headaches subside or disappear, you can then "experiment" by adding back a food item one at a time every three days or once a week. If a headache occurs, you will then know that this food is a headache trigger and should be avoided. Dr. Buchholz cautions that it may take 24 hours after consuming a food for a headache to show up. After you determine which foods trigger headaches you can avoid them. However, he recommends not adding caffeine back into the diet if you have frequent headaches. "Avoid it completely," he says.

• Additionally, as other experts suggest, you may want to try eating more fish as well as a little ginger, which help block headaches in some people.

• If a child has severe headaches and/or epileptic seizures, check out a food allergy. The number-one suspect is milk.

COMMON INFECTIONS
AND BREATHING
PROBLEMS

BOOST IMMUNITY, WARD OFF INFECTIONS

Foods That May Stimulate Immunity: Yoghurt • Shiitake Mushrooms • Garlic • Foods Rich in Beta Carotene and Zinc • A Vegetarian Diet • A Low-Fat Diet

Foods That May Lower Immunity: High-fat Diet, Especially Polyunsaturated Vegetable Oils, Such as Corn, Safflower and Soya bean Oils

---

Nothing makes as much difference to your health as a well-functioning immune system. It can save you from all manner of problems, from minor infections to cancer. To be sure, your genetic makeup mightily influences your immunity, but so do environmental factors. A big one is your diet. Only recently have scientists begun to investigate and unravel the fascinating and complex workings of the immune system, including its dependence on diet. It is increasingly clear that you can manipulate your immunity by what you eat. Foods contain vitamins, minerals and other more exotic compounds that new research shows can broadly stimulate immune functioning, increasing your resistance to various viral and bacterial infections, as well as cancerous growths that flourish or die according to the operation of immune mechanisms.

HOW FOOD CAN INFLUENCE IMMUNITY

What you eat can strongly influence the performance of white blood cells, the frontline warriors against infection and cancer. These are the neutrophils that engulf and kill bacteria and cancer cells, and the lymphocytes that include the T-cells, B-cells and natural killer (NK) cells. The B-cells produce critical antibodies that rush to destroy foreign invaders, such as viruses, bacteria and tumour cells. T-cells direct many immune activities and produce two chemicals called interferon and interleukin that are essential in warding off infections and cancer. Natural killer cells are called the body's first line of defence against the development of cancer; they destroy cancer cells as well as virus-infected cells.

Much research documents that various foods and food components help control the blood concentrations of white cells and their potency. Thus, food acts to stimulate the immune system to action and to boost its current functioning.

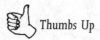 Thumbs Up

THE POWERFUL YOGHURT EFFECT

If you do nothing else for your immune system, eat some yoghurt. It's an age-old fighter of disease, and its reputation in scientific circles is soaring. That yoghurt can kill and disable bacteria has long been appreciated. Now research reveals that yoghurt also works by giving a wide-ranging boost to immune functioning. Recent studies on animals and humans document that yoghurt can stimulate production of gamma interferon, boost activity of natural killer (NK) cells, and rev up production of antibodies. Research in cell cultures a few years ago by Claudio DeSimone, professor of medicine at the University of L'Aquila in Abruzzi, Italy, found that yoghurt was as effective as a synthetic drug, Levaelsole, in enhancing immune functioning.

Dramatic proof in humans comes from research by Georges M. Halpern, M.D., of the University of California School of Medicine at Davis. In the first large-scale study of the immune effects of yoghurt, Dr. Halpern and colleagues found that those eating 1lb (450g) of yoghurt a day for four months had five times more infection-fighting gamma interferon in their blood than non-yoghurt eaters! In that study of 68 persons, age 20–40, one-third got no yoghurt, one-third got yoghurt with active live cultures and one-third got yoghurt that had been heated to destroy the live cultures. Only the yoghurt with live active cultures of *Lactobacillus bulgaricus* and *Streptococcus thermophilus* (standard in yoghurt worldwide) boosted interferon.

More exciting, a year-long follow-up study by Dr. Halpern found that eating only 6oz (170g) of yoghurt daily prevented colds, hay fever and diarrhoea in both young and elderly adults. Hay fever symptoms diminished significantly and colds were down 25 per cent.

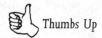 Thumbs Up

EVEN DEAD, YOGHURT FIGHTS ON

In another yoghurt breakthrough, Joseph A. Scimeca, Ph.D., a nutrition scientist at Kraft General Foods, Inc., has shown that yoghurt stim-ulates immunity enough to block lung cancer in mice. Though scientists have long suspected yoghurt has anticancer activity, this is the first good evidence that the two bacterial strains required in common yoghurt might prevent cancer. (Other research suggests that acidophilus culture, optional in yoghurt, may help prevent cancer, notably colon cancer.)

Dr. Scimeca fed mice doses of an ordinary supermarket yoghurt, then injected them with cancer cells. Eating yoghurt reduced the expected number of cancers by one-third. Remarkably, even yoghurt that had been heated, in which 95 per cent of the live cultures were killed, also prevented cancer.

The secret is probably yoghurt's ability to pump up activity of natural killer cells. Dr. Scimeca and others have shown that yoghurt in animals and humans stimulates activity of NK cells that destroy tumour cells.

The yoghurt doses given mice were high, but Dr. Scimeca says the number of bacterial organisms was comparable to what you would get from eating ordinary amounts of yoghurt. It is the concentration of lactobacillus organisms in yoghurt, he says, that spurs natural killer cells toward more ferocious attacks on cancerous cells. Odd as it seems, even dead bacteria, he finds, still exert immune-boosting power. This means even heated yoghurts and frozen yoghurts in which bacterial cultures are often killed could bolster immunity.

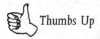 Thumbs Up

HAIL THE ANCIENT SHIITAKE MUSHROOM

To give your immune system a jolt, eat shiitakes − those big, brown, beefy Asian mushrooms now increasingly found in good supermarkets. Practitioners of traditional Chinese medicine have long revered the shiitake's healing powers. In 1960, Dr. Kenneth Cochran, at the University of Michigan, discovered one reason why. He isolated from the shiitake an antiviral substance called lentinan that exhibited strong immunostimulating activity.

A long string of studies finds the shiitake's lentinan a marvel at boosting immunity. Specifically, shiitake's lentinan is known as a biological response modifier and boosts the functioning of macrophages and T-lymphocytes. Research shows it stimulates macrophages to increase production of tumour-fighting interleukin-1, as well as to increase the macrophages' cytotoxic (cell-destroying) activity. The mushroom also stimulates proliferation of T-lymphocyte cells, especially helper cells, and their manufacture of interleukin-2.

New research by scientists at Semmelweis Medical University in Budapest, Hungary, also finds that lentinan can modify cells to resist the colonization or spreading of lung cancer cells. Thus the shiitake may help the immune system combat as well as prevent cancer.

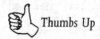 Thumbs Up

THE GARLIC SECRET

Count on garlic to stimulate immune functioning. Part of the explanation for the bulb's reputation as a bacteria, virus and cancer fighter may lie in its ability to augment immune functioning. In particular garlic stimulates the potency of T-lymphocytes and macrophages, key players in immune functions. So found Benjamin H. S. Lau, M.D., of the School of Medicine at Loma Linda University. In lab studies, Dr. Lau documented that garlic extract prodded macrophages to generate more agents to kill microbes and tumour cells. Dr. Lau calls garlic a biological response modifier. Researchers are trying to develop synthetic biological response modifiers as a treatment for cancer.

Several years ago, Tarig Abdullah, M.D., and colleagues at the Akbar Clinic and Research Center in Panama City, Florida, ate large amounts of raw garlic – up to 15 cloves a day – or took Kyolic, a Japanese cold-pressed garlic extract. Others in the study ate no garlic. The blood from the garlic eaters had more natural killer cells. In fact, such NK cells destroyed from 140–160 per cent more cancer cells than did NK cells derived from non-garlic eaters.

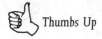 Thumbs Up

VEGETARIANS' IMMUNE ADVANTAGE

Rev up your immune system by eating all kinds of fruits and vegetables. Such plant foods contain a flood of compounds that can boost immunity, including vitamin C and beta carotene. Vegetarians do have more vigorous immune defences. A recent study at the German Cancer Research Center in Heidelberg compared the blood of male vegetarians and meat eaters. They found that vegetarians' white cells were *twice as deadly against tumour cells as those of carnivores*. This means vegetarians needed only half as many white cells to do the same job as meat eaters did. Why vegetarians' white cells are more deadly is not clear. Researchers speculated they may yield greater armies of natural killer cells or more ferocious NK cells. Not surprisingly, the vegetarians also had much higher levels of carotene in their blood; carotene from fruits and vegetables is a documented friend of your immune system.

 Thumbs Up

IMMUNE ARMADAS: FRUITS AND VEGETABLES

Go for spinach and carrots and other fruits and vegetables rich in beta carotene. Studies show such carotene boosts immune defences against both bacterial and viral infections, as well as cancer. In one study of 60 older men and women, average age 56, beta carotene increased the percentage of specific infection-fighting immune cells, such as natural killer cells and activated lymphocytes and T-helper cells, according to research by Ronald R. Watson Ph.D., at the University of Arizona in Tucson. The more beta carotene, the greater the increase in protective immune cells. For example, both 30mg and 60mg of daily beta carotene for two months improved immune cells, but the bigger dose was more powerful. Two months after the beta carotene was stopped, the immune cells sank to pre-experiment levels. Such doses are comparable to eating five to ten carrots or 7–14oz (200–400g) of mashed sweet potatoes a day. Thus, a diet high in carotene foods, such as spinach, kale, sweet potatoes, pumpkin and carrots, could provide these immune-stimulating doses of beta carotene.

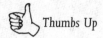 Thumbs Up

ZINC JAZZES UP AGEING IMMUNE SYSTEMS

Be sure to eat foods high in zinc. Your immune system cannot function at top form if you lack zinc. The mineral helps drive many aspects of immunity, including production of antibodies and T-cells, as well as other white-blood-cell activity. Animals deficient in zinc cannot fight off assaults by bacteria, viruses and parasites. Adults and children deficient in zinc, for example, often have more colds and respiratory tract infections.

Zinc may even rejuvenate an ageing immune system, according to Dr. Novera H. Spector, a scientist at the American National Institutes of Health. He explains that zinc may help reverse deteriorating immune functions that decline rapidly after age 60. Beyond middle age, the thymus gland, a major player in our immune defences, begins to shrink drastically. The thymus gland secretes thymulin, a hormone that stimulates production of T-cells. As the thymus gland shrivels up, so does the output of thymulin.

Yet Italian studies in aged mice find that daily low doses of zinc caused a startling 80 per cent regrowth of their thymus glands and a significant increase in active hormones and T-cells that fight off infections.

When Nicola Fabris, Ph.D., at the Italian National Research Center on Aging in Ancona, gave 15mg of zinc daily to a small group of people over age 65, their blood levels of hormones and active T-cells jumped so high as to be equal to levels seen in young people.

The greatest source of zinc is oysters. 3oz (85g) of raw oysters contain 63mg of zinc; 3oz (85g) of smoked oysters have an astounding 103mg. (For a list of other zinc-rich foods, see page 460.)

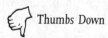 Thumbs Down

FAT BLUNTS IMMUNITY

Go easy on fat. Too much fat, especially of the wrong type, impairs immunity. Evidence in humans shows that excessive fat suppresses natural killer cell activity, immune cells that patrol the body trying to snuff out free radicals and cancer agents before they establish beachheads. One study at the

University of Massachusetts Medical School by James R. Hebert, Sc.D., associate professor of medicine and epidemiology, had young men reduce the fat in their diets on average from about 32 per cent of calories to 23 per cent. Their NK activity shot up about 48 per cent. Those who had had the highest fat diets got the greatest immune boost from the reduction.

Immune vitality also depends on the type of fat. Fish oil (containing omega-3 fatty acids) actually seems to improve immunity. Most worrying are the vegetable polyunsaturated fats (omega-6 fatty acids) predominating in corn, safflower and sunflower seed oils. Eating too much of them can severely disrupt immune functioning. For example, such oils can inhibit formation of lymphocytes, causing a partial shutdown in immune responses.

Additionally, the omega-6 vegetable fats tend to oxidize more quickly, forming oxygen free radicals that attack immune cells. Numerous animal studies find that such vegetable-type fats depress immune functions and free-radical-fighting activity. Feeding corn oil to animals fosters cancer.

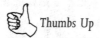 Thumbs Up

WHY WINE DRINKERS ARE MORE IMMUNE TO CERTAIN INFECTIONS

You may unwittingly boost your resistance to some infections by drinking a little alcohol, especially wine. The reason is that it can destroy or disable disease-producing organisms. The ancient Greeks used wine to disinfect wounds. The French used it to help purify polluted tap water in World II. Wine saved countless lives during the raging cholera epidemic of Paris in the late 1800s. A French physician, noticing that wine drinkers were more immune to the scourge, advised people to mix wine into their water as protection. Tests by an Austrian military doctor confirmed that cholera and typhoid germs are quickly killed, within 15 minutes, when exposed to red or white wine, full strength or mixed half and half with water. Later tests have shown that wine consistently kills any number of bacteria, including *Salmonella*, *Staphylococcus* and *E. coli*, common causes of food poisoning. Although wine may have special infection-fighting powers because of compounds formed from grape skins during fermentation, plain alcohol also can destroy unwanted bugs.

Indeed, if you drink alcoholic beverages at the same time you ingest foods contaminated with certain illness-producing bacteria or viruses, you are less likely to become ill, says Karl C. Klontz, M.D., a researcher at the Food and Drug Administration. Dr. Klontz cites studies showing that people who drank a single alcoholic beverage while eating food contaminated with *Salmonella* and staph bacteria were less likely to succumb to food poisoning from the bugs. Further, he found in a recent study that alcohol can almost eliminate the risk of hepatitis from eating contaminated raw oysters.

"With the help of modern science, we are proving what our grandmothers always knew. They used to kill bacteria in fish and fruit by soaking them in wine." – Yves Glories, professor, Institute of Oenology, Bordeaux, France

------

After an outbreak of hepatitis A, caused by eating contaminated raw oysters, Dr. Klontz determined that those who had washed the oysters down with a glass of wine, a cocktail or a shot of spirits did not contract the liver-damaging disease. In fact, the alcohol cut by 90 per cent the risk of developing hepatitis no matter how many contaminated oysters were eaten. Beer drinkers, however, were not protected. Beer does not contain sufficient concentrations of alcohol to disable the virus, says Dr. Klontz. He theorizes that alcohol somehow blocks absorption of the hepatitis virus into the bloodstream, or kills off many of the organisms before they reach the small intestine.

CAUTION: Eating raw oysters, even accompanied by alcohol, is not safe, stresses Dr. Klontz. Alcohol does not knock out the potentially deadly *Vibrio vulnificus* organism, also found in raw oysters; only cooking does so.

IMMUNE-BOOSTING DIET STRATEGIES

- Surely, the best diet to build resistance to infections, as well as cancer, is to eat lots of fruits and vegetables, especially garlic and those rich in beta-carotene and vitamin C.
- Go easy on meat and especially fatty meats.
- Restrict omega-6 fatty acids of the type in corn oil, safflower oil and sunflower seed oil.
- Eat seafood, especially fatty fish and shellfish, as well as other foods high in zinc.
- Eat yoghurt regularly.
- Go easy on sugar. There is some evidence it lowers immunity.

COLDS, FLU, BRONCHITIS, SINUS PROBLEMS, HAY FEVER

Foods That May Help: Chicken Soup • Garlic • Horseradish • Hot Chilli Peppers • Hot Curry Spices • Vitamin-C-Rich Foods • Yoghurt

Foods That May Harm: Milk

It seems almost eerie that age-old food remedies, passed down for centuries by medical sages and grandmothers, have stood the test of scientific inquiry when it comes to respiratory problems, like colds and flu. The doctor who knows most about that is Irwin Ziment, M.D., professor of medicine at UCLA. Dr. Ziment's readings of early medical literature lead him to conclude that foods used to fight respiratory diseases for centuries are very similar to the drugs we now use. They have a common action. They thin out and help move the lung's secretions so they do not clog air passages and can be coughed up or normally expelled. Such foods and drugs are called "mucokinetic" (mucus-moving) agents, and include decongestants and expectorants. Reigning king of the food pharmacy for respiratory diseases is the chilli pepper and other hot, pungent foods. Even Hippocrates prescribed vinegar and pepper to relieve respiratory infections.

HOW HOT FOODS MIMIC DRUGS

Here's how some foods may work by mimicking drugs, according to Dr. Ziment. The mouth-burning stuff in hot red pepper is capsaicin, which has some chemical resemblance to the drug guaifenesin. Guaifenesin is an expectorant, found in about 75 over-the-counter and prescription cough syrups, cold tablets and expectorants, such as Robitussin, Vicks Formula 44D and Sudafed.

Allicin, which gives garlic its flavour, is converted in the body to a drug similar to S-carboxymethylcysteine (Mucodyne), a classic European lung medication that regulates mucus flow.

The main active chemical in horseradish root, a member of the mustard family, is allyl isothiocyanate or mustard oil, which irritates the endings of olfactory nerves, causing tears and salivation.

"A lot of over-the-counter drugs for colds and coughs and bronchitis do exactly what peppers do, but I believe more in peppers. Peppers don't cause any side effects. I am convinced that 90 per cent of all people can tolerate hot food and get a benefit." – Dr. Irwin Ziment, lung specialist at UCLA

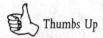 Thumbs Up

WHY YOU SHOULD LIKE IT HOT

Unquestionably, the best mucokinetic foods are hot and spicy. It's not surprising, says Dr. Ziment, that since antiquity, the favoured foods for treating pulmonary and respiratory diseases have been mustard, garlic, and hot chilli peppers. Though the active agents in these foods may work by several mechanisms, Dr. Ziment thinks they most commonly trigger a flash flood of fluids in air passages that thin out mucus so it flows more easily.

As the hot stuff hits the mouth, throat and stomach, it touches nerve receptors that send messages to the brain, which in turn activates the vagus nerve controlling secretion-producing glands that line the airways. The glands instantly release waves of fluids that can make the eyes water and the nose run, as anyone knows who has ever bitten into a hot pepper or a mound of wasabi, a hot mustard served with Japanese sushi. Imagine the same release of watery fluids inside the bronchial passages of your lungs. Breaking up congestion, flushing out sinuses and washing away irritants are common pharmacological traits of all hot, pungent foods, says Dr. Ziment. He prescribes hot foods for any condition in which secretions in the airways are thicker than normal, including sinusitis, a cold with congestion, asthma, hay fever, emphysema and chronic bronchitis.

Dr. Ziment also urges those who already suffer from chronic bronchitis and emphysema to eat hot food regularly, at least three times a week. He says his patients who do so breathe more easily and require less treatment. Further, in surveys, he finds that those who eat more hot spicy cuisine are less likely to develop chronic bronchitis and emphysema, even if they smoke. Smoking is the primary cause of chronic bronchitis and emphysema.

 Thumbs Up

CHICKEN SOUP, ALWAYS CHICKEN SOUP

Why chicken soup for colds? The first authoritative endorsement of chicken soup came from the eminent 12th-century physician, Moses Maimonides. When Sultan Saladin, the mighty Muslim military leader, begged Maimonides for a cure for his son's asthma, the story goes, Maimonides prescribed chicken soup. Never mind that the chicken soup used fat old hens and had no garlic, it probably still did some good, according to Dr. Ziment, for it does have true medicinal properties. Says Dr. Ziment, "Chicken, like most protein foods, contains a natural amino acid called cysteine, which is released when you make the soup. Cysteine bears a remarkable chemical similarity to a drug called acetylcysteine, which doctors prescribe for their patients with bronchitis and respiratory infections." Indeed, acetylcysteine was originally derived from chicken feathers and skin, he notes. Pharmacologically, acetylcysteine, like other mucokinetics, thins down mucus in the lungs, making it easier to expel.

Precisely how chicken soup performs therapeutically against cold symptoms, such as congestion, was revealed in a fascinating experiment by Stephen Rennard, M.D., chief of pulmonary medicine at the University of Nebraska Medical Center. Dr. Rennard tested samples of his wife's Lithuanian grandmother's chicken soup, and discovered that the soup has anti–inflammatory properties, which also makes it a good remedy for asthma, as Maimonides postulated some six centuries ago.

Specifically, Dr. Rennard in rigorous laboratory tests found that chicken soup actually blocked migration of white cells called neutrophils that can lead to inflammation and cold symptoms. Restrained from migrating, the neutrophils "would not accumalate in the lungs," said Dr. Rennard, and therefore, you wouldn't have symptoms of the inflammatory process which in the lungs is cough, production of sputum and general malaise, "in other words, typical cold symptoms". He points out that cold symptoms stem more from the inflammation process than from the original infection itself.

The chicken soup was so therapeutically potent, he said, that it worked even when diluted two hundred times!

"I usually make soup a couple of times a year and keep it in the freezer. That way, if I happen to get a cold, I can pull it out without having to make myself a batch of soup," says Dr. Rennard.

Here's the cold–fighting chicken soup that Dr. Rennard found therapeutic: Put a stewing chicken in a pot with enough water to cover. Bring to the boil and then add the following vegetables either whole or cut up: three large peeled onions, one large peeled sweet potato, three peeled parsnips, two peeled turnips and twelve to fifteen large carrots. Salt to taste. Cook for about one and a half hours. Add six celery stalks and one bunch of parsley. Cook for an hour or until all the vegetables are very soft. Remove the chicken and use for another purpose. Purée the vegetables in a food processor or blender. Return the puréed vegetables to the broth and stir. If you wish, chill or freeze the soup and skim off the fat, then reheat. You can also add matzoh balls.

DR. ZIMENT'S HOT TIPS FOR BREATHING PROBLEMS

"When you're congested, it's better to eat hot salsa than to suck on a menthol cough drop," says Irwin Ziment, M.D., pulmonary specialist at UCLA. Here are Dr. Ziment's other tips for using hot foods to clear up stuffy nose and chest congestion and to help fight sinusitis, bronchitis and emphysema.

- Sprinkle ten to twenty drops of Tabasco sauce in a glass of water and drink it or gargle with it.

- Chew on a chilli pepper.

- Eat a spicy Mexican meal. Do so three times a week if breathing problems are chronic.

- Add whole peeled garlic cloves to your soup. Zapping the garlic in a microwave oven first helps preserve allicin, the primary therapeutic substance.

For a super-congestion-fighting chicken soup, Dr. Ziment advises adding lots of garlic, onions, pepper and hot spices like curry or hot chillies. He calls such soup "the best cold remedy there is". To avoid or fight colds and flu bugs, a bowl of spicy chicken soup every day is Dr. Ziment's prescription. Note: It's better to sip chicken soup than drink it, because the therapeutic effect lasts about a half hour, so you need a continual slow intake of the soup's therapeutic agents.

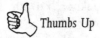 Thumbs Up

SCARE OFF COLDS WITH GARLIC

When you feel a sore throat coming on, eat some garlic or onion to scare off your cold or flu. "If you do it early enough, you may not even get sick," says James North, chief of microbiology at Brigham Young University in Provo, Utah, who confirmed that the two foods, as folk medicine claims, kill viruses responsible for colds and influenza. For example, Dr. North found that garlic extract killed nearly 100 per cent of both a human rhinovirus which causes colds, and parainfluenza 3, a flu and respiratory virus.

Garlic has long been used as a cold medicine throughout the world. It is so common in Russia that it is known as "Russian penicillin". Russian officials once imported 500 tons of garlic to fight an epidemic of influenza, according to reports.

Unquestionably, hundreds of tests show that garlic has strong anti–bacterial and antiviral properties.

"The best home remedy I have found for colds is to eat several cloves of raw garlic at the first onset of symptoms. . . .Cut in chunks and swallow them whole like pills. If it gives you flatulence, eat less. I recommend one or two cloves of garlic a day to people who suffer from chronic or recurrent infections, frequent yeast infections or low resistance to infection." – Andrew Weil, M.D., author of Natural Health, Natural Medicine.

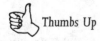 Thumbs Up

DROWN YOUR COLD IN LIQUIDS

Doctors always tell you to drink lots of liquids if you have a cold or flu. One good reason for this is that when you are stuffed up, you breathe through your mouth, and the mucous membranes lining the respiratory tract can get dehydrated. Viruses thrive better in such dried-out environments. Keeping airways moist discourages viruses. Hot fluids are better than cold ones, because there is some evidence that heat per se can debilitate viruses. As Dr. Sackner and others have discovered, the vapours from hot water fight congestion to an extent. Drink six to eight glasses a day of mostly clear liquids, including water but <u>not</u> milk!

"My own remedy is always to eat, just before I step into bed, a hot roasted onion, if I have a cold." – Statement attributed to George Washington

---

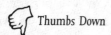 Thumbs Down

CONGESTED OR HAVE SINUS PROBLEMS? SHUN MILK

"Avoid milk if you have a cold," is popular advice. Milk supposedly produces mucus, making you feel more stuffed up. Actually, it doesn't do that, say experts. Still, you should skip milk and dairy products when you are congested.

Here are the facts. Researchers at the University of Adelaide in Australia recently refuted the folklore that milk causes mucus. As a test, they infected 60 healthy adults with a cold virus. Then they collected nasal secretions, comparing the mucus production with milk drinking. Some subjects drank no milk; others drank as much as 11 glasses of milk a day. About one-third said they shunned milk when they had a cold, mostly because it produced phlegm or mucus.

The researchers could find no evidence that milk drinkers produced more nasal secretions. The researchers speculated that milk's slightly viscous consistency makes the throat feel more stuffed up and filled with mucus, even though no more mucus is actually produced in the lungs and nose.

Nevertheless, Dr. Ziment says milk worsens the symptoms of congestion – but not because it causes mucus. Milk, he says, has the opposite action of hot spicy foods. The hot stuff spurs the release of secretions that thin down respiratory mucus, easing congestion. Milk dulls or "sedates" sensory receptors in the mouth and stomach, suppressing that flash flood of watery secretions and prolonging congestion. (Incidentally, that's why milk is a good antidote to the burning sensation in your mouth if you overdose on hot chilli peppers.) "Milk seems to slow down the same secretory reflex that spicy foods help stimulate," says Dr. Ziment. Stay away from milk if you are congested, he advises.

If you have sinus problems, it's also wise to stay away from milk and all milk products, says Dr. Andrew Weil, who teaches at the University of Arizona College of Medicine. He finds that most patients with sinus problems improve dramatically after two months by avoiding milk.

 Thumbs Up

TEAS AND TODDIES FOR SORE THROATS AND COUGHS

Folklore remedies for cold symptoms abound. Here are four that stand up to scientific scrutiny.

Russian Horseradish Toddy. To a glass of warm water, add one tablespoon of grated fresh horseradish, one teaspoon of honey and one teaspoon of ground cloves. Stir. That's a recipe from Dr. Ziment, who says it is an old Russian remedy for sore throat. "Sip it slowly, keep stirring, as the horseradish tends to settle," he advises. You could use it as a gargle. In either event, it soothes and helps heal the throat.

Liquorice Root Tea. Liquorice has an anesthetizing effect; it soothes irritated throats, suppresses coughs. Use liquorice moderately; it can raise blood pressure.

Sage Gargle. German doctors commonly recommend a hot sage gargle for sore throat and tonsillitis, says Michael Castleman, author of The Healing Herbs. Sage's therapeutic benefit comes from its astringent tannins, he says. Here are Castleman's instructions for making a gargle: Use one to two teaspoons of dried sage leaves per cup of boiling water. Steep ten minutes. Don't give medicinal doses of sage to children under age two, he warns.

Onion Cough Syrup. "Put six chopped white onions in a double boiler and add 6oz (170g) of honey. Cook slowly over low heat for two hours and strain. Take at regular intervals, preferably warm." So advise Michael Murray, N.D., and Joseph Pizzorno, N.D., in their book Encyclopedia of Natural Medicine.

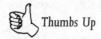 *Thumbs Up*

DR. DUKE'S LARYNGITIS REMEDY

You are hoarse with laryngitis? It's an inflammation of the larynx, accompanied by dryness, coughs and a sore throat. Jim Duke, Ph.D., U.S. Department of Agriculture's expert on medicinal plants, says several foods contain compounds that may help.

"If I had laryngitis," says Dr. Duke, "I would drink pineapple juice with a pinch or so of ginger, nutmeg, rosemary and spearmint and a bit of liquorice as a sweetener." All are laryngitis folk remedies with scientific validity, he says. You could also add thyme and cardamom, which are also therapeutic. If you have high blood pressure, he advises skipping the liquorice.

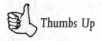 *Thumbs Up*

A SUPER FOOD TO WARD OFF HAY FEVER AND COLDS

Three months before pollen season or cold season, start eating yoghurt. It can build up your immunity, dramatically reducing your suscep–tibility to both these aggravations, says immunologist Georges Halpern, M.D., of the University of California at Davis. In a year-long controlled study of 120 young and elderly adults, he found that eating 6oz (170g) of yoghurt a day significantly reduced the number of days the subjects had hay fever attacks, especially from grass pollens. The yoghurt eaters also had far fewer symptoms of hay fever and allergies. Further, those eating yoghurt daily had about 25 per cent fewer colds during a year than the non-yoghurt eaters.

Yoghurt with live cultures boosts immune functioning by stimulating production of gamma interferon that fights off both infections and allergic reactions. The more gamma interferon, the less of substances called IgE that are the major components of allergic reactions. In previous studies, Dr. Halpern found that gamma interferon jumped nearly fivefold in those eating 1lb (450g) of live-culture yoghurt every day. Thus, although 6oz (170g) is beneficial, Dr. Halpern says you can expect far more protection against colds and hay fever if you eat 12oz–1lb (340–450g) a day. You should start eating yoghurt at least three months ahead of the hay fever or cold seasons, because it takes that long for sufficient gamma interferon to build up in your system, he says. Also, the yoghurt must contain live cultures to be effective. Yoghurt in which bacterial cultures had been killed did not work in Dr. Halpern's tests.

Additionally, eating onions may help relieve hay fever; onions are extremely high in quercetin, recommended by some to quell allergic reactions.

 Thumbs Up

VITAMIN C FIGHTS BRONCHITIS

If you are concerned about chronic bronchitis, buck up the intake of vitamin-C-rich foods in your diet. Eating such foods can help protect the lungs from damage and consequent debilitating bronchitis, declares Dr. Joel Schwartz of the U.S. Environmental Protection Agency. Indeed, chronic obstructive bronchitis, a "smoker's disease" in which the air passages become inflamed and clogged with thick mucus, impairing breathing, may be partly due to a lack of cell-protective antioxidant vitamin C.

A recent major study of 9,000 adults by Dr. Schwartz supports that theory. He discovered that people who ate foods containing 300mg of vitamin C a day were only 70 per cent as likely to have chronic bronchitis or asthma as those eating foods with one-third that much, or about 100mg. The difference is found in one cantaloupe melon or two 8fl oz (225ml) glasses of orange juice.

Dr. Schwartz says a high-vitamin-C diet is especially critical for cigarette smokers who are at high risk for chronic obstructive bronchitis if they smoke long enough. Much research confirms that smokers typically have abnormally low blood levels of vitamin C, presumably because it is used up rapidly by the body in efforts to counteract the toxic oxidative agents in cigarette smoke. In fact, smokers use up so much antioxidant vitamin C that they need three and a half times more vitamin C than nonsmokers just to stay even.

Could it be, speculates Dr. Schwartz, that vitamin C is a missing link – at least a partial explanation of why 10–15 per cent of cigarette smokers succumb to chronic obstructive lung disease but other smokers do not? Perhaps the lucky ones do not wreck their lungs partly because they blunt smoking's effect by taking in more antioxidants in fruits and vegetables. Dr. Schwartz and other experts believe such antioxidants are critical in protecting lung tissue from harm that can lead to chronic obstructive bronchitis and emphysema.

Dr. Schwartz also says a high-salt diet can help bring on respiratory illness, including emphysema. The reason is that too much sodium throws the sodium-potassium ratio out of balance, setting off an exaggerated response by bronchial passages as well as by nervous-system controls that lead to inflammation and lung damage.

OTHER FLU-FIGHTING FOODS

- Ginger destroys influenza viruses.

- A substance called lentinan in shiitake mushrooms fights influenza viruses better than a prescription antiviral drug, according to Japanese tests.

- Quercetin, concentrated in onions, has antiviral and antibacterial activity.

ASTHMA

The idea that food can stave off asthma is very old. The Ebers Papyrus, an Egyptian medical text from 1550 B.C., prescribed figs, grapes, frankincense, cumin, juniper fruit, wine and sweet beer for asthma. Early Chinese medicine recommended tea leaves (*Camellia sinensis*), from which the anti-asthmatic drug theophylline was derived in 1888. Ancient Greek and Roman physicians called for pungent foods like garlic, pepper, cinnamon and vinegar to treat asthma. The famous medieval philosopher-physician Moses Maimonides wrote an entire book, *Treatise on Asthma*, in which he recommended freshwater fish, fennel, parsley, mint, watercress, fenugreek, radishes, figs, quinces, raisins, wine and barley porridge to treat asthma. Of these old-time remedies, those that make scientific sense today are the pungent foods, fruits, vegetables and fish.

FOUR WAYS FOOD CAN AFFECT ASTHMA

Although asthma is still complex and mysterious, knowledge of how food can affect it is much clearer than ever before, based on a new understanding of the origin of asthma. (Incidentally, the number of Americans suffering from asthma has reached an unprecedented high, rising more than 50 per cent from 1980 to a total of 10 million cases in 1990. Deaths have nearly doubled.)

Asthma is characterized by recurrent attacks of wheezing, coughing and shortness of breath that can range from mild to life-threatening. In such attacks, the small airways in the lungs suddenly become clogged with mucus and other secretions; if not cleared the blockage can lead to suffocation. Experts now know that the major long-term underlying cause of asthma is a chronic inflammation and thickening of the bronchial tubes and nasal passages leading to dramatic muscle spasms, constriction of air passages and consequent breathing difficulties. Thus, new therapy is directed primarily at fighting the persistent inflammation.

Eating the right foods may alleviate or prevent asthmatic attacks essentially in four ways: by helping control underlying inflammation of air passages; by dilating air passages; by thinning down mucus in the lungs; and by preventing food-allergy reactions that trigger asthma attacks.

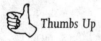 Thumbs Up

ONION THERAPY

Eat onions regularly. The bulbs contain at least three natural anti-inflammatory drugs that strike at the basic cause of asthma. A prominent researcher in the field, Dr. Walter Dorsch of Johannes-Guttenberg University in Mainz, Germany, has discovered strong anti-inflammatory activity in both onion juice and specific onion compounds. In one such test, an onion chemical diphenylthiosulphinate displayed higher anti-inflammatory activity than the popular anti-inflammatory drug prednisolone. Dr. Dorsch has also found that onions do have direct anti-asthmatic effects. In an experiment, guinea pigs were made to inhale histamine, the chemical that induces asthmatic symptoms. Their histamine response jumped 300 per cent. When he also fed the animals onion extract, their histamine response decreased, as did the risk of asthmatic attack.

Onions worked in humans too. When subjects drank onion juice before being exposed to irritants, their bronchial asthma attacks dropped by about 50 per cent! Dr. Dorsch credits thiosulphinates in onions as the major active anti-inflammatory agents. However, onions are the richest of all foods in another powerful anti-inflammatory compound, quercetin, which also can relieve allergies including hay fever. Quercetin, an antioxidant, seems to stabilize membranes of cells that release histamine. In fact, quercetin is chemically similar to cromolyn, an anti-allergic drug that inhibits histamine release.

Dr. Eric Block, of the State University of New York at Albany, has also detected what he calls another "bizarre sulphur compound" in onions that in test tubes helps "prevent the biochemical cascade that leads to asthma and inflammatory reactions".

Another possible explanation of onions' anti-asthma powers is that some asthma may result from a bacterial infection by *Chlamydia pneumoniae*, according to the *Journal of the American Medical Association*. Onions have a fierce reputation for destroying bacteria.

 Thumbs Up

FISH OIL FOR ASTHMA

Absolutely make it a point to eat fatty fish. Fish oil is a good bet as a long-term safe treatment for asthma. A proven anti-inflammatory agent, the oil may help heal inflammation of the air passages, allowing for regeneration of the lining of the airways, restoring easier breathing. That's what British researchers say. Indeed, in tests, they had asthma sufferers take high doses of fish oil, comparable to eating about 8oz (225g) of mackerel daily for 10 weeks. They found that the marine oil cut by 50 per cent the production of inflammation-promoting agents, called leukotrienes. Such leukotrienes are a thousand times more potent in stimulating bronchial constrictions than histamine.

Investigators concluded the test was too short for asthma sufferers to detect an improvement in breathing, saying more time may be needed for fish oil actually to heal the inflamed air passages. However, they contend that regularly eating fish high in anti-inflammatory omega-3 fatty acids, such as salmon, mackerel, sardines, and tuna, may prevent asthma in those who don't have it, as well as help heal it in those who do, by the continual suppression of inflammatory attacks on air passages. It is true that populations, like the Eskimos, who consistently eat lots of seafood have little asthma. A recent study by Joel Schwartz, Ph.D., of the Environmental Protection Agency, found that fish eaters in the United States are less likely to have asthma and other breathing difficulties.

Additionally, a few studies have found some immediate relief of asthma from fish oil. At Guy's Hospital in London, asthma patients who took fish oil had fewer breathing difficulties in the so-called late asthma reaction, an inflammatory condition that is delayed for from two to seven hours after initial breathing problems.

Similarly, French researchers at the Rothschild Hospital in Paris determined in a recent double-blind study that some asthma patients getting fish oil supplements for nine months did improve.

Caution: One study found that fish oil worsened airway obstruction in asthmatics who were also sensitive to aspirin.

 Thumbs Up

ABOLISH WHEEZES WITH FRUITS AND VEGETABLES

If you want to breathe better, eat lots of fruits and vegetables rich in vitamin C. They, too, can help control asthma, probably by subduing inflammation, says Dr. Schwartz. His analysis of the diets of 9,000 adults discovered that Americans who ate the most vitamin-C-packed foods and thus had the most vitamin C in their blood were least likely to have breathing complaints from asthma or bronchitis.

Specifically, eating foods containing at least 300mg of vitamin C daily cut the risk of asthmatic wheezing and bronchitis by 30 per cent. That's the amount in three 8fl oz (225ml) glasses of orange juice or 1lb (450g) of cooked broccoli. Most Americans eat only one-quarter that much vitamin C.

What accounts for vitamin C's anti-asthmatic effects? Dr. Schwartz suspects many reasons, including vitamin C's antioxidant activity which can, among other things, neutralize oxygen free radicals that may stimulate inflammation. Vitamin C can also accelerate histamine metabolism (histamine is formed during allergic reactions) and affect smooth muscle involved in bronchospasms. Additionally, vitamin C affects prostaglandins that help control inflammation. In other tests, high doses of vitamin C – from 500–1,000mg a day – have staved off asthma attacks and improved breathing functions by relieving bronchial constriction.

 Thumbs Up

NON-MEAT EATERS BREATHE BETTER

Fruit and vegetable power against asthma may be more complicated than just vitamin C. There's evidence that embracing vegetables totally and giving up all animal products helps relieve asthma. In a study of 25 patients, fully 71 per cent improved after four months without meat and dairy foods; after a year, 92 per cent had improved! That meant no meat, fish, eggs or dairy products. Why did it work? Doctors say maybe because the diet deprived patients of possible allergens – agents in food that could trigger asthma. Another possibility is that a major cause of inflammatory responses is leukotrienes and these are made from arachidonic acid, a fatty acid found in animal foods.

 Thumbs Up

TRY FIERY PEPPERS

Eat hot, pungent foods to get immediate relief from asthma. Hot chilli peppers, spicy mustard, garlic and onions can all make breathing easier for asthmatics by opening up air passages, says Irwin Ziment, M.D., a pulmonary disease expert at UCLA. He explains that such foods have "mucokinetic" (mucus moving) activity that thins out the viscous mucus that otherwise would plug up the small airways, making breathing difficult for asthmatics.

One way fiery foods work, Dr. Ziment believes, is by stimulating nerve endings in the digestive tract that order a release of watery fluids in the mouth, throat and lungs. These secretions help thin down the mucus, so it does not clog airways and can be expelled, allowing normal breathing.

Additionally, spicy foods have other anti-asthmatic properties. It's been found that capsaicin, the hot stuff in chilli peppers, has anti-inflammatory activity when eaten; when inhaled, it acts as a bronchodilator in those with mild asthma. Onions, as well as garlic, have anti-inflammatory properties.

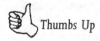 Thumbs Up

JAVA – GOOD MEDICINE

To dilate bronchial tubes, try caffeine. During the 1800s caffeine was a prime anti-asthmatic drug, but in the 1920s it was replaced by theophylline, which is still commonly prescribed. Yet, there is evidence that caffeine can help prevent and treat asthma symptoms. For one thing, coffee drinkers appear to have less asthma. A major study of 72,284 Italians over age 15 concluded that regular long-term use of coffee, presumably because of caffeine, both reduced the intensity of bronchial attacks and prevented their occurrence. In regular one-cup-a-day consumers, asthma odds dropped 5 per cent; for two-cup-a-day drinkers, the odds fell 23 per cent, and for drinkers of three or more cups, the risk went down 28 per cent. There was no significant additional benefit from drinking more than three cups a day. The doctors said the caffeine in three cups of coffee had about the same bronchodilating effect as a standard dose of theophylline.

"One of the commonest and best reputed remedies of asthma is strong coffee." – Dr. Hyde Salter, *Edinburgh Medical Journal,* 1859

Similarly, Harvard researcher Scott T. Weiss, M.D., recently suggested that drinking coffee regularly could eliminate about two million cases of asthma in the United States. Dr. Weiss, who analysed government health data on 20,000 Americans, found that regular coffee drinkers had about one-third fewer asthma symptoms than non-coffee drinkers. Coffee users were particularly less likely to suffer attacks of wheezing, as well as bronchitis and allergies. Once again three cups a day seemed more protective than two cups a day, although even one daily cup did some good. Dr. Weiss notes that coffee and tea are the oldest known bronchodilators, drugs that open airways, making breathing easier. One study deemed caffeine roughly 40 per cent as potent as the drug aminophylline, a common bronchodilator. Theoretically, caffeine breaks down in the body into other compounds, particularly theophylline, which relaxes the muscles surrounding the bronchial tubes.

A couple of cups of strong black coffee is also good emergency treatment for an asthma attack – just as effective as theophylline – according to researchers at the University of Manitoba.

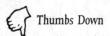 Thumbs Down

ASTHMA IN THE PEPSI GENERATION

Some foods can provoke sudden, acute attacks of asthma, especially in children. Such common food allergy triggers are eggs, fish, nuts and chocolate. Even colas, for unknown reasons, may generate asthma symptoms in youngsters, British researchers at Hammersmith Hospital in London discovered. Ten children, between the ages of 7 and 17, all said they typically wheezed and coughed immediately after drinking a cola, and that the effect lasted from an hour to a couple of days. To find out whether there was an actual physical reason, scientists had the youngsters drink colas one day and soda water or plain water on other days. Then their breathing was measured. Sure enough, although there was no gross change in airway function, nine of the ten children did display increased airway sensitivity to histamine within 30 minutes after drinking the cola compared with the other drinks.

The researchers blamed the wheezing and coughing on the colas. "We believe this is the first time that cola drinks have been shown to cause symptoms of asthma," they concluded.

BEWARE DELAYED FOOD-TRIGGERED ASTHMA ATTACKS

An asthma attack induced by a food commonly happens within minutes or an hour or so after eating the offending food, but some asthmatic reactions take a day or more to appear. A study from the Netherlands of 118 asthmatics found that some food-instigated attacks were "late-onset," occurring 32–38 hours after eating the food, and lasting 48–56 hours. Avoiding the incriminating foods for six months to a year reduced bronchial complaints in 93 per cent of the cases.

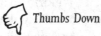 Thumbs Down

ASTHMA FROM COW'S MILK

Suspect milk. It is another common culprit in asthma. Going on milk-free diets can cause considerable improvement in some asthmatics. Though children are most likely to have asthmatic reactions to milk, it can also happen in adults.

A 29-year-old man suddenly began to suffer from bronchospasms two or three times a week; each attack lasted for one or two hours. Every day he seemed to have a dry cough and some breathlessness after breakfast. His asthma became so severe that on a couple of occasions he had to go to a hospital emergency room. Then one day he drank a cold glass of milk, and 20 minutes later found himself in the emergency room with a major bronchospasm and hives all over his body. He was treated with drugs and within an hour he had recovered but his doctors in Madrid, Spain, kept him for further tests.

Milk was the villain. When asked to drink 2fl oz (60ml) of milk, he suffered a bronchospasm. When given dried casein from milk) he had an attack of wheezing and abdominal pain within 20 minutes.

There were no warning signs leading up to this sudden and severe allergy, reported the doctors. He had no other food allergies. As long as he stayed away from milk, his asthma symptoms did not return.

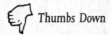 Thumbs Down

CHINESE RESTAURANT ASTHMA

Beware MSG. Typically, people who are sensitive to MSG have headaches, a burning sensation along the back of the neck, chest tightness, nausea and sweating. However, MSG can also trigger an asthmatic attack. Further, such a connection can be hard to spot because it may not show up immediately; it may be a delayed reaction appearing six to twelve hours later. So found Australian researchers when they tested 32 asthmatics, many of whom appeared to have MSG-induced asthma.

After a five-day additive-free diet, the subjects were given various doses of MSG. More than 40 per cent responded with asthma. Seven had asthma along with symptoms of "Chinese restaurant syndrome" one to two hours after taking MSG. In six subjects the asthma symptoms did not appear until six to twelve hours later. "These studies confirm that MSG can provoke asthma, that the higher the dose, the more likely the attack, and that MSG is not safe for some individuals," concluded the researchers.

DIET STRATEGIES AGAINST ASTHMA

- Concentrate on eating anti-inflammatory foods that have a good chance of preventing and alleviating inflammation of the linings of the air passages. Such foods promise to ward off new damage as well as lead to a healing of air passages and restoration of proper breathing. Try to include these foods in your everyday diet: onions, garlic, fatty fish, fruits and vegetables, especially those high in antioxidant vitamin C.

- Also critical: Avoid vegetable oils, such as corn oil and safflower and sunflower seed oils, which are high in omega-6 fatty acids. These promote inflammation and counteract the benefits of the anti-inflammatory foods, especially the fish oil.

- Restrict or avoid meat and all animal fats; they also promote inflammation.

- Eat hot peppers and spicy foods, both to prevent and alleviate asthma attacks. They make breathing easier by unplugging air passages.

- You can use coffee in an emergency to relieve an asthma attack. You could also try drinking one to three cups a day to prevent asthmatic symptoms if the coffee does not cause any adverse effects.

- Avoid any foods that seem to make your breathing worse or that trigger asthmatic attacks.

BLADDER INFECTIONS

Foods That May Help Prevent or Relieve Bladder Infections:
Cranberries • Blueberries • Lots of Fluids

Foods That May Worsen Symptoms: Caffeine • Chocolate

Bladder infections plague women more often than any health problem except colds. You have the urge to urinate frequently, and there is usually burning and pain and sometimes blood in the urine when you do. Such urinary tract infections or bladder infections, also known as cystitis, are usually caused by common *Escherichia coli* bacteria that get into the upper urinary tract, the urethra and bladder. (It's also possible to have cystitis symptoms without an infection if the bladder becomes irritated.) Men, too, have bladder infections, but much less frequently.

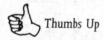 *Thumbs Up*

CRANBERRIES AND BLUEBERRIES: A STICKY NEW THEORY

Drink cranberry juice to ward off recurring bladder infections. It's centuries-old advice with new credibility. For years physicians thought cranberries worked by creating an acidic urine that killed infection-causing E. *coli* bacteria but new findings reveal a much more ingenious cranberry plot against bacteria. Cranberries, as well as blueberries, possess unique compounds that block infectious bacteria from clinging to the cells lining the urinary tract and bladder. E. *coli* bacteria, normally existing in the gut, creep into the urinary tract where, using tiny hairlike appendages, they anchor themselves to bladder cells and proceed to spread infection. The cranberry compound cripples the "landing gear" appendages of the bacteria, so they are washed away in the urine, their attempts to establish an infectious beachhead defeated.

Anthony Sobota, Ph.D., a microbiology professor at Youngstown State

University in Ohio, first discovered the cranberry mechanism in 1984. Then in 1991, Israeli scientists at the Weizmann Institute of Science made a splash in the *New England Journal of Medicine* by announcing they had detected at least two compounds, present in both cranberries and blueberries, that incapacitate the molecules by which E. *coli* germs attach to the surface cells of the urinary tract. The Israeli scientists tested several juices, including grapefruit, mango, guava, orange and pineapple. Only blueberry and cranberry juice had the right chemical stuff to fight and effectively disable the stick-em ability of the infectious germs. The scientists think the two berries are unique. Blueberries belong to the same shrub genus (*Vaccinium*) as cranberries.

How much cranberry juice is needed? Studies show anywhere from 4–16fl oz (115–455ml). A classic, often-cited 1966 study by Prodromos N. Papas of Tufts University School of Medicine found that 16fl oz (455ml) of cranberry juice a day for three weeks prevented infections in 73 per cent of a group of 60 patients. When they stopped drinking the juice the infections reappeared in about half of them within six weeks. Even a daily 4–6fl oz (115–170ml) of cranberry juice cocktail (30 per cent cranberry juice), taken for seven weeks, prevented urinary tract infections in about two-thirds of 28 elderly men and women, according to a 1991 study.

THE CRANBERRY ACID MYTH

Some doctors have suggested that cranberry juice is not such a good remedy because it creates highly acidic urine that might irritate the bladder, worsening symptoms in some people. Such fears seem ill-founded. The long-time medical assumption that eating cranberries makes urine acidic enough to destroy or inhibit bacteria is probably mistaken. "Any acidic effect of cranberries is very mild, not likely to be harmful or irritating to the bladder:' says William Graham Guerriero, M.D., professor of urology at Baylor College of Medicine in Houston. Ara Der Marderosian, Ph.D., of the Philadelphia College of Pharmacy and Science, says studies show a person must drink six or more glasses of cranberry juice daily before the urine becomes acid to any degree. Thus, contrary to popular medical opinion, cranberries do not seem to make the urine acidic enough to kill bacteria, to cause irritation of the bladder or to act as the primary mechanism by which cranberry juice thwarts bladder infections.

DIET PRESCRIPTION TO PREVENT BLADDER INFECTIONS

• If you have recurring urinary tract infections, try a daily dose of an 8oz (225ml) glass or two of cranberry juice or cranberry juice cocktail. There's a good chance it will work to prevent future infections if the responsible bacteria are common E. coli.

• Also try eating blueberries, which contain similar bacteria-adhesion blockers.

• Drink lots of fluids – at least 3 pints (1.7 litres) a day.

• Avoid caffeine and chocolate during an active infection; they may be irritating to inflamed tissues.

Important: Cranberry juice may help prevent recurring urinary tract infections, but don't rely on cranberry juice to cure such infections. Prescription antibiotics may be necessary.

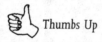 Thumbs Up

THE FLUID CURE

Drink lots of fluids, including water, to prevent and help cure bladder infections. Fluids dilute concentrations of bacteria in the urine, and promote frequent urination that gets rid of bacteria. Since E. coli multiply rapidly, the longer urine remains in the bladder, the more bacteria it contains and the greater the pain, burning sensations and other symptoms. Fluids of all types promote urination, flushing away the bacteria. Thus, cranberry juice does a super double-duty job of flushing and crippling the bacteria at the same time.

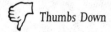 Thumbs Down

BEWARE CAFFEINE AND CHOCOLATE

Typically, tissues in the urinary tract are inflamed during a bladder infection; thus, certain foods may be irritating and make symptoms worse. A big culprit is caffeine, according to Dr. Guerriero. He advises avoiding caffeine and chocolate (another potentially irritating food to some) if you have a bladder infection.

THE HERPES VIRUS

THE THREE **WORST** FOODS TO EAT IF YOU ARE PRONE TO HERPES

- Chocolate

- Nuts

- Foods containing Gelatine

Do you have facial cold sores or "fever blisters," canker sores (ulcers inside the mouth), genital blisters, shingles (a painful inflammation of the sensory nerves) or infectious mononucleosis, also called Epstein-Barr disease? If so, you, like thirty million Americans, are tormented by the herpes virus. You may be able to help control the outbreaks by what you eat. Although the virus lies dormant in 90 per cent of us, diet may well determine whether the virus becomes reactivated and explodes into herpes symptoms, according to Richard S. Griffith, M.D., professor emeritus of medicine at Indiana University School of Medicine and an infectious disease specialist.

FEAST OR FAMINE CAN CONTROL HERPES FLARE-UPS

Here is Dr. Griffith's explanation. Molecules of what you eat end up in your cells. Whether you present the virus with a banquet or slim pickings at that cellular meeting may determine whether the rascal revives to torture you. If you feed the herpes virus enough of the right stuff, it may grow ferociously, prodding the body to make cold sores, genital blisters and other symptoms. On the other hand, you can starve the virus, subduing it so it can't cause much trouble.

There are food "good guys" and "bad guys" in the herpes drama. In the 1950s, Dr. Griffith says, it was discovered that amino acids found in food can either stifle or encourage the growth of the herpes virus. Adding the amino acid arginine to the herpes virus in cell cultures made it grow like crazy. Adding the amino acid lysine halted the growth and spread of herpes viruses in cells. One theory is that lysine wraps a protective coat around the cell, barring the virus from penetrating and eviscerating the cell. If that's the case, doesn't it make sense to feed the herpes virus a diet low in the growth-stimulant arginine and rich in the growth-inhibitor lysine? Letting the virus feast in the opposite manner could be foolhardy.

That's what Dr. Griffith thinks. So for about 20 years he has been telling herpes patients to provide a starvation diet for the virus by eating foods high in lysine and low in arginine. What counts, he says, are the relative amounts of these two amino acids in your cells. It's the "balance of power" between the two amino acids that determines whether the virus takes over cells and flourishes in your body. At that juncture, you want lots of lysine and little arginine to keep the virus in check.

THE ARGININE EXPERIMENTS

As a test of how arginine can prod the herpes virus into acting up, Dr. Griffith gave patients high doses of arginine — 500mg four times a day — and restricted their lysine intake. Three out of five quickly developed such severe herpes outbreaks that he stopped the study. One subject who ordinarily had cold sores only on his lip developed them under his eye. A little girl broke out with herpes all over her mouth. The severe outbreaks happened overnight after taking the arginine.

And how much would you have to eat to get the amount of arginine used in the study. *A mere 2oz (55g) of peanuts or chocolate!*

At the same time, eating enough lysine-rich foods can help override the threat of a high-arginine diet. Foods high in lysine are: milk, soya beans, meat, including beef and pork. (Lysine is often added to animal feed, thus it can be high in meat.) "I've noticed that herpes patients don't seem to drink much milk," says Dr. Griffith. Further, infants commonly have a first attack of herpes infection right after they are weaned and taken off high-lysine milk, he notes.

HERPES-PROMOTING FOODS

It's not just the amount, but the balance between arginine and lysine in foods. The following foods have high ratios of arginine to lysine and thus tend to stimulate growth of the herpes virus, according to Dr. Richard Griffith.

Absolutely Avoid:
Almonds
Brazil nuts
Cashews
Hazelnuts
Peanuts
Pecans
Walnuts
Chocolate
Gelatine

Restrict if you eat lots of them:
Coconut
Barley
Corn
Oats
Wheat, including wheat bran, wheat germ, and gluten
Pasta
Brussels sprouts

"BUT I EAT NUTS AND DON'T GET HERPES"

Not everyone, however, gets herpes symptoms from eating high-arginine foods. Nor does cutting out arginine-rich foods curb all herpes attacks. Some people can eat all the nuts they want without disturbing the virus. Why? For the same reason that not everybody's blood pressure goes up from eating salt, says Dr. Griffith. It's a highly individual matter.

You can use a low-arginine, high-lysine diet both to prevent and heal herpes outbreaks, says Dr. Griffith. "The worst thing you can do if you already have a herpes sore is to eat high arginine foods like nuts. That perpetuates the growth of the virus," he says. Not all experts agree with Dr. Griffith's finding but there's no risk in the diet, and the alternative may be expensive drugs with potentially hazardous side effects, and/or little therapeutic benefit.

HOW TO TELL IF FOOD TRIGGERS HERPES OUTBREAKS

"All you have to do is experiment," says Dr. Griffith. If food high in arginine, like nuts, chocolate and gelatine is causing herpes flareups, you can tell overnight, he insists. It's this simple: Eat a lot of peanuts and/or chocolate and gelatine and see if you feel the beginnings of the sores, blisters or pain the next day. All some people have to eat is a handful of peanuts to experience herpes outbreaks. For others it takes more, but a small snack pack, or 3½oz (100g) of nuts – is usually enough for a test.

"It's fairly easy to get most of the arginine out of your diet by leaving out nuts, chocolate, and gelatine. Chocolate-covered nuts are a double threat." – Richard S. Griffith, M.D.

If you don't have a herpes reaction, such foods are probably not at fault, says Dr. Griffith, so don't worry about them. For those who are susceptible to food-induced herpes outbreaks, they know it every time. "If you break out once from eating nuts, you do it each time you eat nuts," he says. "The response is very consistent."

Stop it early. Once the herpes infection explodes into full-blown blisters or sores, healing it with the high-lysine, low-arginine method is more difficult. The sooner you take action against the virus, the better. The dietary measures are most effective in preventing recurrence of herpes outbreaks or in thwarting the herpes symptoms in the initial stages – right after you first feel the stinging and pain of an emerging herpes attack. It's at that point you should cut out arginine-rich foods.

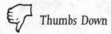 Thumbs Down

THE CASE OF THE PEANUT BUTTER SANDWICH

If you're trying to avoid food-aggravated herpes attacks, don't forget peanut butter is essentially ground-up peanuts, and consequently high in arginine, a threat to be avoided. So found one patient who was highly vulnerable to genital herpes, especially around the time of her menstrual period. The distress was exceedingly severe and painful.

Dr. Griffith put her on a low-arginine diet and prescribed lysine supplements, 500mg twice a day. Her herpes attacks lessened and virtually disappeared for more than a year. Then they came back. The reason was that she started eating peanut butter sandwiches for lunch, feeding her cells lots of arginine. After she cut out peanut butter, her herpes outbreaks once again vanished. She has remained free of the herpes attacks for the last five years, says Dr. Griffith.

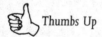 Thumbs Up

SEAWEED VS. HERPES

Another way to curb herpes may be to eat seaweed. When the herpes virus meets certain edible seaweeds, it shrivels and retreats. That's what two researchers at the University of California's Naval Biosciences Laboratory in Berkeley discovered in test tube studies. They put extracts of eight different kinds of seaweed from the red algae family into test tubes with human cells that had been infected with either herpes simplex virus 1 (which causes cold sores) or virus 2 (which causes genital herpes). The spread of the virus was slashed by 50 per cent. More impressive, when the scientists first exposed the human cells to the seaweed extracts and then added the viruses two hours later, the viruses did not thrive at all, blocking pro-herpes activity 100 per cent.

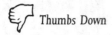 Thumbs Down

SHINGLES AND CHOCOLATE

Shingles can be one of the most painful conditions, and shows up frequently in the elderly. One estimate found that about half of people over age 80 have had shingles. It happens, explains Dr Griffith, when the herpes virus which has been present for a long time in the body revives, possibly because immune resistance declines with age. It gets into nerve cells, causing painful blisters on the skin; even after these heal, the pain remains in about 5 per cent of the cases because of what is called postviral neuralgia.

Shingles are a serious condition, requiring medical attention. However, as a preventive, Dr. Griffith advises staying away from foods high in arginine. An example: One elderly patient kept a large chocolate Easter rabbit as a table decoration; then one day she ate most of it. The next day she came down with shingles. If you already have postviral neuralgia, Dr. Griffith recommends taking two 500-mg lysine tablets three or four times a day as a test to see if it helps.

TIPS TO COMBAT COLD SORES, CANKER SORES, GENITAL HERPES, SHINGLES AND EPSTEIN-BARR DISEASE

If you are tortured by herpes outbreaks, try cutting out high-arginine nuts, chocolate and gelatine. When you have a herpes outbreak or feel the beginnings of one, stop eating arginine-rich foods right away. The quicker you take action, the more likely you are to benefit, says Dr. Griffith. Such action can't hurt, and you may be pleasantly surprised to see the herpes outbreak recede.

Generally he finds that cutting down on high-arginine foods is enough to thwart the virus. If it does not work, he recommends taking one or two 500-mg lysine tablets a day for as long as the herpes infection tends to recur.

Such measures won't work for everyone, but you may be one who gets some relief. It is worth trying.

JOINT AND BONE
PROBLEMS

RHEUMATOID ARTHRITIS

Foods Most Likely to Trigger or Aggravate Arthritis: Corn •
Wheat • Milk • Meat • Omega-6 Vegetable Oils (Corn, Safflower,
Sunflower)

Foods That May Relieve Arthritis: Fatty Fish • Vegetarian Diet •
Ginger

Old-time medical texts and popular polemics are overflowing with
dietary cures for arthritis and rheumatism: Avoid tomatoes, potatoes and
other "nightshade" plants; lay off meat, spicy or acidic foods, citrus, coffee, white sugar, cereals; eat more kelp, devil's claw, yucca and
ginseng. As early as 1766, an English medical text prescribed cod liver oil
to treat chronic rheumatism and gout. By the mid-1800s cod liver oil was
routinely prescribed for various diseases of the joints and spine, according
to the 1907 *Dispensatory of the United States*. More recently, Dale Alexander
popularized the use of cod liver oil in a best-selling book, claiming the oil
helped "lubricate the joints". His explanation was simplistic, but modern
science now understands why the idea was not so far off the mark.

IT'S NO LONGER FOOD FOLKLORE

The notion that food has anything to do with arthritis, particularly
rheumatoid arthritis, has long been rejected as dangerous medieval
nonsense – pure quackery. Some who have not kept up with medical
advances may still believe that. However, new medical discoveries reveal
food's ability to literally rev up or cool down inflammation – the key
process in arthritis, which literally means "fire in the joints". Leading
arthritis specialists now acknowledge that diet can soften the symptoms
of arthritis and, in some cases, may be the sole or prime instigator of the
suffering. To be sure, the tendency to arthritis may be inherited, and other
factors, even a virus, may be involved, but there is strong new evidence

that diet can be a very real aggravator or combatant of arthritis.

There's even scientific support for the idea, long held in primitive folk medicine, that specific foods are like demons that invade and wreck the bodies of certain susceptible individuals and that nothing short of an exorcism of that food from your diet will save you. Furthermore, your favourite food could be your worst tormentor. If that sounds like a plot from "The Twilight Zone," consider the remarkable case of the British Ms. X.

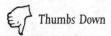 Thumbs Down

"I WAS CRIPPLED BY MY CHEESE CRAVINGS"

Sophisticated readers might guffaw with skepticism if they read that headline in a cheap tabloid but physicians didn't laugh when the same story appeared under the sober headline: "Rheumatoid Arthritis and Food: a Case Study" in the sedate and serious British Medical Journal.

Poor Ms. X. A mere 38 years old, she had been riddled with rheumatoid arthritis for 11 years. The joints of her arms, legs and hips were severely inflamed and swollen. She had no hand grip to speak of and she could barely move without excruciating pain. She was extremely fatigued and stiff for several hours every day.

Nothing helped. She had already been treated to all of modern science's heavy artillery – salicylates, nonsteroidal anti-inflammatory agents, gold, penicillamine, prednisone, even blood exchanges. They brought little or no relief; in fact, their toxic side effects made her sicker.

Then her rheumatologists at Hammersmith Hospital in London began to inquire about her cheese cravings. Yes, she confessed, since her early twenties, she had had a passion for cheese. So fierce were her cravings that she sometimes ate 1lb (450g) a day. The doctors noticed that she also had multiple drug allergies; even taking aspirin upset her stomach.

Could it be a food allergy? Could all this pain and suffering be self-induced by some substance that her body recognized as foreign, thus alerting the immune system to dispatch armies of antibodies to fight the hapless invader, inadvertently destroying her joints and body in the process? Would this virulent arthritis vanish if they could find such a culprit? It was worth a shot. They persuaded her to cut out all dairy products – milk, butter and cheese.

HOW FOOD CAN AFFECT RHEUMATOID ARTHRITIS

It's now known that diet can squelch rheumatoid arthritis in at least two entirely different ways. One: Specific food components, notably fat, can regulate the functioning of hormonelike bodily agents, called eicosanoids, which help control inflammation, pain and other arthritic symptoms.

Two: Rheumatoid arthritis in some people may be a striking and overwhelming allergic-type reaction to specific foods. Thus, in one case, you might treat symptoms by eating certain foods that, in fact, act as drugs to relieve the pain, swelling, fatigue and stiffness of arthritis. In the other case, avoiding one or more foods may provide an instant and permanent cure, vanquishing the disorder forever.

Nobody knows why certain people may be more vulnerable to food-triggered arthritis. One speculation is that some arthritis sufferers have abnormally penetrable or "leaky" gastrointestinal tracts, letting food or bacterial antigens (allergy triggers) pass more readily into the bloodstream, where they set off inflammation and other havoc. Another theory is that bacteria in the gut feed on particular foods and then produce toxins that cause symptoms.

Then again, such food-precipitated rheumatoid arthritis may not be the classical disease at all. Dr. Richard Panush, a prominent arthritis researcher, suggests "allergic arthritis" may be an entirely separate disorder from conventional rheumatoid arthritis.

Nevertheless, the case for diet-connected arthritis grows steadily stronger.

Within three weeks, her joint swelling and morning stiffness diminished, and over the next few months, completely disappeared. Her grip came back and the pain went away. Blood analyses showed that her frightening immune system dysfunction had also returned to normal. After more than a decade of crippling pain unrelieved by modern medicine's best, she was cured − not just of symptoms but of the disease at its genesis.

Then one day she ate some dairy products by mistake. Twelve hours later, the arthritic symptoms returned with a vengeance.

The doctors did a final, confirming test. In medical jargon it's called a "challenge" − a deliberate reintroduction of the offending food.

After Ms. X had had full mobility and very little arthritic disease for fully ten months, the doctors summoned her back to the hospital and watched while, during three days, she bravely ate 3lb (1.4 kg) of cheddar cheese and drank seven pints of milk. Within twenty-four hours, her body was undergoing transformation. The armies of destructive antibodies were on the march again – the rheumatoid arthritis was back complete with weakened grip, morning stiffness, swollen fingers (one finger's ring size doubled), and allergic immune disturbances. Tests were positive for IgE antibodies to both milk and cheese protein. The destructive antibodies were at their peak twelve days after Ms. X stopped eating the cheese and milk. Not surprisingly, the strongest reaction was to the cheese.

As far as anyone knows, Ms. X's crippling arthritis did not come back as long as she refrained from eating cheese and milk.

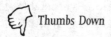 Thumbs Down

SUSPECT CORN: ANOTHER CRIPPLER

Spurred by publication of the case incriminating cheese, another doctor was inspired to report an equally dramatic case of food-caused arthritis. This time the culprit was corn. "The most impressive patient in my own experience had had active rheumatoid arthritis 25 years, was taking azathioprine and soluble aspirins . . . had already had a plasma exchange and was slowly but steadily going downhill," Dr. Ronald Williams, a London physician, wrote in the *British Medical Journal*.

It turned out she had an allergy to corn, which, ironically, was also used as a "packing," or filler, in her medication. She excluded all corn from her diet and her improvement in one week was "dramatic," said Dr. Williams. Alas, after six weeks, her arthritis flared badly, and Dr. Williams thought that, sadly, the placebo effect of a new treatment had worn off. Then it was discovered that during that week, corn-flour thickening had been added to her gravy without her knowledge. When that was eliminated, she continued to improve rapidly. "She is now . . . feeling and looking better than she has done for over 10 years," wrote Dr. Williams.

"No one would be foolish enough to claim that every case of rheumatoid arthritis is associated with a food allergy, but if only one in 20 is — and I suspect that it is considerably more — I question whether we have the right to withhold such a simple, safe, brief and noninvasive investigation [of food allergy] in a disease of such appalling chronicity." — Ronald Williams, M.D., London

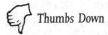 Thumbs Down

BEWARE CEREAL, TOO

Italian investigators at the University of Verona tell of a patient who recovered from rheumatoid arthritis when she stopped eating cereals. Despite corticosteroid shots and oral gold salts, she got constantly worse until the physicians discovered that she had an allergic reaction to cereals.

Consequently, they eliminated cereals from her diet for three weeks and she got dramatically better. As a test, she again deliberately ate cereals and her joint pain, morning stiffness and all other signs of rheumatoid arthritis returned. She banned cereals from her diet and the flare-ups stopped; she had had no signs of arthritis for an entire year at the time of the report.

Cereals are indeed a common trigger of rheumatoid arthritis flare-ups. A British study declared cereals, specifically corn and wheat, the number one culprit among a group of rheumatoid arthritis patients sensitive to food. More than half got arthritis symptoms after eating these grains. The critical pro-arthritis agent in wheat is believed to be gluten.

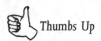 Thumbs Up

GO ON A FAST FOR QUICK RELIEF

If rheumatoid arthritis sufferers go on a fast or limit themselves to a few foods, there's plenty of medical evidence they usually feel better; joint pain and stiffness diminish. That's convincing proof that diet helps regulate the body's agents of inflammation — and that avoiding certain foods can effect a kind of cure. To be sure, food reactions are highly individual and could come from almost any food you can think of but prime suspects are meat and meat fat.

Many people have found relief in spartan vegetarian-type diets, including the Dong Diet, created by San Francisco physician Collin H. Dong and popularized in a 1973 best-selling book, *The Arthritis Cookbook*. The Dong Diet forbids meat as well as tomatoes, dairy products, peppers, alcohol, hot spices and chemical additives, especially MSG. Such foods, Dr. Dong argues, can provoke arthritis-triggering allergies. It's certainly possible.

When Richard Panush, M.D., a rheumatologist and chairman of the department of medicine at Saint Barnabas Medical Center in New Jersey, prescribed the Dong Diet for 26 of his patients with long-standing, progressive rheumatoid arthritis, five of them markedly improved. However, so did others eating a placebo diet that restricted different foods. About 20 per cent on both diets had less morning stiffness, better grip strength, and fewer swollen and tender joints. Stopping either diet brought renewed flare-ups in many patients. Dr. Panush, until then a dedicated skeptic about a diet-arthritis connection, conceded that "an occasional patient might be sensitive to certain foods". In further tests, Dr. Panush confirmed that one of the patients had severe arthritis reactions to milk, another to shrimp and a third to nitrite, a preservative in cured meats.

THREE REASONS TO GIVE UP MEAT IF YOU HAVE RHEUMATOID ARTHRTIS

1. Meat contains the type of fat that stimulates production of inflammatory agents in the body.

2. Meat may produce "allergic" reactions that incite arthritis flare-ups because of individual reactions, probably inherited.

3. Some meats, particularly cured meats, such as bacon, ham, hot dogs and processed cold meats, contain preservatives and other chemicals that trigger allergic arthritic reactions in some individuals. This is in addition to the inflammatory properties of the meat's fat.

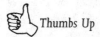 *Thumbs Up*

THE CASE FOR VEGETARIANISM

Give up meat and your arthritis may go away. So declared a widely acclaimed, groundbreaking study in 1991 by Norwegian researchers, documenting that meatless diets relieved rheumatoid arthritis symptoms in nine out of ten patients! The diets were therapeutic, not just because of allergic reactions to meat but also because animal fat itself incites joint inflammation, said researchers.

Jens Kjeldsen-Kragh, M.D., of the Institute of Immunology and Rheumatology at the National Rheumatism Hospital of Oslo, found that switching to a vegetarian diet resulted in better grip strength and much less pain, joint swelling and tenderness and morning stiffness in about 90 per cent of a group of arthritic subjects, compared with controls eating an ordinary diet. The subjects noticed improvement within a month, and it lasted throughout the entire year-long experiment.

For the first week, to rid their bodies of residual food triggers, the subjects ate a "fasting" liquid diet of herbal teas, vegetable broth, and juices from carrots, beetroot, celery and potatoes. For the next three to five months, they were put on a vegan diet (no animal products, including meat, fish, milk and eggs). They also avoided gluten (wheat), refined sugar, citrus fruits, strong spices and preservatives – all of which could possibly trigger symptoms. Then they began the process of gradually adding back foods, one by one – first, a "new" vegetarian food, and later, dairy products and wheat products. If a flare-up occured within 2–48 hours after eating the food, they rejected it, waited a week and tried again. If, on the second try, the food caused symptoms, they scratched it entirely.

Dr. Kjeldsen-Kragh concluded that about 70 per cent of the patients improved because they avoided fats, notably meat fat, likely to instigate the inflammation process. The others, he suspects, felt better because they excluded "allergic" foods from their diets.

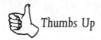 Thumbs Up

PROOF THAT A VEGETABLE CURE IS STRONGER THAN DRUGS

One woman's longstanding arthritis vanished after she embraced a vegetarian diet, ending her dependence on potent drugs, according to her New Jersey physician, Joel Fuhrman. Writing in a recent medical publication, Dr. Fuhrman says that although it "might seem preposterous that anything as simple as diet might benefit arthritis," it can be so remarkably effective that it seems "perhaps irresponsible" not to advocate it. Here is his description of the case:

A 62-year-old woman with severe rheumatoid arthritis and other problems was on nine different medications – Altace, Azulfidine, Beclovent, Digoxin, Ecotrin, Nasalcrom, Organidin, Prednisone and Seldane. She hadn't been able to close her hand to make a fist in 10 years and had pain in multiple joints.

We decided to begin a fast, followed by a plant-based vegetarian diet. After the medically supervised fast, the arthritis was gone. . . . She is still on the vegetarian diet now, five months later. She has continued to remain free of symptoms. She no longer requires any of the nine medications she had needed before coming to my office six months ago. She has regained physical strength and movement that was lost over 10 years ago.

TWENTY FOODS MOST LIKELY TO AGGRAVATE ARTHRITIS

Here are the foods that provoked rheumatoid arthritis symptoms in the greatest percentages of patients, according to a recent study by British authority L. Gail Darlington. Corn and wheat were the worst culprits, triggering symptoms in more than half of those tested.

Food	Percentage
Corn	56
Wheat	54
Bacon/pork	39
Oranges	39
Milk	37
Oats	37
Rye	34
Eggs	32
Beef	32
Coffee	32
Malt	27
Cheese	24
Grapefruit	24
Tomato	22
Peanuts	20
Sugar (cane)	20
Butter	17
Lamb	17
Lemon	17
Soya	17

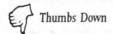 Thumbs Down

IS ARTHRITIS A MILK ALLERGY?

If you have arthritis, give up milk and dairy products for a week and see if your symptoms ease up. That's a quick, simple test, and it may bring surprising results. There is much proof that dairy foods are arthritis instigators in some people. For example, Dr. Richard Panush once tested a 52-year-old woman who blamed her rheumatoid arthritis partly on milk. Sure enough, when she downed unmarked capsules of freeze-dried milk powder (equal to an 8oz (225ml) glass of milk), she was in misery; her joints became swollen and tender, and she suffered up to 30 minutes of morning stiffness. The symptoms were worst within 24–48 hours of drinking the milk, and disappeared in a day or two. She was able to control her arthritis simply by staying away from dairy foods. In a further indictment of milk, Dr. Panush was able to produce inflammatory synovitis in the joints of rabbits merely by switching them from water to milk.

Could arthritis also somehow be related to lactose intolerance or common "milk allergy"? Yes, Israeli scientists suspect, especially if you are a woman, although they don't know why. In a study of 15 women and eight men with arthritis, they discovered that seven patients had more than a 50 per cent reduction in pain, swelling and a consequent reduction in medication, when they stayed off milk. Interestingly, all the patients were women and all of them were deficient in lactase, the enzyme that helps digest the milk sugar lactose. In other words, they were lactose intolerant, "allergic" to cow's milk. So, if you are a woman with lactose intolerance, be exceptionally aware that your arthritis could be milk related.

THE MYSTERIOUS TOMATO PHOBIA

What about tomatoes? The tomato and other members of the nightshade family, including white potatoes, aubergines and sweet peppers, have villainous reputations as triggers of arthritis symptoms. Avoid these awful nightshades, and supposedly your arthritis will diminish or disappear; this is frequently voiced folk wisdom.

The idea prospers mainly because of the experience of Norman F. Childers, Ph.D., now a professor of horticulture at the University of Florida. After Dr. Childers developed disabling disorders, including severe joint pains and stiffness, he observed his diet closely, and concluded that the arthritic symptoms came several hours after he ate tomatoes. He knew that nightshade plants had a shadowy past. At one time, for example, tomatoes were considered deadly, and weeds of the nightshade family (containing solanine) had been implicated in rheumatic disorders in livestock.

HOW COMMON IS FOOD-INSPIRED ARTHRITIS?

Nobody really knows how widespread food-instigated "allergic arthritis" might be. It's virtually anybody's guess and estimates are wide-ranging since no definitive studies have been done. Dr. Panush puts the figure at no more than five percent of all patients with rheumatoid arthritis. His one-time co-researcher, Dr. Robert Stroud of the University of Florida, thinks the figure is more like 20 to 30 percent.

Dr. James C. Breneman, then at the University of Cincinnati Medical Center, who chaired a committee formed by the American College of Allergists to look into the association between arthritis and food allergies, put the estimate much higher. He said: "I think it's reasonable to estimate that somewhere in the neighborhood of 60 to 80 percent of arthritis sufferers would benefit from dietary manipulation." One double-blind challenge test even concluded that between 85 and 90 percent of patients have symptoms exacerbated by certain foods.

One by one, Dr. Childers says, he eliminated all nightshades from his diet and all his aches and pains vanished. He has received testimonials from thousands of others, he claims, attesting to similar relief. Dr. Childers contends the nightshades contain toxins that attack the cells of susceptible individuals, which he estimates to be 10 per cent of the population.

Some experts find the abuse heaped on tomatoes bewildering, for there are no controlled scientific studies incriminating nightshade foods as prominent allergic triggers of arthritis. Indeed, a British study ranked tomatoes fourteenth out of twenty foods likely to trigger arthritis symptoms; tomatoes affected 22 per cent of the study subjects. No other nightshade plant was on the list. Food-arthritis authority Dr. Panush suggests that some people, by rejecting a wide spectrum of nightshade foods, may accidentally exclude one that triggers their arthritis symptoms. Is there any reason to think the nightshade family is more disreputable – any more likely to attack your joints than other foods? So far, the evidence is weak, although many people are still convinced giving them up brings pain relief Such passionate belief and personal testimony cannot be disregarded, but at the moment, neither can it be scientifically confirmed. If there is a biochemical reason to condemn tomatoes widely or universally, its discovery is lurking somewhere in the future.

● BOTTOM LINE ● *Unfortunately, you cannot rely on one universal, simplistic, so-called "correct" diet to solve your arthritis woes. You must tailor-make your own anti-arthritis diet to find which of a wide range of foods is your particular nemesis.*

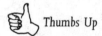 Thumbs Up

DOES A HERRING A DAY KEEP RHEUMATOLOGISTS AWAY?

It's a good bet, so is a piece of salmon, mackerel, tuna, a tin of sardines or other fish rich in omega-3 fatty acids. Several centuries of folklore were right. Fish oil is a bona-fide anti-inflammatory agent, according to Dr. Alfred D. Steinberg, an arthritis expert at the American National Institutes of Health. The oil can help quench the fires of inflammation. Moreover, marine oil acts directly on the immune system, suppressing 40–55 per cent of the release of compounds called cytokines that help destroy joints.

At least half a dozen well-conducted double-blind studies show that eating moderate amounts of fish oil reduces symptoms of arthritis, says pioneering researcher Joel M. Kremer, M.D., associate professor of medicine, Albany Medical College in New York. In one such study by Dr. Kremer, all three patients had multiple swollen and tender joints, fatigue and morning stiffness lasting more than a half hour. When they took fish oil capsules for fourteen weeks, their symptoms let up. For example, their joint tenderness subsided by more than a third, and they were free of fatigue for two and a half hours longer every day.

Dr. Kremer also found that the marine fat suppressed production of leukotriene B4, an inflammatory substance considered mainly responsible for arthritis symptoms. The greater the drop in leukotriene B4, the fewer the number of tender joints. Other research finds that fish oil significantly decreases leukotrienes within just one month! Further, leukotriene production picks up again within a month of discontinuing fish oil. It usually takes a month of fish oil eating to see improvement, says Dr. Kremer. After that, relief is rapid and more intense, the longer you continue getting the fish oil.

How much do you need? The daily amount used in the study was about the same as eating a 7oz (200g) serving of salmon or a couple of tins of sardines. A British expert says 3½oz (100g) of herring provide as much active EPA-type oil as the typical arthritis treatment doses of fish oil supplements.

The point is it takes more fish oil to subdue active rheumatoid arthritis than to prevent it. You may never be plagued with arthritis in the first place if you consistently eat small portions of fatty fish over many years, say researchers.

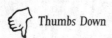 Thumbs Down

BEWARE CORN OIL AND COUSINS

If fish-fat is good for arthritis, other fats are not. Don't stoke the fires of arthritis by eating too much of the land-based fats. These fats, in fact, tend to cancel out the anti-arthritic medicine in fish. That means if you eat a nice hunk of salmon along with a salad doused in corn-oil dressing, or sardines with the typical mayonnaise, or fish fried in safflower oil, or even meat with your fish, you tend to defeat your good intentions and leave your joints to suffer. The worst enemies are the polyunsaturated fats high in so-called omega-6s, found in abundance in corn oil, safflower oil and sunflower oil and in the meat of animals fed such fats. Many experts worry increasingly about these fats.

The problem: Too much omega-6 type fatty acids, in comparison with omega-3 type fish fatty acids, dominates cell biochemical activity, spurring production of substances that trigger inflammation and other detrimental consequences. This does not happen because of any idiosyncratic "allergy" to such oils. The effect is universal, posing a potential hazard to everyone.

"Cut back on vegetable oils with omega-6s, if you suffer from any kind of chronic inflammatory disease," warns Harvard's Dr. George Blackburn. Such pro-inflammatory fats are also a primary reason eating meat can stimulate arthritis. The cooking oil with the best ratio of omega-3 to omega-6 fatty acids is rapeseed oil. Olive oil is all right also. (For a rundown of omega-3 and omega-6 fatty acids in oils, see page 463.)

 Thumbs Up

THE GINGER REMEDY

Try ginger to relieve your rheumatoid arthritis. The spice, too, is an anti-inflammatory agent, says Dr. Krishna C. Srivastava of Odense University in Denmark, an internationally known medical researcher on spices. Ginger has been used for thousands of years in Ayurvedic medicine, India's system of traditional medicine, to treat various rheumatic and musculoskeletal diseases. After mapping out theoretically how the spice works, Dr. Srivastava tested small daily doses on a group of arthritis patients for three months. Most had less pain, swelling and morning stiffness and more mobility.

He tells of one 50-year-old Asian auto mechanic who started taking ginger within a month of being diagnosed with rheumatoid arthritis. Every day he ate about 1¾oz (50g) of fresh ginger lightly cooked with vegetables and meats. His symptoms diminished after a month. After three months of ginger eating, the man was "completely free of pain, inflammation or swelling," and has remained so for ten years, says Dr. Srivastava.

Dr. Srivastava recently treated 50 patients successfully with ginger over a two-year period. The dose he routinely recommends to his arthritis patients is either ⅙oz (5g) of fresh ginger or ½g of ground ginger (about a third of a teaspoonful), taken three times a day. The fresh ginger can be incorporated in cooking, as can the ground ginger. If taken alone, the ground ginger is best dissolved in liquid or taken along with food so it does not burn your mouth. In such modest therapeutic doses, ginger appears to have no side effects, experts say.

 Thumbs Up

SPICES BEAT SOME ANTI-ARTHRITIS DRUGS

Ginger, in fact, is superior to the widely prescribed anti-arthritis drugs known as NSAIDs (non-steroidal anti-inflammatory drugs), says Dr. Srivastava. These NSAIDs bring relief mainly by blocking formation of hormone-like substances that induce inflammation. All NSAIDs have major side effects, including inducement of stomach ulcers, discouraging their prolonged use.

In contrast, ginger works through at least two and probably more mechanisms. It blocks formation of both prostaglandins and other inflammatory substances called leukotrienes. Further, Dr. Srivastava suggests ginger's antioxidant activity breaks down inflammatory acids in the joints' synovial fluid.

Ginger is not the only arthritis-fighting spice. Dr. Srivastava notes that turmeric and cloves also combat inflammation. Turmeric has proved anti- inflammatory in animal tests, and curcumin, a prime compound in turmeric, improved morning stiffness, walking time and joint swelling in 18 patients with rheumatoid arthritis. In fact, 1,200mg of curcumin had the same anti-arthritis activity as 300mg of the anti-inflammatory drug phenylbutazone.

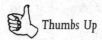 Thumbs Up

FISH AND GARLIC VS. OSTEOARTHRITIS?

Osteoarthritis is the so-called "wear and tear" arthritis that results in knobby fingers as we age, and is by far the most common type. Since osteoarthritis also involves inflammation, fish oils might have an anti-inflammatory effect here too. In a small preliminary study of 26 patients, British researchers at St. George's Hospital Medical School in London found that small doses of fish oil, added to regular medication, did alleviate pain and made physical activity easier.

Dr. Srivastava has also found powered ginger effective in combating pain and swelling from the inflammation of osteoarthritis. In one test, three-quarters of those stricken who took a third of a teaspoon of powered ginger three times a day for up to two and a half years got considerable relief.

FOUR FOOD WAYS TO BEAT RHEUMATOID ARTHRITIS

• Look for allergic food triggers of arthritis. Be most suspicious of cereals and grains, notably corn and wheat, as well as dairy products and meats. Authorities suggest that you not try a wholesale elimination and reintroduction of foods in attempts to ferret out arthritis-triggering foods, without a physician's supervision. You can, however, eliminate a suspected food from your diet to see if symptoms let up. Wait for at least a couple of days to a week for symptoms to subside before eating the food again. If the symptoms return, you may want to stop eating the food.

• Forgo meat, especially bacon, pork and beef. You may have an intolerance of certain meats. Also, saturated meat fats can stimulate the inflammatory process. Try a meatless diet to see if it helps.

• Eat oily fish, such as salmon, herring, mackerel, sardines or tuna three or more times a week. Such fish oils are anti-inflammatory agents. Try a little daily ginger, another anti-inflammatory agent.

• At the same time, cut back on omega-6 type fat, concentrated in corn oil, safflower oil, sunflower oil and margarines made from these oils. They can undo the benefit from the fish oils and also upset the chemical balance of fatty acids in cell membranes, fostering inflammatory attacks on tissue and joints. Meat fats do the same thing.

If you have osteoarthritis, it's also wise to restrict the polyunsaturated oils of the omega-6 type, that is, corn oil and relatives, that can promote inflammation.

An intriguing possibility is garlic. Physicians in India noticed during a study of garlic's impact on heart disease that garlic eaters often got relief from joint pain, in particular those with osteoarthritis. During the test, subjects ate two to three raw or cooked garlic cloves every day. Garlic is known to affect prostaglandins that help control inflammation, but the bulb has not been tested specifically on arthritis sufferers.

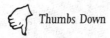 Thumbs Down

PLAIN OLD JOINT PAIN AND FOOD "ALLERGY"

If you have unexplained attacks of plain old joint pain, and yet no signs of arthritis, suspect a food allergy. Certain foods can trigger joint pain, inflammation and swelling, even though you do not have underlying arthritis. So says D. N. Golding, a rheumatologist at Princess Alexandra

Hospital in Harlow, Essex. He has documented what he calls "allergic synovitis," an inflammation of a synovial membrane that secretes fluid in the joint cavities to keep the joints lubricated and moving smoothly. With inflammation come joint pain and swelling, especially during bone movement. People most often stricken are those with various allergies, especially rashes, hives and hay fever.

Fascinating, says Dr. Golding, was the case of a 49-year-old woman with recurring hives and severe pain in various joints – fingers, wrists, knees, ankles, feet. At first doctors mistakenly thought she had rheumatoid arthritis, and put her on strong painkillers and anti-inflammatory drugs. The real culprit turned out to be milk and dairy foods.

Doctors looked on in amazement as she proved her predicament by drinking a glass of milk. Within a few hours her knee was swollen. Proof positive came when synovial fluid drawn from the knee joint showed signs of severe inflammation. Dr. Golding has also linked joint pain and synovitis with allergic reactions from eating eggs and cheese. He notes that acute or episodic attacks of joint pain are common and often unexplained, especially among allergy sufferers. In fact, an early study, done in 1943, found that 20 per cent of allergic patients had such rheumatic attacks. It's a clue worth pursuing if you have unexplained attacks of joint pain.

OSTEOPOROSIS

Foods That May Help: High-Calcium Foods • Nuts and Fruits • Pineapple Juice • Vitamin D

Foods That May Harm: Excessive Caffeine, Sodium, Alcohol

Everybody knows that getting your calcium (otherwise known as drinking your milk) helps build strong bones. And keeping strong bones can help save you from osteoporosis, that progressive bone-thinning disease that haunts over 2 million people in the UK. One in three women and at least one in twenty men are affected by osteoporosis resulting in 30 per cent of orthopaedic beds being taken by osteoporosis fracture patients. Every 10 minutes in this country someone has a fracture as a result of osteoporosis, including some 50,000 hip fractures, 50,000 wrist fractures and 40,000 spinal fractures, resulting in 40 deaths every day.

Although heredity is the number one determinant of whether you develop the bone disease, diet and other factors, like exercise, account for some of the risk, according to noted authority Robert P. Heaney, M.D., of Creighton University in Omaha, Nebraska. He cites new research showing the importance of lifelong calcium intake in combating the crippler. New evidence also suggests there's more to strong bones than wolfing down calcium. Other foods may help knock out the calcium you think you're storing up, and scientists have discovered that other nutrients are also essential for guarding against bone loss.

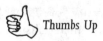 Thumbs Up

BORON FOR BONES

It's an unexpected new finding: An obscure trace mineral called boron can have a mighty influence on your prospects for osteoporosis. If you don't eat fruits and nuts, you don't get enough boron. That lack can hamper calcium metabolism, making your bones more brittle. New research shows that boron dramatically boosts blood levels of the hormone oestrogen and other compounds that prevent calcium loss and bone demineralization. In other words, boron acts as a mild "oestrogen replacement therapy".

Without adequate boron, your body cannot retain critical calcium, according to Dr. Forrest H. Nielsen at the U.S. Department of Agriculture's Human Nutrition Research Center in North Dakota. He discovered that postmenopausal women on low-boron diets were more likely to lose calcium and magnesium, bone-strengthening minerals. When they got 3mg of boron a day – easily obtained in food – their calcium losses dropped by 40 per cent.

Boron seems to work, says Dr. Nielsen, by boosting steroid hormones in the blood. In his studies, boron caused the most active form of oestrogen, *oestradiol 17B* to *double*, reaching levels found in women on oestrogen replacement. Blood levels of testosterone, the precursor to oestradiol, more than doubled.

Unfortunately, the average American gets only half the boron found effective in the studies. Dr. Nielsen suspects that boron deficiencies might explain why Americans who eat lots of high calcium dairy products are still prone to osteoporosis. It might also explain why vegetarians have less osteoporosis. Boron is richest in fruits, especially apples, pears, grapes, dates, raisins and peaches; in legumes, notably soya beans; in nuts, including almonds, peanuts and hazelnuts, and also in honey.

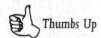 Thumbs Up

PINEAPPLE PROTECTION

To keep your bones strong, try drinking pineapple juice or eating other foods high in the trace mineral manganese. So advises Dr. Jeanne Freeland-Graves, professor of nutrition at the University of Texas at Austin. Manganese, like boron, is implicated in bone metabolism. Animals deficient in manganese develop severe osteoporosis, says Dr. Freeland-Graves. She also suspects the same thing is true in humans. Indeed in one study she discovered that women with osteoporosis had about one-third less manganese in their blood than healthy women. Further, when given manganese the diseased women absorbed twice as much, showing that their bodies needed it.

"Pineapple is full of manganese. When we want to up the content of manganese in the diet, we tell women to eat pineapple or drink pineapple juice," says Dr. Freeland-Graves. Manganese from pineapple, especially the juice, is readily absorbed, she observes. Other good sources of manganese are oatmeal, nuts, cereals, beans, whole wheat, spinach and tea.

 Thumbs Up

THE CALCIUM CONNECTION

The best known mineral with clout to ward off osteoporosis is calcium. It both builds strong bones and helps keep them from disintegrating in later years. Your best bet is to load up on calcium to create strong bones while you are young. Researchers at Indiana University recently studied identical twins, ages, 6–14. They found that the twin who got double the calcium up until the time of puberty had bones that were up to five per cent denser than the twin who merely ate about 900mg a day, a little more than the recommended daily allowance. This definitely gives the high calcium-consuming kids the edge, said researchers. Such youngsters have about a 40 per cent lower risk of fractures in later life.

A string of studies shows that eating calcium when you are young equals stronger bones and fewer fractures when older. But what if you goofed in childhood and did not get enough calcium? Eating calcium will not build bones, that is, increase their mass any, probably after age 30, says Dr. Heaney. Getting enough calcium after young adulthood is still critical because it helps retard bone loss, preventing fractures. Women should enter menopause with the strongest, heaviest bones possible. At that time, when oestrogen shuts down, calcium begins to drain from bones at dramatic rates. The idea is to keep bones strong by eating enough calcium to slow the losses. A recent study of 300 postmenopausal women found that raising calcium intake from 400mg (found in ½ pint (285ml) of milk) to 900mg a day (found in just over 1 pint (570ml) of milk) "abolished age-related bone loss in women six or more years past menopause". Another new study showed that women and men who ate more than 760mg of calcium a day had 60 per cent fewer hip fractures than those eating less than 400mg.

How much calcium is enough? Postmenopausal women can probably get full bone protection from 900–1,000mg of calcium per day, says Dr. Heaney. He cautions that calcium does not have magical properties to prevent or reverse bone loss and fragility due to other factors. That is, eating lots of calcium cannot overcome a genetic predisposition to osteoporosis. All calcium can do is correct a calcium deficiency, that does contribute to osteoporotic fractures, says Dr. Heaney. The National Osteoporosis Society based in Radstock, Avon now recommend 1000mg daily for everyone over the age of 12 raising to 1200mg for pregnant and nursing women and 1500mg for pregnant and nursing teenagers or women over 45 years of age not on HRT.

If milk disagrees with you, don't despair. There are many excellent calcium sources besides dairy foods, including kale and tofu. In fact, you absorb calcium from kale much better than from milk, says Dr. Heaney. Interestingly, women in Asian countries have very little osteoporosis, although they consume low amounts of milk and other dairy foods. By far, most of their bone-protective calcium comes from non-dairy foods, such as green leafy vegetables and soya beans. (See page 457–8 for a list of foods high in calcium.)

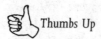Thumbs Up

VITAMIN D STRENGTHENS BONES

Be sure to get enough vitamin D, especially if you are an older woman. Without enough vitamin D, bones grow weaker. Postmenopausal women need 10 per cent more than the RDA for the vitamin to prevent calcium loss, according to a study of 333 such women by Elizabeth A. Krall, Ph.D., at the U.S. Department of Agriculture's Research Center at Tufts University. Worse, she says, most women don't come close to getting the RDA for vitamin D. The average intake in her study was only 112 international units (IU); the RDA is 200 IU. She says older women need at least 220 IU, because they lose the ability to absorb vitamin D as they age.

New Zealand researchers at the University of Otago also found that women taking vitamin D for two or three years had fewer fractures than women who got only calcium. The vitamin D was more therapeutic for those in the early stages of osteoporosis than in the advanced stages.

An excellent source of vitamin D is fatty fish. 3½oz (100g) of canned salmon contain 500 IU of vitamin D. The same amount of canned sardines contains 300 units. Eel is especially high with 5,000 IU per 3½oz (100g). An 8fl oz (225ml) glass of milk has 100 IU. The problem is worse in winter. Since sunlight is a good source of vitamin D, human levels of the vitamin fall in winter, even among people living in the South. (For a list of foods high in vitamin D, see page 461.)

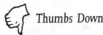 Thumbs Down

SALT – THE CALCIUM THIEF

Too much salt could help destroy your bones by robbing them of calcium, especially if you are elderly. New Zealand researchers first put elderly women on a low-salt diet (1,600mg of sodium daily), then switched them to a high salt diet (3,900mg of sodium daily). They ate the same amount of calcium on both diets. Yet, on the high salt diet, about 30 per cent more calcium was flushed out of the body, diverting it away from bones. The researchers say this could be detrimental at any age, but especially to elderly women at high risk of osteoporosis and bone fractures.

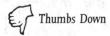 Thumbs Down

CAN DRINKING COFFEE BREAK YOUR HIP?

Drinking up to three cups of coffee a day seems safe, says Dr. Heaney. One fear is that caffeine fosters osteoporosis by promoting excretion of calcium, robbing bones of the mineral. Some studies have suggested dangers. A look at 3,170 older men and women who participated in the famous Framingham Heart Study indicated that two or more cups of coffee a day boosted the chances of breaking a hip by about 50 per cent, although a single cup seemed safe.

Now Dr. Heaney and colleagues have amassed new-evidence from a rigorously controlled double-blind study of premenopausal women, in which some got caffeine in capsules, comparable to drinking about three cups of coffee a day, while the rest got placebos. All ate about 600mg of calcium a day. For 24 days of the study they were hospitalized in a metabolic unit where their diet was controlled and their blood was analysed every day. The surprising finding was that the caffeine did not significantly reduce calcium absorption or excretion. "We don't see any evidence moderate caffeine intake is detrimental," said Dr. Heaney. What about higher doses? Maybe.

Indeed, a recent Harvard study of 84,000 middle-aged women found that those who drank more than four cups of coffee a day were about three times more likely to suffer hip fractures than women who drank little or no caffeine or coffee. Tea exhibited no detrimental effect. A high-caffeine intake combined with a low-calcium intake is particularly risky.

DIET PRESCRIPTION TO PREVENT OSTEOPOROSIS

The best prevention is to get adequate levels of critical nutrients that build and preserve bone density, such as calcium, boron, manganese and vitamin D, during your entire lifetime.

• After menopause and the loss of oestrogen, eating certain foods with oestrogenic activity, such as soya beans and high-boron foods, may help boost oestrogen levels, helping protect against development of osteoporosis.

• If you are a young woman, eat sufficient fat or cholesterol to maintain normal body fat and oestrogen levels to sustain normal menstrual periods.

• Go easy on foods and beverages that steal calcium. Keep coffee intake below three cups a day. Restrict sodium, which can flush calcium out of the body, weakening bones.

• If you drink alcohol, a drink a day may help bones; heavy drinking destroys them.

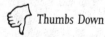 Thumbs Down

BONE-BREAKING BOOZE?

The surprising truth is that a little alcohol, from three to six drinks a week, can actually raise oestrogen levels in postmenopausal women, helping prevent osteoporosis, according to University of Pittsburgh researchers. Larger doses of alcohol, however, do not boost oestrogen further and can be very harmful to your bones as well as the rest of your health.

There's evidence excessive alcohol intake fosters osteoporosis by directly attacking and destroying bone cells. At autopsy, alcoholics have bones that look like those of people 40 years older, says Dr. Heaney. The recent Harvard study found that drinking alcohol, especially beer and spirits, raised the odds of breaking both a hip and a forearm. The more alcohol consumed, the greater the risk. Women drinking two to three beers a day more than doubled their chances of breaking a hip compared with nondrinkers. More than four daily drinks of spirits boosted chances of a broken hip seven times!

The bone-safe dose – about the same as that recommended for other health conditions: no more than one or two drinks a day.

REPRODUCTIVE
FUNCTIONS

SEX, HORMONES AND FERTILITY

Foods That May Be Beneficial: Fruits and Vegetables • Foods High in Vitamin C and Folic Acid

Foods That May Be Damaging: High-Fat foods

It may surprise you to find out that food contains sex hormones and has the power to manipulate hormone concentrations in your body, influencing all sorts of functions including sex drive, reproduction, menopausal symptoms, cardiovascular disease and susceptibility to hormone-dependent cancers, such as breast cancer and prostate cancer. In fact, scientists now know that at least 300 plants, many of them edible, possess "oestrogenic activity". That is, they help regulate the female hormone oestrogen. Eating wheat bran, cruciferous vegetables (cabbage, Brussels sprouts, cauliflower, broccoli), legumes, and alcohol can cause oestrogen levels to fluctuate. Further, how much fat you eat helps regulate both female and male hormones. A fatty diet may play havoc with a man's hormones and thus, his sex life.

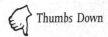 Thumbs Down

SHOULD RAMBO EAT HAMBURGERS OR PASTA?

What a shock! Although it's popular to portray real he-men as eating meat, presumably for virility, physical performance and courage in battle, meat, it turns out, may be more likely to create wimps. Eating meat with its accompanying fat does not seem the best way for men to boost their supplies of male hormones. In fact, several studies find that eating fatty meals may actually dampen sex drive by sending blood stores of the male hormone, testosterone, plunging.

A recent study by A. Wayne Meikle, professor of endocrinology and metabolism at the University of Utah School of Medicine in Salt Lake

City, found that blood testosterone levels plunged by about 50 per cent in a group of eight men after they downed fatty milk shakes containing 57 per cent of their calories in fat, 9 per cent in protein and 34 per cent in carbohydrates. In contrast, testosterone levels did not sink in the same men after they drank low-fat shakes in which 73 per cent of the calories came from carbohydrates, 25 per cent from protein and a mere 1 per cent from fat.

What does it mean? That a high-fat diet over time may curb a man's interest in sex, says Dr. Meikle.

"We looked only at the immediate result of one high-fat meal, though it may be hypothesized that after some time a high-fat diet could weaken a man's sex drive." – A. Wayne Meikle, M.D., University of Utah

---

There may even be a "double whammy" effect on sex drive from eating a steady diet of high-fat cheeseburgers, fried chicken, chips, cheese and ice cream, he says. Fatty foods make men fat, and men with higher body fat have sunken testosterone levels also. Additionally, a high-fat diet may eventually thwart erections. Eating fat helps clog the arteries that send blood to the penis, causing an erection, just as it clogs other arteries. Arterial blockages are a major cause of impotence.

FATTY FOODS AND OESTROGEN

The amount of fat women eat influences oestrogen levels. A high-fat diet boosts oestrogen. Thus cutting back on fat seems to deter breast cancers, and perhaps other hormone-dependent cancers, by giving them less oestrogen to feed on. Several studies show that both premenopausal and postmenopausal women who cut back significantly on fat, say from 35–40 per cent of calories to 20 per cent, have significant drops in blood oestrogen levels.

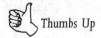 Thumbs Up

REJUVENATING AGED SPERM

If a man's sperm do not succeed at impregnation, there may be several reasons. They could be too few in number and volume, abnormal, or poor quality or too sluggish; they may tend to clump together, a condition called agglutination, so they can't move quickly. All these problems worsen with age. Swifter, more potent sperm belong to the young. In fact, sperm definitely begin a downslide in men starting around age 24. In one study, men age 45, when compared with men age 18, had a 30 per cent lower sperm count and sperm motility, 50 per cent more abnormal sperm and a 50 per cent drop in sperm viability. Consequently, three-quarters of the older men were infertile.

 Thumbs Up

A YOUTH ELIXIR FOR OLD AND TIRED SPERM

There is a sperm elixir of youth, so common as to be almost stunning — vitamin C. Solid studies indicate that getting enough vitamin C can perk up sperm, giving them new life and agility. Animal studies decidedly show that a vitamin C deficiency severely harms the testes, resulting in deficient sperm. In humans, bucking up vitamin C intake restores fertility. It's well known that men with sperm agglutination measurements in excess of 25 per cent cannot produce babies. When Dr. William A. Harris, a professor of obstetrics and gynaecology at the University of Texas Medical Branch in Galveston, gave such men 1,000mg of vitamin C per day for 60 days, the results were startling. Their sperm counts jumped by nearly 60 per cent; the sperm were 30 per cent more frisky, the per cent of abnor-mal sperm dropped – and, as supreme proof, all of the men getting the vitamin C had impregnated their wives at the end of the two-month trial. None of the "controls," those not taking vitamin C, managed to do so.

How much vitamin C is needed to rejuvenate ageing sperm? That was the focus of another study by Dr. Harris and University of Texas colleagues Dr. Earl B. Dawson and Leslie C. Powell. They tried two daily dosages, 200mg and 1,000mg. Their subjects were 30 men between ages 25 and 45, all in good health, but infertile. The doctors concluded that the higher dose of vitamin C worked faster, but after a couple of weeks the lower 200mg dose was just as effective at bringing sperm up to fertile quality. Thus both doses work, says Dr. Dawson, but "the higher dose just works about three times as fast".

The theory is that vitamin C works primarily because it is an antioxidant that protects semen from being degraded by attacks from renegade molecules called oxygen free radicals. For example, sterility-inducing clumping seems induced by oxidative damage. Scientists have documented that a substance called "nonspecific sperm agglutinin" (NSA) protects sperm by attaching to the surface of the spermatozoa but if the NSA is oxidized by the free radicals, it can no longer affix to sperm. Consequently, they clump together, paralyzing their forward march or motility.

It's impossible to define a sperm rejuvenation dose for all men, because how much vitamin C is needed to keep sperm functioning properly depends greatly, says Dr. Dawson, on how much a man is exposed to toxic compounds such as air pollutants, heavy metals, petrochemicals and cigarette smoke. Such toxins, Dr. Dawson believes, accumulate over the years in the tissues of the seminal gland where semen is produced. Thus a man who works in an oil refinery or smokes two packs of cigarettes a day needs more vitamin C to keep his sperm detoxified than a man who is not so chemically exposed. Such accumulation also helps explain why men become more infertile with age. Dr. Dawson estimates that 16 per cent of all men over age 25 suffer from sperm agglutination, signifying vitamin C deficiency and infertility. Dr. Dawson has documented that heavy smokers can improve the quality of their sperm in all ways by getting at least 200mg of vitamin C per day.

This proven effective dose is easy to get in food. Further, lower doses may also work, although it's unknown, because they have not been tested. Dr. Dawson suggests that men once exposed to noxious chemicals might want to take 1,000mg of vitamin C per day for a couple of months to cleanse their semen of toxic chemicals, hastening a return to fertility. After that, lower doses, supplied in the diet, could maintain sperm quality.

Dr. Dawson cautions that vitamin C restores fertility only in men who do not have other specific physical problems that prevent conception. A physician should rule out such possibilities before you put full faith in the powers of vitamin C, he advises.

A SPERM-ALERT DIET

It's easy to get a sperm enlivening dose of vitamin C through diet. The mere 200mg of the vitamin shown to restore sperm to normal functioning are found in each of the following foods:

- one and a half red peppers (212mg)

- 8oz (225g) fresh cooked broccoli (200mg)

- three kiwi fruit (222mg)

- one cantaloupe melon (226mg)

- three oranges (210mg)

- two 8fl oz (225ml) glasses of orange juice (208mg)

- 13oz (370g) cooked fresh cauliflower (204mg)

- 12oz (340g) raw strawberries (200mg)

There's a bonus from getting vitamin C in food instead of from a bottle. Food contains other substances that can also help block sperm deterioration, tests show. One is the antioxidant glutathione, concentrated in green leafy vegetables, asparagus and avocado.

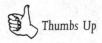 Thumbs Up

AN ORANGE A DAY KEEPS DEFECTIVE SPERM AWAY

Men who lack vitamin C are also more likely to pass on genetically damaged sperm that can cause birth defects. So found Bruce Ames, Ph.D., of the University of California, Berkeley. He analysed sperm from 24 men: 15 had subnormal levels of vitamin C; and of these, eight had high levels of genetic damage to their sperm. Such damaged sperm boosts the chances of birth defects in offspring. Amazingly, most men could get enough vitamin C in a single orange a day to protect their sperm from the genetic damage.

Dr. Ames explains that sperm cells are continually damaged by oxygen free radicals. Vitamin C, an antioxidant, blocks the damage. At the same time, cells work continually to repair this damage to the sperm but if the body's repair system becomes overloaded, partly because there is not enough counteracting vitamin C, a birth defect may get through. "It increases your probability. We don't know by how much," says Dr. Ames.

However, the margin of safety is tiny. In Dr. Ames' tests, the genetic damage to sperm occurred when vitamin C levels were only slightly below the RDA (recommended dietary allowance) of 60mg of vitamin C a day. A single orange contains 70mg of vitamin C, enough to counteract the damage. Smokers, however, need at least twice as much sperm-protecting vitamin C, because cigarette smoke annihilates so much of the vitamin's antioxidant powers, notes Dr. Ames.

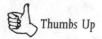 Thumbs Up

FOOD ANTIDOTE FOR SERIOUS BIRTH DEFECTS

Neural-tube defects, such as spina bifida and anencephaly, which can leave an infant with brain damage and paralysis, are heartbreaking. Yet women can dramatically slash the odds of these deformities by simply getting 0.4mg a day of folic acid, a B vitamin. Evidence of folic acid's amazing protection has been accumulating for a decade. A recent international eight-year study of 1,817 women by physicians at the Medical College of St. Bartholomew's Hospital in London clinched the case. All the women had previously given birth to babies with neural-tube defects. However, those who took 0.4mg of folic acid a day cut their odds of having another infant with such deformities by 72 per cent!

Although women who have had an infant with such a deformity are more likely to have another, most of the neural-tube deformities are first-time occurences. Thus, all foetuses are potentially at risk.

To keep your foetus safe, you must get enough folic acid before you get pregnant, says Dr. Godfrey Oakley of the Centers for Disease Control and Prevention. There is no time to act afterward because the defect occurs in the first 28 days after conception, before most women realize they are pregnant. Sufficient folic acid must be in your system for a month before conception as well as during the first three months of pregnancy, say experts.

ANTI-BIRTH DEFECT DIET

A daily 0.4mg-dose of folic acid found to prevent neural-tube birth defects can be obtained in an ordinary diet. For example, eating all of the following in a day would meet the requirement:

- 8fl oz (225ml) orange juice (0.07mg)

- 1oz (30g) All-Bran cereal (0.1mg)

- 3¼oz (90g) cooked spinach (0.13mg)

- 2¼oz (65g) cooked dried beans (0.12mg)

• BOTTOM LINE • *All women capable of getting pregnant should get 0.4mg of folic acid daily as a precaution against neural-tube defects. You can get that in several daily servings of fruits, vegetables (especially green leafy ones), cereals (many of which are fortified with folic acid) and legumes. For a list of foods high in folic acid, see page 458–9.*

MENSTRUAL PROBLEMS

> **Foods That May Alleviate Menstrual Problems:** Yoghurt and High-Calcium Foods • Carbohydrates • High-Manganese Foods • Soya beans • Other "Oestrogenic" Foods
>
> **Foods That May Aggravate Menstrual Problems:** Caffeine • A Very-Low-Fat Diet

If you have menstrual problems, you may be able to alleviate them with diet. Scientists have long known that food can influence the female hormone oestrogen, affecting menstruation, and that carbohydrates are strongly linked to premenstrual syndrome (PMS). Now research reveals surprising new clues about how certain food and nutrients, including calcium, manganese, and especially dietary fat and cholesterol, may influence menstruation.

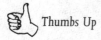 *Thumbs Up*

CALCIUM SUBDUES MOOD SWINGS

An extra glass of skimmed milk or serving of greens a day may help cure and prevent mood swings and physical pain before or during your period. The reason is that you would be getting twice as much calcium as the average American woman gets – 1,300mg a day instead of the average 600mg daily. This much seems to alleviate such menstrual discomfort, according to James G. Penland, Ph.D., a psychologist at the U.S. Department of Agriculture.

Dr. Penland had a small group of women with typical menstrual cycles take either 600mg or 1,300mg of calcium a day for six months. The women getting the low dose calcium showed decidedly more signs of PMS, notably in the week before their menstruation. They were subject to greater mood swings, characterized by irritability, anxiety, crying and depression. Their work performance and efficiency also dropped just prior to and during menstruation. Additionally, they also had more headaches, backaches, cramps and muscle stiffness during menstruation. Why eating less calcium had these detrimental consequences, and precisely how calcium fits into the complex puzzle of PMS, is unclear, said Dr. Penland.

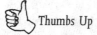 *Thumbs Up*

THE TEA AND TOAST CURE FOR HEAVY FLOW

Concerned about heavy menstrual flow? It could be largely due to skimping on foods rich in manganese. So says Phyllis Johnson, Ph.D., of the U.S. Department of Agriculture's Human Nutrition Research Center in Grand Forks, North Dakota. She made the discovery during a study of 15 young women who were on low-manganese diets for five and half months. They ate a mere 1mg of manganese per day – about half the national average. To Dr. Johnson's surprise, the women's menstrual flow increased in volume by about 50 per cent. The increased blood loss also swept away between 50 and 100 per cent more iron, copper, zinc and manganese.

Why the bleeding was so much heavier is a mystery but "it's the first time research has turned up any kind of dietary effect on menstrual flow," Dr. Johnson says. To help prevent such abnormally heavy menstruation losses, eat more foods rich in manganese, such as fruits (especially pineapple) and vegetables, whole grains, nuts and seeds. "Tea also has a great deal of manganese," she adds.

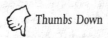 *Thumbs Down*

TOO LITTLE FAT TO MENSTRUATE

One of the greatest threats to menstruation and reproductive functioning is a deficiency of fat both in the diet and in the body. In fact, if women do not have sufficient levels of LDL cholesterol, traditionally called the "bad fat," they may not menstruate normally, says Laurence M. Demers, Ph.D., professor of pathology and medicine at Pennsylvania's Milton S. Hershey Medical Center. It's ironic, he says, that some young women, through fanatic exercise and ill-advised dieting, try to get their body fat and LDL blood cholesterol as low as possible, thereby wrecking their menstrual cycles, making them temporarily infertile and susceptible to fragile bones and osteoporosis in later years.

Dr. Demers explains that the female hormone oestrogen, which regulates menstruation, is partly derived from fat and cholesterol. "People think the ovary makes oestrogens, but the fat tissue also makes oestrogens. That is an important source for overall levels of oestrogen. When your body is starved of fat, it shuts down reproductive functions. Therefore, you need a certain percentage of body fat to bring about normal hormone production for normal menstrual regularity." You also need a critical amount of LDL cholesterol, he adds, because oestrogen is synthesized from the precursors of LDL cholesterol. Young women with very low levels of LDL cholesterol put themselves in a hazardous situation, says Dr. Demers. For unknown reasons, vegetarian women are especially susceptible to irregular menstrual periods, regardless of their fat intake.

The solution: Eat enough fat to keep body fat stores and cholesterol at sufficiently high levels to support normal regular menstruation. Monounsaturated fat, as in olive oil, is a good bet.

PMS – ARE SWEETS A CAUSE OR A CURE?

Do some women with PMS crave carbohydrates as a "self medication" to help relieve their symptoms? Or does eating too many sweets help bring on symptoms of PMS? In other words, are carbohydrates, including sugar and chocolate, a cure or a cause of PMS? If you suffer with PMS should you eat more carbohydrates or less?

Recent evidence comes down on the side of eating carbohydrates to stave off symptoms of PMS. Compelling research by MIT's Judith Wurtman has found that women with PMS symptoms often recover quickly when they eat carbohydrates, but not other foods. In one test, Dr. Wurtman had women with PMS live at an MIT Research Center for a few days during the premenstrual and postmenstrual parts of their cycle. At first, they were allowed to eat whatever they wanted. Invariably, women with the most severe PMS chose the most carbohydrates, including both sweets and rolls, pasta and potato salad – but only when they were premenstrual.

As a clincher, Dr. Wurtman then did a test in which she had women, both PMS sufferers and nonsufferers, eat a specific dose of carbohydrates – 1½oz (40g) of cornflakes with low-protein artificial milk. The PMS sufferers were typically depressed, angry, hostile fatigued and irritable.

Within an hour of eating the carbos, the women's spirits had lifted dramatically. "It was just like taking a Valium," exclaimed Dr. Wurtman. On mood-assessment tests the women reported 43 per cent less depression, 38 per cent less confusion, 47 per cent less fatigue, 42 per cent less tension and 69 per cent less anger. Cornflakes did not alter the moods of non-PMS sufferers (controls) or PMS sufferers in their post–menstrual week. Dr. Wurtman believes carbohydrates produce higher concentrations of the neurotransmitter serotonin, elevating mood.

Women with PMS should not deny a craving for carbohydrates, such as desserts, sweets, bread, potatoes, rice, pasta and cereals, insists Dr. Wurtman. "That craving represents a cure for PMS not a cause," she says.

Deborah J. Bowen, Ph.D., a psychologist at the University of Washington, agrees. Her studies have found that women who cater to food cravings report fewer menstrual problems, such as cramp and sluggishness, than women who don't.

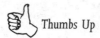 Thumbs Up

NEW CARBO DIET FOR PMS

Some British doctors also agree that carbohydrates are good medicine for PMS, and have even come up with a high-carbohydrate diet to relieve PMS symptoms. They have found that eating a small portion of starchy carbohydrates (bread, potatoes, pasta, oats or rice) every three hours and within one hour of going to bed or getting up combated PMS symptoms. In a study of 84 women with severe PMS, they discovered that typically seven hours passed between consumption of starchy carbohydrate foods during the day and 13 hours overnight. So they asked the women to go on an every-three-hour starch regimen – or six small meals a day. The three-hour carbo regimen was dramatically successful, relieving symptoms in 70 per cent of the women. Nearly one-quarter of them were able to control PMS symptoms with diet alone

British researchers have a differing explanation for effectiveness of the carbo-treatment. They suggest that regularly eating carbos helps maintain a steady blood sugar level throughout the waking day. Long intervals between carbohydrate intake results in dips and rises of blood sugar with the release of adrenaline that prevents full utilization of prog-esterone, a female hormone. Sugar and carbo binges, common in women with PMS, may be attempts to get blood sugar up, bringing progesterone back to proper levels, relieving symptoms, they theorize.

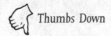 Thumbs Down

ANOTHER THEORY: BLAME CAFFEINE

If PMS is so disabling it upsets your life, try giving up caffeine beverages for a couple of months to see if the symptoms let up. So advises Dr. Annette Rossignol, an associate professor of public health at Oregon State University. Dr. Rossignol first noted that women in China who drank one-half to four cups of tea a day were twice as likely to have PMS as non-tea drinkers. Drinking from four and a half to eight cups a day increased their PMS incidence about tenfold.

Dr. Rossignol then followed up with a study of 841 female American students. Here, too, caffeine seemed to be a culprit. Those consuming at least one cup of a caffeine-containing beverage per day, such as coffee, tea or soft drinks, were more prone to PMS. The more caffeine they consumed, the more severe their PMS symptoms. Not all individuals had their PMS worsened by caffeine; some may be more sensitive to caffeine's effects than others, suggests Dr. Rossignol. You can find out fairly quickly if you are so affected. "You can tell within two or three months of giving up caffeine whether it is contributing to PMS," says Dr. Rossignol. How caffeine might promote PMS is unknown.

CAN FOODS REPLACE OESTROGEN AFTER MENOPAUSE

When women stop making oestrogen, they enter into menopause, sometimes suffering side effects, such as hot flushes and mood disturbances. The lack of oestrogen may also boost the risk of heart disease and osteoporosis in later years. Is it possible to help overcome oestrogen depletion by eating foods that boost the body's supply of oestrogen, thus softening the symptoms of menopause? "Yes, that is a definite possibility," says Mark Messina, Ph.D., a nutritionist formerly with the American National Cancer Institute. To what extent is unknown and depends on women's individual responses, but some research suggests that eating soya beans, as well as flaxseed, can stimulate oestrogen in postmenopausal women.

Fascinating studies by Mark L. Wahlqvist, professor of medicine at Monash University in Victoria, Australia, revealed oestrogenic activity from eating soya beans and flaxseed. Dr. Wahlqvist's group studied 25 postmenopausal women not taking oestrogen replacement. They ate their regular diet for two weeks. Then for two weeks in turn they ate a diet rich in soya flour (1½oz (40g) a day), red clover sprouts or flaxseed (about 1oz (30g) a day). All of these have produced oestrogen activity in animals.

Both soya flour and flaxseed did raise oestrogen levels and activity. According to Dr. Wahlqvist, a sensitive indicator of oestrogenic activity is vaginal cell maturation. Vaginal smears revealed significantly increased oestrogenic activity in the women eating soya and flaxseed. A couple of weeks after the women went off their special diets, their cell measurements returned to normal.

Only high-protein soya bean products have oestrogenic activity. That means soya beans, textured soya protein, tofu, soya milk and tempeh, but not soya sauce and soya bean oil.

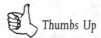 Thumbs Up

THE FRUIT-AND-NUT CHEMICAL BOOSTS OESTROGEN

Eating foods rich in the mineral boron can boost oestrogen levels in postmenopausal women to a stunning degree – as much as taking oestrogen replacement therapy does, according to studies by U.S. Department of Agriculture researcher Dr. Forrest Nielsen. Boron seems to work, he says, by boosting steroid hormones in the blood. He documented that in women getting adequate amounts of boron, the most active form of oestrogen – oestradiol 17B – doubled, reaching levels found in women on oestrogen replacement.

The diet of the average American contains about half the boron found effective in the studies. High levels of boron are found in fruit, especially apples, pears, grapes, dates, raisins and peaches; in legumes, especially soya beans; in nuts, including almonds, peanuts and hazelnuts; and in honey. You could get the doses used in the study by eating a couple of apples a day and 3½oz (100g) of peanuts.

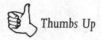 Thumbs Up

BEER AND BOURBON BOOST OESTROGEN

Surprisingly, a beer, a shot of spirits, a glass of wine or other alcoholic beverage imbibed every other day, can raise oestrogen levels in older women, possibly alleviating menopausal problems, as well as warding off heart disease and osteoporosis. So says Judith Gavaler, Ph.D., associate research professor of medicine at the University of Pittsburgh. Her recent studies of postmenopausal women suggested that three to six drinks a week boost natural oestrogen levels about 10–20 per cent as much as oestrogen replacement therapy does. Moreover, the alcohol effect equalled oestrogen replacement in reducing the risk of heart disease. Dr. Gavaler emphasizes, however, that more than six drinks a week does not further raise oestrogen.

Alcohol itself can boost oestrogen, says Dr. Gavaler, possibly by stimulating the activity of an enzyme that converts androgens into oestradiol. But interestingly, oestrogen boosts from alcoholic beverages do not come entirely from the alcohol. Dr. Gavaler found that both alcohol-free beer and bourbon concentrate, derived mostly from corn, also spiked oestrogen production in animals and postmenopausal women. Thus, some oestrogenic activity stems from natural hormones in grain, hops and other plants used to make alcoholic beverages. She has isolated two such plant oestrogens in beer. Dr. Gavaler favours a comprehensive screening of common foods for oestrogenic activity – something that has never been done – so women can know which foods affect oestrogen levels.

A question: Could eating foods that boost oestrogen promote breast cancer? Dr. Stephen Barnes, at the University of Alabama, answers that often-asked question by noting that soya beans, for example, have an odd oestrogenic effect that actually appears to counter breast cancer. He theorizes that soya beans work much like the anti-breast-cancer drug tamoxifen. Paradoxically, he says, the soya bean hormones protect breast cells from cancer, and if soya beans do perform like tamoxifen, they can be expected also to help prevent osteoporosis and bone loss, as tamoxifen does, he says. However, much more research is needed to sort out the very complex consequences for both women and men of eating foods that can manipulate hormones.

OESTROGEN IN AMERICAN YAMS? A MAJOR MYTH

Some doctors tell postmenopausal women to eat yams as a partial substitute for oestrogen replacement. A letter in the *Journal of the American Medical Association* even suggested that women could get some oestrogen from uncooked yams if they ate large quantities of them, possibly alleviating vaginal dryness and helping prevent osteoporosis.

Don't count on it, say experts. Dr. Norman Farnsworth, an authority on plant hormones at the University of Illinois in Chicago, notes that the small orange-type yams, more accurately called sweet potatoes, found in good supermarkets have insignificant oestrogenic activity. True yams, which contain diosgenin, a steroid that was the source of the original birth control pill, are tropical or Mexican wild yams. (Common edible American yams do not contain diosgenin.) Even so, such wild yams are virtually inedible, says James Duke, the U.S. Department of Agriculture's expert on medicinal plants, because the yam's oestrogenic compounds or phytosterols "are so soapy and bitter tasting".

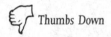 Thumbs Down

HOT FLUSH TRIGGERS: HOT DRINKS AND ALCOHOL

As logical as it may seem, many women do not consider that drinking hot fluids and/or alcohol can bring on hot flushes. That they can was proved decidedly by physicians at Withington Hospital in Manchester. Dr. K. A. McCallum, in tests of women in menopause and men receiving therapy for prostate cancer, found that quickly drinking a hot cup of tea or coffee was likely to bring on hot flushes – defined as a feeling of rising heat in the upper body accompanied by a sensation of general heating with visible reddening of the face and neck, sometimes along with profuse sweating and palpitations. In fact, the greatest number of flushes developed within ten minutes after drinking tea or coffee and lasted about a minute and a half. Drinking a shot of 40-proof whisky also produced nearly as many flushes. Both the hot drinks and the whisky produced many more flushes than did sitting close to a heater.

The researchers concluded that the hot coffee, tea and whisky all caused a "thermogenic insult on body temperature control mechanisms," which then triggered an exaggerated physiological response to try to maintain body temperature.

When subjects in the study reduced the temperature of their hot drinks the frequency of flushing dropped, in some cases by half.

DIABETES AND OTHER FOOD CONNECTIONS

DIABETES

In 1550 B.C., the famous Ebers Papyrus advised treating diabetes with high-fibre wheat grains. Not much has changed. Plant foods are still the drug of choice, but now scientists have much more sound reasons for thinking they work. Through the centuries more than 400 plants have been prescribed as diabetes remedies. In Europe, Asia and the Middle East, raw onions and garlic have long been favourite anti-diabetic drugs. Ginseng is popular in China. The common edible mushroom is widely used in some parts of Europe to control blood sugar. Barley bread is a common treatment in Iraq for diabetes. Cabbage, lettuce, turnips, beans, juniper berries, alfalfa and coriander seeds turn up as diabetes treatments in many cultures.

The surprising fact is such food remedies do have an anti-diabetes rationale. Modern tests confirm that all of them, or compounds isolated from them, can lower blood sugar and/or stimulate insulin in animals, humans or cell cultures.

WHAT DIABETES IS AND HOW FOOD CAN AFFECT IT

Diabetes is essentially too much sugar in the blood. It happens when your pancreas produces either no insulin or insufficient or ineffective insulin, the hormone that stimulates cells to absorb and store glucose (sugar). If the insulin can't handle glucose, blood sugar levels rise abnormally, causing much havoc, including excessive urination and thirst, weakness, fatigue and cardiovascular and kidney damage.

There are two main types of diabetes. The more severe, less common Type I diabetes strikes children and sometimes young adults, usually under age 35. Since cells of the pancreas that secrete insulin are gradually destroyed, presumably by some sort of immune reaction, Type I diabetics must take insulin injections because their pancreas produces virtually no insulin. Type I is also known as insulin-dependent diabetes or juvenile diabetes.

A far wider threat to most Britains is Type II diabetes, which almost always develops after age 40. Ironically, people with this type diabetes often have lots of insulin, but it doesn't perform well because cells are "resistant" to it. Such diabetes, also called noninsulin-dependent or adult-onset, accounts for 75 per cent of all cases, afflicting some one million Britains, perhaps as many as a quarter who do not know they have it.

Since what you eat has a major impact on blood sugar and insulin, food is a prime player in triggering, exacerbating and controlling diabetes.

Here are some ways food can affect diabetes:

• Overloads of certain foods that cause sharp spurts of blood sugar put burdens on insulin; restricting such foods keeps blood sugar levels more even.

• Certain foods contain compounds that stimulate the activity and potency of insulin or act directly to regulate blood sugar.

• Antioxidants in food, such as vitamins C and E, may ward off free radical attacks on beta cells that worsen inflammation and other damage. Such antioxidants also counteract oxidation of diabetics' LDL cholesterol, which is more susceptible to harm than that of nondiabetic individuals. Type II diabetics are two to three times more vulnerable to heart disease than nondiabetics.

• Especially intriguing is the prospect that the onset of Type I diabetes may be fostered by very complex delayed "allergic reactions" to food constituents, such as proteins in milk.

"It's incorrect to say that sugar causes diabetes. The real cause is insufficient or ineffective insulin – the hormone that controls how the body metabolizes sugar. To blame sugar is to put the cart before the horse." – Dr. Gerald Bernstein, American Diabetes Association.

DIET CAN BE THE CATCH

The development of diabetes is complex and ill understood. But current theory holds that you are born with a vulnerability to diabetes, and then something in the environment, including diet, sets in motion events that trigger overt symptoms of disease.

Diet and diabetes have always been intimately connected, perhaps not surprisingly, because diabetes is a disorder of the pancreas, the gland that produces insulin, which is required to turn foods into energy. First, your stomach breaks down carbohydrates into glucose, a common sugar. The pancreas responds by turning out insulin needed to transport the glucose from the bloodstream into muscles, where it is stored or converted to energy. At one time eating too much sugar was thought to cause diabetes, but no longer. The development of diabetes is far more complex and still very mysterious but it does not happen overnight. It usually takes years to develop. During that critical phase, your food choices can help defeat a genetic susceptibility to diabetes.

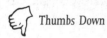 Thumbs Down

MILK: A CAUSE OF JUVENILE DIABETES?

Don't give infants cow's milk, especially if there is a history of diabetes in the family. As fantastic as it may seem, drinking cow's milk during infancy may trigger Type I diabetes years later in genetically prone youngsters. This suggests juvenile diabetes is a vicious type of "food allergy". It also means that keeping infants away from dairy foods in the first year of life, probably the most critical period, might save numerous children from the fate of diabetes.

Evidence that milk can incite juvenile diabetes is mounting. Here's how experts think it happens. Certain proteins in cow's milk provide the antigen (foreign substance) that fools the immune system into attacking its own tissue – in this case, the crucial beta cells in the pancreas, destroying those cells' ability to make insulin. Indeed, a new study by Hans-Michael Dosch and colleagues at the Hospital for Sick Children in Toronto has discovered antibodies, indicating an immune reaction to specific milk proteins, in the blood of 100 per cent of a group of children with Type I diabetes. Only 2.5 per cent of nondiabetic children in the study had such antibodies. The researchers have no doubts that the proteins could have triggered allergic immune reactions leading to diabetes. In laboratory rats, milk proteins decidedly trigger diabetes by destroying insulin-secreting beta cells.

Further, infants who are breast-fed and deprived of cow's milk for longer periods are much less likely to develop diabetes. In another incriminating new study, researchers at Children's Hospital in Helsinki compared early exposure to cow's milk with later risk of diabetes. They found that exclusively breastfeeding infants during the first two to three months of life slashed their chances of developing diabetes by age 14 by 40 per cent! Withholding cow's milk for longer periods also further reduced diabetes odds. Infants not given supplemental cow's milk-based formulas until four months of age had a 50 per cent lower risk of developing diabetes.

Swedish researchers at Karolinska Institute in Stockholm have also found that youngsters from birth to age 14 who eat more high-protein, high-complex-carbohydrate foods and foods containing nitrosamines are more likely to develop diabetes. They theorize that certain proteins may directly attack the beta cells of the pancreas; for example, foods rich in complex carbohydrates, such as bread, are also often rich in wheat gliadin, a protein shown to harm beta cells in rats. Nitrosamines, cancer-causing agents sometimes found in cooked bacon, may also be toxic to beta cells, they speculated.

"We know that genetic factors predispose certain people to diabetes. But all of the data suggests that lifestyle factors, particularly diet and exercise, can determine whether those genetic factors actually manifest in the disease." – James Barnard, Ph.D., professor of physiological science, UCLA

AVOIDING DIABETES' SNEAK ATTACK

Type II diabetes can sneak up on you. You may not have diabetes now, but you could be on the verge of developing it. Being overweight is a formidable threat. Most people with such diabetes are overweight, and losing weight is usually a powerful deterrent or remedy. However, another hazard may be lurking to draw you into full-fledged diabetes. You may be one of the many normal-weight people who have insulin resistance or insulin sensitivity, as it is called. This means that your insulin is no longer able to perform as it should. Insulin resistance is a hallmark sign of Type II diabetes; it is also common in obesity. More alarming, it can foreshadow the development of diabetes. Insulin resistance frequently exists in people who are diagnosed with diabetes a decade or so later.

Here's how it can happen. Your cells become sluggish and inefficient in responding to insulin's instructions to take up glucose. Your pancreas, then, has to churn out more insulin constantly to keep blood sugar normal. Tired and overworked, the pancreas may finally become exhausted and unable to produce enough insulin, forcing your body to capitulate to full-fledged Type II diabetes. Many experts are convinced that what you eat through the years can help avert that final surrender. Insulin resistance is probably inherited, but remains hidden until it is triggered by an environmental happening, most likely diet.

Much research on diet is directed toward preventing the long march from insulin resistance, or glucose intolerance, to full-blown diabetes. Eating certain foods can help keep diabetes away.

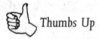 Thumbs Up

FISH FORESTALLS DIABETES

Eating fish may cut in half your chances of developing Type II diabetes. That startling fact comes from Dutch researchers at the National Institute of Public Health and Environmental Protection. They tested 175 normal healthy elderly men and women to be sure they were free of both diabetes and impaired glucose tolerance, a condition that often foreshadows diabetes. Four years later when they repeated the tests, they found many cases of impaired glucose tolerance but interestingly, only 25 per cent of those who regularly ate fish had developed the problem, compared with 45 per cent of non-fish eaters.

The researchers concluded that fish eaters were only about half as likely to develop diabetes as non-fish eaters. The clear message is that something in fish, perhaps the omega-3 type fat, seems to protect the body's ability to handle glucose, staving off diabetes. The amount of fish needed for protection was extremely small – a mere 1oz (30g) a day of lean, fatty or canned fish.

Caution: Diabetics should not take fish oil capsules except under a doctor's supervision. They have proved troublesome in glucose regulation for some diabetics.

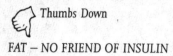 Thumbs Down

FAT – NO FRIEND OF INSULIN

Restrict fat; it can quicken your descent into diabetes. A recent study at the University of Colorado Health Sciences Center found that eating an extra 40g of fat a day (as found in a 4oz (115g) fast-food hamburger and large fries) triples your odds of developing diabetes! Excessive fat in the diet, especially saturated animal fat, seems to damage insulin's effectiveness. Researchers at the University of Sydney in Australia took cells from the muscles of older nondiabetic men and women undergoing surgery. They measured the saturated fatty acids in the cell membranes and tested the patients for insulin resistance. They found that the more saturated fatty acids in cells, the greater the insulin resistance. On the other hand, higher tissue levels of polyunsaturated fats, particularly fish oil, indicated better insulin activity and less resistance.

In fact, the researchers also reported that feeding animals omega-3 fish oils effectively overcame their insulin resistance.

In another study, eating fat diminished the efficiency of insulin, promoting abnormally high levels of blood sugar. Jennifer Lovejoy, Ph.D., an assistant professor at Louisiana State University, studied the eating habits and insulin activity of 45 nondiabetic men and women; about half were obese and half were normal weight. Both being obese and eating more fat increased insulin resistance. This means, says Dr. Lovejoy, that even normal individuals who eat lots of fat, notably animal fat, decrease their insulin efficiency and boost their vulnerability to diabetes.

• BOTTOM LINE • *Cutting down on saturated dairy and animal fats and eating more fatty fish may help stave off diabetes.*

"Potatoes are like sweets as far as a diabetic is concerned." – Phyllis Crapo, an associate professor at the University of California at San Diego, who discovered that mashed potatoes cause greater surges in blood sugar than ice cream does.

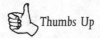Thumbs Up

THE ALLIUM MEDICINE

Eat onions. They have an ancient and respected place in medicine as a treatment for diabetes. Modern studies show that onions do have powers to lower blood sugar and at levels found in the diet. For example, Indian researchers fed subjects onion juice and whole onions (in doses of 25–200g) and found that the greater the dose, the more the blood sugar was depressed. It made no difference whether the onion was raw or boiled. The investigators postulate that the onions affect the liver's metabolism of glucose, or release of insulin, and/or prevent insulin's destruction.

The probable active hypoglycemic agents are *allyl propyl disulphide* and *allicin*. Indeed, as early as 1923, scientists detected blood-sugar depressors in onions, and in the 1960s, investigators isolated anti-diabetic compounds from onions that are similar to the common anti-diabetic pharmaceutical known as tolbutamide (Orinase) that stimulates insulin synthesis and release. In rabbits, the onion extract was 77 per cent as effective as a standard dose of tolbutamide.

Thumbs Up

BROCCOLI – THE BLOOD SUGAR WONDER

Eat broccoli; it is a super source of chromium, a trace mineral that seems to work wonders on blood sugar. If you have Type II diabetes, chromium can help regulate blood sugar, often reducing medi–cation and insulin needs. If you are on the verge of diabetes, chromium may save you from a plunge into full-fledged disease. Indeed, if your glucose tolerance is borderline, as it is in about a quarter of ordinary Americans, chromium can fix it. Even if your blood sugar is low instead of high, chromium can yank it back up to normal. Whatever the blood sugar problem, chromium tends to normalize it, says Richard A. Anderson, Ph.D., at the U.S. Department of Agriculture's Human Nutrition Research Center in Beltsville, Maryland. Dr. Anderson blames soaring rates of Type II diabetes partly on a deficiency of chromium in the diet and cites some 14 studies done during the 1980s, showing that chromium improved glucose tolerance.

Chromium seems to increase insulin's efficiency so you need less to do the job. How is a mystery, but Dr. Anderson notes that in test-tube experiments, biologically active chromium attaches tightly to insulin, enhancing by up to one hundred times the hormone's main mission of oxidizing glucose into carbon dioxide.

Yet, about 90 per cent of Americans get less chromium than the recommended 50–200 micrograms a day. Some high-chromium foods are nuts, oysters, mushrooms, whole grains, wheat cereals, beer, wine, rhubarb, brewer's yeast – and broccoli! One analysis found that 5oz (140g) of broccoli contained 22 micrograms of chromium, ten times more than any other food. Barley is also rich in chromium, perhaps helping explain the grain's longtime use in Iraq as a diabetes remedy. In animal experiments, barley helps suppress insulin surges.

 Thumbs Up

THE POWER OF CURRY SPICE

Don't overlook the power of fenugreek seeds, long used in the Middle East and India to treat several diseases, including diabetes. Now there's evidence the seeds may indeed help control diabetes.

Scientists at India's National Institute of Nutrition recently ground up fenugreek seeds and gave the powder to Type I diabetics. Their fasting blood sugar fell, their glucose tolerance improved, and their blood cholesterol went down. This caused the researchers to conclude that ground-up fenugreek seeds could be a useful anti-diabetic agent.

Israeli scientists at Hebrew University of Jerusalem also have shown that fenugreek seeds can lower blood sugar and cholesterol in both diabetics and healthy people. Additionally, they have identified an active ingredient of fenugreek seeds. It is a gel-like soluble fibre called *galactomannan*. In animal studies, the fenugreek gel binds up bile acids, lowering cholesterol, much the way common drugs do.

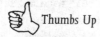 Thumbs Up

THE CINNAMON DRUG

Add spices to boost insulin activity. It may be more than our taste buds that inspire us to use cinnamon and cloves frequently to spice up sweet foods, such as pumpkin pie. Such spices actually have drug-like properties that help us handle the sugar in such sweets. The USDA's Dr. Anderson discovered that various spices help stimulate insulin activity, which means the body can process sugar more efficiently and therefore needs less insulin. Dr. Anderson did some test-tube experiments in which he measured insulin activity in the presence of certain foods. Although most showed no effect, three spices and one herb tripled insulin activity: cinnamon, cloves, turmeric and bay leaves. Cinnamon was the most potent.

Only a little cinnamon, such as the small amounts sprinkled on toast, can stimulate insulin activity, he says. A dash of cinnamon on any number of appropriate foods may help keep blood sugar in check.

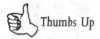 Thumbs Up

BRING ON THE BEANS

Eat high carbohydrate, high-fibre foods, like legumes, to keep diabetes away and under control. That's mainstay advice for anyone concerned about diabetes, according to experts such as James Anderson, M.D., at the University of Kentucky College of Medicine. He insists that the same foods that lower cholesterol and fight heart disease are excellent fare for diabetics, who are at high risk of heart disease. That especially means foods high in soluble fibre. (For a list of such foods, see page 50–51.) Dr. Anderson says more than 50 studies show that such high-fibre foods significantly hold down blood sugar along with triglycerides and cholesterol.

High-fibre diets work so well that many patients on such diets have decreased or eliminated their need for supplemental insulin and other anti-diabetic medications.

WHICH IS WORSE – CARROTS OR CANDY?

Eat foods that don't incite sharp long-lasting spurts in blood sugar. Such foods rank low on the so-called "glycemic index," a relatively new concept. For years it was assumed that simple carbohydrates (sugar) were far and away the major villain in boosting blood glucose and that complex carbohydrates (fruits, vegetables, grains and legumes, such as potatoes and carrots), which are slowly absorbed, were neutral or beneficial. In the late 1970s and early 1980s, that concept got a violent shaking up when several scientists, including Phyllis Crapo, R.D., of the University of California at San Diego, and David J. A. Jenkins, M.D., of the University of Toronto, measured blood sugar after feeding subjects a variety of foods. To virtually everyone's surprise, the most rapid rises in blood sugar were stimulated not by ice cream and candy bars, but by carrots, potatoes and processed cereals! The notion that complex carbohydrates are automatically safer for diabetics than simple carbos turned out to be myth.

A 10-year scientific argument has ensued over whether this sugar-boosting potential of individual foods, now called the "glycemic index," is of any practical significance. When you mix foods up in your stomach, does it really matter? Dr. Jenkins insists it does. His research indicates that eating foods low on the glycemic index improves overall blood sugar control in patients with both types of diabetes. Moreover, he stresses, the diets lower triglycerides.

FOODS MOST LIKELY TO BOOST BLOOD SUGAR

Here is the glycemic index, or impact on blood sugar, of common foods when compared with glucose, which produces the most potent blood-sugar rises. The higher the percentage, the greater the food's ability to spike blood sugar.

100 per cent: Glucose

80–90 per cent: Corn flakes, carrots, parsnips, potatoes (instant mashed), maltose, honey

70–90 per cent: Bread (wholemeal), millet, rice (white), broad beans (fresh), potato (new)

60–69 per cent: Bread (white), rice (brown), Muesli cereal, shredded wheat, water biscuits, beetroot, bananas, raisins, Mars bar

50–59 per cent: Buckwheat, spaghetti (white), sweetcorn, All-Bran, oatmeal biscuits, peas (frozen), yams, sucrose, potato crisps

40–49 per cent: Spaghetti (whole wheat), oatmeal, sweet potato, beans (navy), peas (dried), oranges, orange juice

30–39 per cent: Butter beans, lima beans, haricot beans, black-eyed peas, chickpeas, apples (Golden Delicious), ice cream, skimmed and whole milk, yoghurt, tomato soup

20–29 per cent: Kidney beans, lentils, fructose

10–19 per cent: Soya beans, peanuts

Source: Dr. David J. A. Jenkins

Both Dr. Jenkins and others point out that even people without diabetes benefit from eating foods low on the glycemic index. For one thing, such foods help prevent surges in insulin that may create insulin resistance, leading to diabetes. Also, new research shows that high levels of insulin in the blood are undesirable and may have other consequences, such as acting as a growth factor to promote cancer. Eating low-glycemic foods helps keep blood sugar down and hence insulin levels needed to process it.

WHAT DIABETICS SHOULD EAT AND DO EAT

Here's the best anti-diabetic diet, according to most experts in the United States and the United Kingdom: Eat 50–60 per cent of your calories in carbohydrates, less than 30 per cent in fat (less than 10 per cent in saturated fat) and 30–40g of fibre a day. According to a recent survey few diabetics meet the recommendations. Only 3 per cent of 92 patients studied ate 50 per cent or more of their calories in carbohydrates; in most the figure was about 40 per cent. Only 14 per cent kept their fat intake below 35 per cent of total calories; most ate 60–80 per cent more saturated fat than was deemed good for them. They found that 40 per cent of the men but only 10 per cent of the women got the advisable dose of fibre.

The researchers explained the disheartening situation by saying that "many diabetic patients had not seen a dietitian for years" and were possibly following outdated advice that once curbed carbohydrates.

 Thumbs Up

CALL IN ANTIOXIDANT VITAMINS

If you have diabetes, be extra sure to eat foods high in antioxidants, such as vitamins E and C and beta carotene, advises James Anderson, M.D., of the University of Kentucky College of Medicine. The reason is that the artery clogging process appears abnormal and more severe in diabetics. Specifically, diabetics' bad-type LDL cholesterol is more susceptible to oxidation, and thus more likely to become "toxic". In turn, such oxidized LDL is theoretically more likely to clog arteries. This might help explain why the risk of heart disease is two to three times higher in diabetics, says Dr. Anderson.

What causes the dangerous oxidized cholesterol? Probably diabetics' sustained high levels of sugar in the blood. As sugar is metabolized, it releases the oxygen free radicals that tend to make cholesterol toxic. You may help counteract them by zapping them with antioxidants.

ANTI-DIABETES DIET STRATEGIES

• To help prevent Type I diabetes, avoid giving dairy foods to infants for at least the first year of life.

• To ward off Type II diabetes, eat more fish, legumes, nuts and high-chromium foods such as grains and broccoli and lose excessive weight Also restrict fat, for it promotes insulin resistance.

• If you have diabetes, the diet recommended by most experts is a high-fibre, high-carbohydrate starchy diet, heavy in whole-grain breads, pasta, rice, oats and especially legumes, which are extremely low on the glycemic index. It takes such high-fibre starches longer to break down, so they are more gradually absorbed into the blood.

• Especially recommended are foods high in water-soluble fibre, such as legumes and oats. Such fibre turns into a gel in the digestive tract, stretching the time required for the absorption of sugar in foods and preventing dangerous post-meal blood sugar surges.

• The best all around advice is to eat the same diet as the one that helps prevent heart disease — foods that are low in fat, especially animal fat, and rich in high-fibre carbohydrates such as beans, oats, whole grains, nuts, fruits and vegetables.

OTHER FOOD CONNECTIONS

ACNE

If you fear that eating chocolate gives you acne or pimples, you are not alone. It is a common belief, but it's a medical myth. Dermatologists at the University of Pennsylvania proved it by persuading 65 acne-plagued adolescents to overdose on chocolate. Every day for a month they ate the amount of chocolate in 1lb (450g) of plain chocolate. For another month, they ate a dummy chocolate bar. The acne did not worsen when the kids binged on the real chocolate.

McIodine Threat

On the other hand, if you are acne-prone, beware of regularly eating too much iodine. Excessive iodine can irritate pores, bringing on acne flare-ups. You get iodine in iodized salt, of course but high amounts have also surprisingly been detected in fast foods and milk. Consumer's Union once found that the average iodine content of a fast-food meal was more than 30 times the recommended dietary allowance (RDA) of 150 micrograms daily – or an astonishing 4,500 micrograms of iodine per meal! A recent analysis of milk samples collected from 175 dairy herds throughout Wisconsin averaged 466 micrograms of iodine per litre; 11 per cent of the samples contained more than 1,000 micrograms of iodine per litre. The iodine gets in the milk through contaminated milking equipment and medication given to cows.

Among foods, seaweed, including that used to wrap Japanese sushi, is exceedingly high in iodine. Kelp – brown seaweed – is the highest source of iodine known, with a whopping 1,020 parts per million. Shrimp and shellfish are moderately high in iodine.

How much iodine it takes to raise pimples depends on an inherited sensitivity to iodine, says James E. Fulton, Jr., M.D., head of the Acne Research Institute in Newport Beach, California. "In some who are acne-prone, I'd say 1,000 micrograms or one milligram of iodine a day could be a problem." Other research showed that eating two kelp tablets a day, each containing 225 micrograms of iodine, triggered acne flare-ups.

There's also Swedish evidence that acne sufferers often have a zinc deficiency. The best sources of zinc? Shellfish, especially oysters and lobster, wheat germ, whole-grain cereals, peanuts, pecans, legumes, liver and turkey.

AIDS

There is no concrete evidence in humans that the HIV virus (the reputed cause of AIDS) can be prevented, slowed down or stopped by food substances but there are some intriguing possibilities from lab experiments. Certain foods and food compounds may help boost immune functioning, helping ward off some of the other diseases and infections associated with AIDS.

Vegetable Virus Stoppers
In test tubes, two food compounds have blocked the spread of the HIV virus – vitamin C and glutathione, a strong antioxidant, concentrated in fruits and vegetables. One astonishing experiment, by Dr. Alton Meister at Cornell University Medical College, found that glutathione blocked 90 per cent of the spread of the AIDS virus. Dr. Meister stimulated human cells to produce the AIDS virus in petri dishes. When he added glutathione, the virus replication slowed down dramatically, and the more glutathione added, the greater the effect. Dr. Meister says AIDS patients have exceptionally low levels of glutathione, and that a glutathione deficiency may contribute to the spread of AIDS. Glutathione is an antioxidant concentrated in fruits and vegetables. (See page 429.)

Immune-Boosting Mushroom
Any foods that bolster the immune system might help. One test found some amazing results from extracts of shiitake mushrooms. Japanese tests found shiitake more effective against the HIV virus than the common anti-AIDS drug AZT.

Infection-Fighting Garlic
Natural antibiotics such as garlic might be beneficial against the potentially devastating "opportunistic infections" that flourish when the immune systems of AIDS patients become depressed. Such common infections are tuberculosis and fungal infections of the lungs. In folklore and even in mainstream medicine, large amounts of garlic have been used to help cure such lung infections. For example, garlic was widely used by physicians to treat tuberculosis in the 1920s and 1930s before

the advent of modern drugs. Some physicians are investigating garlic's powers against opportunistic infections associated with AIDS.

• BOTTOM LINE • *Even though there is no human evidence that specific food compounds can fight or prevent AIDS, it still makes sense to take advantage of the known benefits of certain food compounds on immunity and infections. That means eating lost of fruits and vegetables, full of antiviral glutathione and carotenoids, including beta carotene, which have been shown to boost immune functioning. Garlic can't hurt either, and may help against opportunistic infections.*

BENIGN BREAST DISEASE

Small, noncancerous, but often painful lumps in the breast are known as benign breast disease or fibrocystic breast disease. You may be able to discourage these lumps by avoiding a family of food chemicals, called methylxanthines, of which caffeine is best known. John Minton, M.D., at Ohio State University, first raised the issue in 1979. He found that the benign lumps disappeared in 65 per cent of a group of women who gave up coffee, tea, colas and chocolate that contained the methylxanthines caffeine, theobromine and theophylline.

A large-scale 1985 study by Italian researchers at the "Mario Negri" Institute for Pharmacological Research found that the more coffee women drank, the greater their risk of benign breast lumps. One or two cups a day doubled the chances. Three or more cups a day nearly quadrupled the vulnerability to the lumps. However, after five cups a day, the risk leveled off.

Still, many studies have detected no connection. After a look at 3,400 women, the largest study ever done on the issue, the American National Cancer Institute weighed in with its opinion: There is no connection between methylxanthine intake and risk of fibrocystic breast disease.

• BOTTOM LINE • *Nevertheless, many women find that the pain in their breasts is relieved by cutting down on or cutting out caffeine sources and chocolate. Since it can't hurt and may help, it makes sense to try it. If it works for you, that's all that counts.*

Another possibility is cabbage. New research suggests that eating more cruciferous vegetables — cabbage, broccoli, cauliflower — may help curtail fibrocystic breast disease by speeding up metabolism to dispose more quickly of oestrogen that aggravates breast lumps, according to Jon Michnovicz of the Institute for Hormone Research in New York City.

BREAST-FEEDING

Mothers, to stimulate a nursing infant's appetite, eat a little garlic an hour before starting breast feeding. Yes, oddly, the strong flavour and odour of garlic in breast milk does just that, according to a study done at the Monnel Chemical Senses Center in Philadelphia.

To test the theory, researchers gave half of a group of nursing mothers a garlic capsule and the other half, an inactive pill.

A whiff of the milk taken from the garlic-eating mothers confirmed its pungent odour. Yet the babies liked it. They attached to the breast longer, sucked more and tended to drink more milk when it smelled of garlic.

One way to discourage your baby from taking more milk is to take a nip of alcohol before breast-feeding. That contradicts folklore belief that it spurs milk production and improves the infant's appetite. On the contrary, the infants drank "significantly" less milk from mothers who had downed orange juice spiked with alcohol.

The researchers think strong flavours in general whet a baby's appetite, and that alcohol either depresses it or impairs sucking ability or milk production.

CATARACTS

Eating vegetables, especially spinach, may save you from cataracts that often develop as you age. A cataract is a clouding of the lens of the eye that can cause loss of sight. According to a study in the British Medical Journal, spinach stood out as the food most likely to prevent cataracts in a group of elderly women. A probable reason is spinach's rich stores of antioxidants, including beta carotene. Indeed, the investigators found that women who ate the most beta carotene in fruits and vegetables were only 40 per cent as likely to develop cataracts.

The theory is that cataracts are believed to be partly caused by oxidation of the lens, for example, by sunlight striking the lens over the years. Thus, keeping the lens supplied with lots of protective antioxidant appears to counteract or delay cataract development.

Indeed, studies show that those who skimp on fruits and vegetables are much more likely to develop cataracts. For example, researcher Paul Jacques, at the U.S. Department of Agriculture, has found that people who eat less than three and a half servings of fruits and vegetables a day are four times more likely to get cataracts. Eating less than a serving and a half of fruits and vegetables hiked cataract odds six times!

Further, Dr. Jacques found that those with the lowest blood levels of vegetable carotenoids were seven times more likely to develop age-related cataracts, and those with scant vitamin C in their blood were 11 times more likely to have a certain type of cataract! Low levels of folic acid, found in green leafy vegetables such as spinach and broccoli, as well as legumes, also predicted cataracts. Drinking tea, packed with antioxidants, also appears to deter cataracts.

And Asparagus, Too

An ancient herbal formula called *hachimijiogan* has long been touted to prevent the progression of cataracts. Now research finds that the remedy actually increases levels of the antioxidant glutathione in the lens which is severely lacking in nearly all forms of cataracts. Such low levels may contribute to their formation. You get glutathione in many fruits and vegetables, including asparagus, avocado, watermelon and oranges. This mechanism may help account for vegetables' good showing against cataracts. (For a list of foods rich in antioxidants, see page 428.)

CHRONIC FATIGUE

If you or anyone you know has chronic fatigue, which may or may not be diagnosed as chronic fatigue syndrome, be aware that all that suffering could be caused by a delayed food allergy. The condition known as chronic fatigue syndrome is difficult to treat and is characterized by extreme fatigue and depression, which are often debilitating. However, Talal Nsouli, M.D., an allergist and associate clinical professor at Georgetown University School of Medicine, has found that food allergies are responsible in about 60 per cent of the patients who come to his clinic suffering from chronic fatigue. "It's almost unbelievable," he says. "When they avoid the foods, they recover fully."

The three most common culprits incriminated in chronic fatigue, he finds, are wheat, milk and corn.

If a food allergy is confirmed by a skin test and/or the common blood test, known as RAST, Dr. Nsouli then has the patient avoid the suspect food for three weeks. If there is improvement, the patient then does a "food challenge," eating the food again to see if symptoms return within a few days. If they do, that is convincing evidence the food is at fault.

In one case, an 18-year-old girl, diagnosed with chronic fatigue syndrome, was under psychiatric care for severe depression and was on antidepressant medication. She turned out to be allergic to wheat. "She went on a wheat-free diet and within three weeks the symptoms began to disappear. She stopped seeing the psychiatrist and quit taking the antidepressants and is doing fine," says Dr. Nsouli. Since remnants of the food may circulate in the body for a long time, it usually takes three to four weeks before you can expect to see improvement, he stresses.

CROHN'S DISEASE

Crohn's disease is an inflammatory disease of the colon that most often strikes children and young adults. The cause is unknown. But there is evidence of food intolerances. A group of British physicians at Addenbrookes Hospital in Cambridge have been treating active Crohn's disease successfully, they say, with diet for several years. They first determine which foods are linked to Crohn's flare-ups, then these foods are stricken from patients' diets. The treatment has worked as well as surgery and drugs, claims Dr. John O. Hunter. He says X-rays have often shown striking improvements; indicators of inflammation have become normal again.

"Patients who develop a satisfactory diet have overall relapse rates of less than 10 per cent a year, which matches the success of surgery," says Dr. Hunter. The diet is even more successful than typical medication, he claims. Foods most likely to induce Crohn's symptoms, Dr. Hunter finds, are wheat, dairy products, cruciferous vegetables (cabbage, broccoli, cauliflower, Brussels sprouts), corn, yeast, tomatoes, citrus fruits and eggs.

Eating yeast, indeed, proved detrimental to Crohn's patients in a recent test at Ninewells Medical School in Scotland. Adding a little yeast to the diets of those with Crohn's for a month stirred up more disease activity and flare-ups. When patients went on a low-yeast diet, their disease activity dropped dramatically. The worst flare-ups occurred in patients who exhibited antibodies to yeast, indicating a decided immune or "allergic" reaction. Yeast, of course, is found most notably in bread. The researchers speculated that some Crohn's patients have an abnormal immune response to certain foods that fosters inflammation.

Additionally, it's wise for Crohn's patients to eat more anti-inflammatory fatty fishes and shun pro-inflammatory animal fats and omega-6 vegetable oils. This should help mute inflammation.

A high sugar intake has also been linked to Crohn's.

EAR INFECTIONS

If your infant or child has chronic ear infections, be sure to investigate diet before resorting to expensive, hazardous and possibly unnecessary antibiotics and medical procedures. Amazing as it may seem, such persistent ear infections are often due to food allergies.

How could a youngster get ear infections because his food disagrees with him? Here's how it happens. A food allergy can trigger a chronic inflammation and swelling of the middle ear, leading to a stagnation of fluids that become overrun with bacteria. The result is a full-blown infection, medically known as *serous otitis media*, also popularly called "glue ear". If not properly treated, the infection can damage the bony structures of the ear, causing hearing loss and consequent learning problems.

Incredibly, new research shows that most chronic ear infections may be due to eating the wrong foods. In a recent major test, allergist-immunologists Talal M. Nsouli, M.D., and J. A. Bellanti, M.D., at Georgetown University School of Medicine, did food allergy tests on 104 children, ages one and a half to nine years old, with chronic ear infections. *An astonishing 78 per cent showed sensitivities to various foods.* More important, the ear infections cleared up in fully 86 per cent of youngsters when they stopped eating allergy-producing foods for 16 weeks. Not surprisingly, when they went back on their normal diets, ear infections reappeared in nearly all of them. The most common culprits: milk, wheat, eggs, peanuts and soya products.

According to Dr. Nsouli, most of these youngsters had seen numerous specialists and were on the verge of undergoing surgery to insert fluid-draining tubes into their ears. Fortunately, most were saved from the surgery when the real food cause was discovered. Allergies usually disappear within days or weeks after the offending food is discontinued but it takes ear infections several months to clear up, says Dr. Nsouli.

• BOTTOM LINE • *If your child has chronic ear infections, skin or blood allergy tests by a qualified allergist as well as food challenges can be critical. Be especially suspicious if other family members have allergies. If the underlying cause is a food allergy, giving up the food is a quick, cheap way to cure the infection permanently.*

GLAUCOMA

A surprising new way to prevent glaucoma may be to eat fish and fish oil, says Prasad S. Kulkarni, Ph.D., of the University of Louisville, in

Kentucky. In new research, rabbits, commonly used in studies of the eye, when fed food soaked in cod liver oil, displayed considerable drops in intraocular pressure, which is elevated in those with glaucoma. "If it works as well in humans as it does in healthy animals, this could be a good prophylactic against glaucoma," said Dr. Kulkarni. When normal rabbits ate the fish-oil-soaked food, their intraocular pressure dropped 56 per cent. Off the cod liver oil, the animals' eye pressure returned to pre-experiment levels.

Dr. Kulkarni got the idea from surveys of Eskimos indicating they have very low rates of open-angle glaucoma. He suspected the reason was the Eskimo's marine diet, rich in fish oil. The theory still, of course, needs testing on humans but eating fish is a good health idea in any event. Dr. Kulkarni believes fatty fish, when consumed regularly might help deter glaucoma.

GUM DISEASE

If you don't get enough Vitamin C, your gums rot. Scientists know for sure that happens from long-ago descriptions of the scourge known as scurvy, which was rampant from the 1300s until the early 1800s, especially among sailors who went to sea for months without fresh fruit. One graphic description of the ravages of scurvy noted, "Their mouths became stinking, their gums so rotten that all the flesh did fall off, even to the root of the teeth." The cure for scurvy, discovered by British naval physician James Lind in 1747, turned out to be fresh fruit, namely citrus fruits; the active agent was later identified as vitamin C.

Modern tests confirm that low intake of vitamin C produces bleeding gums and other signs of gingivitis. When monkeys and other animals are deprived of vitamin C, their gums swell and haemorrhage, collagen degenerates, and their teeth get loose. Deprived humans react the same way. Canadian investigators, for example, deliberately deprived subjects of vitamin C, and then gave them supplements of 60–70mg a day, the amount in an orange. They showed that vitamin C biochemically pepped up the gums. Bleeding decreased; white blood cell formation increased; collagen-producing fibroblasts increased; the gums showed biological signs of better health. This does not mean, however, that megadoses of vitamin C push the gums into greater health. Vitamin C seems to improve gums only in those who lack it.

Further, a large-scale United States government analysis showed that Americans who ate more vitamin C foods were less likely to have gum diseases.

The clear message is for healthy gums, eat fruit and vegetables rich in vitamin C.

INCONTINENCE

If you have a tendency to incontinence – frequent and urgent impulses to urinate – drinking tea or coffee may make it worse. It is not just because caffeine is a diuretic that increases the amount of urine. Recently researchers at St. George's Hospital in London uncovered another caffeine trick. Caffeine can exert pressure on the bladder by causing muscles surrounding it to contract, increasing the need to urinate in some incontinent individuals. Researchers studied 20 incontinent women with frequent urges to urinate and ten normal controls. All took 200mg of caffeine, the amount in a couple of cups of weak coffee.

Tests showed that within 30 minutes after drinking the caffeine the bladders of the women with the frequent urges to urinate were filling up rapidly. The bladder contractions of the incontinent women were about twice as strong as those of normal women. The caffeine had no such effect on the normal women.

Alcohol is also a diuretic that can promote incontinence. Despite claims to the contrary, there is no evidence other foods (beside caffeine and alcohol) have any influence on incontinence, according to the *Harvard Health Letter*.

LUPUS

Lupus is an autoimmune inflammatory disorder with various symptoms, including weakness, chronic fatigue, a bright red skin rash, as well as pain and soreness in the joints. Diet may help alleviate the symptoms. Critical, as with other inflammatory disorders, is the type of fat you eat. As a general rule, avoid animal fats and omega-6 type polyunsaturated oils, such as corn, safflower and sunflower-seed oils. Such fats promote inflammation. Eat oily fish such as sardines and salmon that fight inflammation.

A recent British test of 27 lupus patients showed that those taking fish oil capsules improved significantly while those taking placebo pills got worse or stayed the same during a 34 week trial. Andrew Weil, M.D., of the University of Arizona Medical School, advises lupus patients to eat sardines packed in sardine oil (sild oil) three times a week.

Strange Alfalfa Lupus

It also makes sense for those with lupus to restrict legumes and certainly alfalfa sprouts. There's evidence lupus may be tied to adverse food reactions. Six months into an experiment, researchers at the Oregon Health Sciences University in Portland noted that monkeys eating alfalfa became sick. Tests surprisingly revealed medical signs of lupus! Deprived of alfalfa, the monkeys partially recovered. Put back on the alfalfa, they again fell severely ill and one died. In further tests, more commonly eaten alfalfa sprouts had the same sad effect. The culprit in alfalfa, researchers determined, was an amino acid called l-*canavanine*. Straight l-canavanine fed to monkeys also produced lupus-like symptoms.

Unquestionably, it can happen in humans. One 50-year-old man who ate alfalfa seeds in a cholesterol-lowering experiment developed lupus symptoms; he recovered fully after he stopped eating the alfalfa seeds.

MACULAR DEGENERATION

It's true. Eating a carrot a day may save you from going blind in old age. Through the years, the macula, a tiny central part of the retina, is constantly ravaged by exposure to reckless gangs of oxygen free radicals from sunlight and other environmental factors. Eventually, the macula may deteriorate, causing diminished vision, even blindness. Macular degeneration affects about 10 million Americans over age 50 and 30 per cent over age 75. Yet, feeding the eyes steady low doses of antioxidants through the diet may help the macula fend off the years of vision-destroying assaults by free radicals.

Indeed, people who eat the most fruits and vegetables high in beta carotene are less likely to be stricken by age-related macular degeneration. When researchers at the University of Illinois at Chicago analysed the diets of about 3,000 older Americans in 1988, they discovered that eating a mere carrot a day – or any other beta-carotene-rich fruit or vegetable – cut the odds of macular degeneration by 40 per cent compared with eating such foods less than once a week. Further, the more often the folks ate beta-carotene foods, the more their risk dropped. The study suggested that foods high in vitamin C, another antioxidant, also deter macular degeneration. Blueberries may pack a particular wallop in preserving vision. Blueberry extract, high in compounds called antho-cyanosides, has been found in clinical studies to slow down visual loss.

And Eat Your Oysters
Older people often have a zinc deficiency, and that, too, may promote macular degeneration. Zinc stimulates an enzyme critical to the functioning of retinal cells. If the enzyme gives up, as it often does with age, possibly from a lack of zinc, the cells may become abnormal, fostering macular degeneration. In test-tube studies, zinc revs up the crucial enzyme's activity by as much as 190 per cent. Further, high doses of zinc supplements, taken under a doctor's supervision, have curbed the progression of macular degeneration in some individuals.

• BOTTOM LINE • *To prevent macular degeneration, eat a fruit or vegetable rich in beta carotene every day. Best bets: sweet potatoes, carrots, spinach, kale and pumpkin. Also be sure to get adequate zinc. Oysters are by far the richest zinc source. One 3oz (85g) tin of smoked oysters has as much zinc as that found to retard macular degeneration in studies. (For a list of other zinc-rich foods, see page 460.)*

METABOLISM

Eating hot spicy foods such as mustard and hot peppers can actually speed up metabolism, burning off calories. In one test, British investigators added about three-fifths of a teaspoon of hot chilli sauce or ordinary yellow mustard to a meal. The hot stuff caused average metabolism in 12 subjects to shoot up 25 per cent burning off 45 extra calories in the next three hours. Mustard and hot sauce caused one person to burn off 76 calories − or 10 per cent of the calories in a 760-calorie meal.

A new Australian study shows that ginger may also rev up metabolism, burning off calories. Biochemists applied both fresh and dry ginger extracts to the tissue of animals and found that the spice induced tissues to use up about 20 per cent more energy than normally. Most responsible for the increased activity was gingerol, the chemical that gives ginger its pungent taste.

To what extent ginger might work in humans is unknown. Some researchers believe that many pungent spices and foods tend to spur thermogenesis, the burning of calories.

MULTIPLE SCLEROSIS

Multiple sclerosis is a mysterious neurological disease with symptoms varying from mild to gravely disabling. Lately, researchers are pursuing a dietary link with new zest. Some clues are that populations that eat a lot of fat, notably dairy fat, have high rates of MS while fishing communities seem oddly immune to the disorder. This raises suspicions that peculiar abnormalities in digesting fat may be partly at fault.

Indeed, neurologist Roy Laver Swank, M.D., at the Oregon Health Sciences University in Portland, has long been treating multiple sclerosis quite successfully with a low-saturated-fat diet. Writing in the British medical journal The Lancet in 1990, Dr. Swank chronicled the astonishing success of his MS diet. He tracked 144 MS patients for 34 years. Decidedly, those who cut saturated fat to under 20g a day had much less deterioration and lower death rates than those who ate more saturated fat.

Most dramatic benefits showed up in those who started the low-fat diet before they became significantly disabled. "If we got them on the diet before disability set in, 95 per cent lived for 30 years without disability. All who did not go on the diet went downhill and most died within 20 years," says Dr. Swank. He now finds that eating even less saturated fat – no more than 15g daily – yields greater and faster improvement. Dairy fats appear most destructive to those with multiple sclerosis. Number two is meat fat.

At the same time, MS patients may need more omega-3 type marine fat. In a recent study, Ralph T. Holman, Ph.D., of the University of Minnesota and Emre Kokmen, M.D., of the Mayo Clinic documented that MS patients have very abnormal patterns of blood fatty acids, characterized by a severe lack of omega-3 fatty acids.

Dr. Holman blames the fatty-acid imbalance mostly on a defect in metabolizing fat, and suggests it can be partly overcome by eating oils rich in omega-3 fatty acids. "Fish oil is more potent," he says, but plant oils, mainly rapeseed oil and flaxseed oil, may also help. Nor does it take "astronomically high levels of oils" to correct the deficiency, says Dr. Holman. "We are talking about a few teaspoons a day."

In a recent British test, fish oil reduced the severity and frequency of relapses among 312 MS patients during a three-year period.

DR. *SWANK'S LOW-FAT MULTIPLE SCLEROSIS DIET*

Here are the highlights of Dr. Swank's MS diet:

- No red meat the first year, including dark meat chicken and turkey. After that, no more than 3oz (85g) of red meat a week, the leanest possible.

- No dairy products with 1 per cent or more butterfat. You can eat any amount of nonfat milk, skimmed milk, buttermilk (without cream or butter bits added), evaporated skimmed milk, nonfat dry milk powder, rinsed low-fat cottage cheese, dry curd cottage cheese, very-low-fat cheeses and yoghurt.

- No processed foods with saturated fat.

- Not more than 15g or 3 teaspoons of saturated fat per day. 8fl oz (225ml) of whole milk contains 5g of saturated fat, one tablespoon of butter, 7g, and 1oz (30g) of cream cheese or cheddar cheese, 6g.

- A minimum of four teaspoons and a maximum of ten teaspoons per day of unsaturated fat, such as sunflower seed oil, corn oil, cottonseed oil, soya bean oil, sesame oil, wheat germ oil, linseed oil, groundnut oil and olive oil.

- One teaspoon of cod liver oil daily, as well as fish a couple of times a week, or an average 1oz (30g) of seafood a day.

NEURALGIA

Finding any kind of dietary relief would be a godsend for some 15,000 Americans who every year develop trigeminal neuralgia, also known as tic douloureux, a nerve disorder of excruciating and episodic pain that often comes suddenly, lasts less than a minute and then rapidly disappears. The pain centers around the mouth, teeth and nose, and can be triggered by merely chewing, smiling, talking or touching the face. Common therapy calls for drugs and sometimes nerve-severing surgery to relieve the pain, possibly with side effects and complications including loss of facial sensation and motor control.

Some hope for alleviating this condition with diet comes from researchers at the University of Oklahoma Health Sciences Center in Oklahoma City. They reported the case of a woman who eliminated the pain of neuralgia by giving up caffeine. It was her own idea to try the diet therapy. She was 45 when the first severe episodic pain came on the right side of her face. So awful was the condition that even a light breeze on her cheek or an attempt to smile would trigger the pain.

She regularly drank three to four cups of instant coffee a day, and drank more when the pain was particularly bad. Wondering if caffeine might be partly at fault, she switched to decaf. Remarkably, after two or three weeks the severe pain lessened, and she could touch her face without eliciting the excruciating pain. For a whole year she remained free of episodes of pain by avoiding caffeine. Then, as a test, she drank a couple of cups of hot cocoa for a week; the following week the neuralgic pain was back. Later she noticed that a mere one cup of caffeinated coffee was enough to trigger a week-long episode of "moderately intense" pain.

For two years she has been able to keep the pain in check with a low-caffeine diet. She now eats only a trace of caffeine, at most 10mg of caffeine a day compared with as much as 380mg during the previous painful days.

Stephen Glore, Ph.D., assistant professor of clinical dietetics at Oklahoma University, who reported the case, suggests caffeine might somehow stimulate the firing of the sensitive trigeminal nerve in certain individuals. Dr. Glore stresses there's no evidence that everyone with this disorder would benefit from shunning caffeine. Still, the possibility makes it well worth a try for anyone.

Good-bye Nuts and Chocolate

The herpes virus might be implicated in this type of neuralgia, says Richard Griffith, M.D., professor emeritus at Indiana University School of Medicine. Thus, he suggests cutting out high arginine foods, such as chocolate and nuts, to help curb the herpes virus. One patient, a compulsive eater of nuts and chocolate who was scheduled for surgery for this condition, followed Dr. Griffith's advice. His facial pain disappeared "virtually overnight," eliminating the need for surgery, says Dr. Griffith. One patient does not a study make, but there is little harm in giving Dr. Griffith's method a try before resorting to more dire treatments.

PARASITES

Anyone can get an intestinal parasite, and it's much more likely if you travel to developing countries. One of the most common parasites worldwide is *Giardia lamblia*, often picked up in drinking water, and it can play havoc with your stomach. One study found that such parasitic intestinal upset is frequently mistaken for irritable bowel syndrome – with symptoms of abdominal pain, constipation, diarrhoea and nausea. A New York physician recently noted that about *half* his patients complaining of irritable bowel problems were actually infected with the *Giardia lamblia* parasite!

One solution is antibiotic drugs, which often must be taken for long periods and can have serious side effects. Another answer is garlic, a common folk medicine for intestinal disorders.

Garlic proved superior in a recent test by Egyptian doctors at Ain Shams University in Cairo. Low doses of fresh garlic, as well as garlic capsules, virtually wiped out symptoms of *Giardia lamblia* infection in 26 children within one day! Stool examinations showed that all were completely cured within three days. In contrast, the doctors say drugs for giardiasis must be taken for a week and sometimes for ten days, "with possible undesirable side effects".

The researchers prepared the fresh garlic remedy by whipping up about thirty peeled fresh garlic cloves with a little water in a blender at short bursts until it was homogenized. They kept the garlic mixture chilled. Then they gave doses of one part garlic mixed into twenty parts distilled water – or about 5 tablespoons (75ml) of the garlic solution – twice a day to the children.

The garlic also worked against another parasite called *H. nana*, the doctors found. Symptoms improved in eight out of ten children infected with this worm within two days, and disappeared in three days. The other two children completely recovered in five days.

• BOTTOM LINE • *Eating garlic regularly may make your stomach and intestines a lethal environment for these and other parasites, giving you constant protection. As a crude treatment, you could also simple nibble on a raw garlic clove or mix crushed garlic in a little cold water and drink it immediately.*

There's also scientific evidence that eating pumpkin seeds kills intestinal worms, as folk medicine claims.

PARKINSON'S DISEASE

If you don't eat enough of certain foods early in life, it may cause problems many years later. The stage for Parkinson's disease, a progressive nervous system disorder, may be set earlier in life by a deficiency of antioxidant vitamin E. That is a theory explored by Lawrence Golbe, M.D., a neurologist at the University of Medicine and Dentistry of New Jersey.

In a study of 106 Parkinson's patients he found that women with the disease were less likely as young adults to have eaten peanuts and peanut butter, high in vitamin E. Men patients had skimped on salads with dressings earlier in life. The oil in salad dressing is rich in vitamin E. Another study showed that people free of Parkinson's said as young adults they ate more seeds, nuts and salad oils, rich in vitamin E. Thus, researchers speculate that too little vitamin E foods earlier in life might somehow leave the brain vulnerable to the onset of Parkinson's years later. There's even preliminary evidence that massive doses of vitamin E (800 to 3,000 units daily) may slow progression of the disease. More extensive tests of vitamin E therapy for Parkinson's are ongoing.

PROSTATE PROBLEMS

If you have that common male condition, enlargement of the prostate gland, which affects about half of all men over age 50, eating pumpkin seeds may help. According to Dr. James Duke of the U.S. Department of Agriculture, a daily handful of pumpkin seeds is a popular folk medicine for this condition in many parts of the world — notably Bulgaria, Turkey and the Ukraine — and there is a scientific rationale. Pumpkin seeds are rich in the amino acids alanine, glycine and glutamic acid. In a controlled study of 45 men, these amino acids in pure form reduced the major symptoms of prostate enlargement. For example, they relieved or reduced night-time urination by 95 per cent, the urgency of urination by 81 per cent and frequency of urination by 73 per cent.

Surprisingly, 2½oz (70g) of pumpkin seeds contains five times more of the amino acids than the daily amount found effective in the study, says Dr. Duke. Thus, he figures that pumpkin seeds may work as well as the pure amino acids alone or as well as certain drugs specifically designed to treat the condition.

Other potential remedies for prostate swelling, according to Dr. Duke, are cucumber seeds, watermelon seeds, sesame seeds, carob, soya beans, flaxseed, almonds, walnuts, Brazil nuts, peanuts and saw palmetto fruit (a dwarf prickly palm from south eastern U.S.) Dr. Duke suggests that such foods, along with pumpkin seeds, could be ground together into a peanut-butter-like spread he calls "Prosnut Butter". 1oz (30g) a day, or about two tablespoons, would provide therapeutic amounts of the amino acids and other useful substances, he says.

PSORIASIS

There's intriguing evidence that fish oils may help prevent and relieve the symptoms of psoriasis, an inflammatory skin disease characterized by red, dry, scaly skin, pain and itching. For example, a British study by researchers at Royal Hallamshire Hospital in Sheffield found that a dose of fish oil, equal to eating 5oz (140g) a day of an oily fish such as mackerel, "significantly" alleviated symptoms, particularly itching, within eight weeks. In another study, Vincent A. Ziboh, a dermatologist at the University of California at Davis, found that 60 per cent of a small group of patients had mild to moderate improvement – less redness and itching – after eight weeks of taking fish oil capsules. Other studies, however, have not found much, if any, improvement from fish oil.

Still, since psoriasis is an inflammatory disorder, and fish oil is an anti-inflammatory, it makes eminent sense to eat more oily fish. Over time, such tiny infusions of the oil may do some good. The part of fish oil most effective is eicosapentaenoic acid (EPA), which is particularly concentrated in salmon and mackerel.

Additionally, as with any inflammatory disease, it's wise to cut back on pro-inflammatory animal fats and omega-6 type vegetable oils, such as corn, sunflower and safflower oils and margarines and shortenings made from them.

RECTAL ITCHING AND BURNING

If you have rectal itching or burning, it could be something in your diet. Some possible itching culprits, according to physicians at the Mayo Clinic, are caffeine, nuts and chocolate. If you think such foods may play a role, they suggest you avoid them for a few weeks to see if it helps.

Overeating hot chilli peppers can lead to rectal burning during defecation in some people. Doctors at the University of Texas even coined a name for the condition, "jaloproctitus," after studying participants in a jalapeño-eating contest. Each contestant had eaten three to thirteen jalapeño peppers. The hot capsaicin from the peppers was incorporated into the faeces, causing a burning sensation as they passed through the anus.

SLEEP

One of food's best sleeping pills is something sweet or starchy. Honey has long been used in folk medicine as a soporific. So if falling asleep or staying asleep is a problem, try eating 1oz (30g) or so of sweet or starchy stuff about half an hour before going to bed. "For most people this is as effective as a sleeping pill, but without the side effect of morning grogginess and the potential for abuse inherent in sleep drugs," says Judith Wurtman, Ph.D., a nutrition researcher at MIT and an expert on the subject.

Her suggestions: low-fat foods with little or no protein, such as breakfast cereal without milk, caramel-coated popcorn, fig bars, gingersnaps, or a waffle with one tablespoon of maple syrup. All have a sedative effect on the brain.

What about that old folklore standby – a glass of warm milk to fight insomnia? Countless people swear by it. However, modern science has disputed it. Experts have insisted that milk does not work because it does not contain nearly enough of the sleep-inducing chemical tryptophan which converts in the brain to the "sleep chemical" serotonin. Indeed, scientists at MIT insist that drinking milk is more likely to wake most people up.

New research, however, has discovered natural opiates called caso-morphins in milk that may give some validity to the folklore remedy. Such casomorphins theoretically could make you drowsy says Purdue University authority Varro Tyler, Ph.D. "I think milk does work in some people, especially if it's warm, for some unknown reason," he says. "Perhaps it is the casomorphins." Arizona physician Andrew Weil agrees that milk helps some people overcome insomnia, saying he has seen many people who do get a sedative effect from drinking milk at night.

The only advice until science sorts this out is to follow the dictates of your own body; if milk helps you sleep, use it.

Beware Baby's Milk Insomnia

On the other hand, milk is a very real threat to the sleep of some infants. Babies who consistently wake up in the night for no apparent reason may be suffering from "cow's milk insomnia," according to a Belgian study. Researchers at University Children's Hospital in Brussels studied 17 children, ranging in age from two months to 29 months, who had severe sleeping problems that could not be traced to common causes such as nightmares and colic.

When the youngsters were put on a diet free of cow's milk, the change was dramatic. All but one began sleeping like babies should. Instead of waking up an average five times per night as they did when drinking cow's milk, they usually woke up only once. Instead of a mere five hours sleep per night, they got 13 hours.

The researchers speculate that natural substances in milk may stimulate some infants' nervous systems, keeping their brains alert, or trigger an allergic reaction that makes them restless.

It's True About Caffeine

The biggest dietary antagonist to sleep is caffeine. As almost everyone knows, caffeine can keep you awake when you would rather snooze, especially if you are not used to caffeine and/or if you are elderly. Typical is one study at Vanderbilt University School of Medicine, showing that consuming caffeine a half hour to an hour before sleep dramatically disturbed the sleep of some individuals. They took longer to fall asleep and did not sleep as long or as well. However, least affected were heavy caffeine consumers, who perhaps had developed a tolerance to caffeine's effects on sleep. Those who did not regularly use caffeine suffered the most sleep distress from caffeine.

SMOKING

If you are trying to quit smoking, some foods may dampen your cravings for the addictive nicotine that keeps you hooked.

Try Oats

Yes, eating oats, as in oatmeal and oat bran, may help you stifle nicotine cravings and kick a cigarette habit. Boiled oats have long been used in India's Ayurvedic system of medicine to treat opium addiction. Then, someone noticed that the recovered addicts often lost interest in cigarettes as well. That led researcher C. L. Anand at Ruchill Hospital in Glasgow, to do a double-blind, placebo-controlled experiment published in the scientific journal *Nature*.

He took committed cigarette smokers and gave one group an extract of fresh oats and others a placebo. A month later the oat eaters had diminished cravings for cigarettes and were smoking only one-third as many cigarettes as they had before the test or as the non-oat-eating controls. In fact, five of the 13 oat eaters stopped smoking entirely; seven cut back by 50 per cent. Only one continued to smoke as before. Further, the craving was suppressed for as long as two months after the smokers stopped eating the oats! A later study in mice identified a compound in the oats thought to be the active anti-smoking ingredient.

IF YOU'RE TRYING TO WEAN YOURSELF FROM CIGARETTES

Foods That May Make It Easier by Increasing Body Alkalinity: Spinach, beet greens, raisins, figs, dried lima beans, dandelion greens, almonds.

Foods That May Make It Harder by Increasing Body Acidity: Alcohol, red meats, liver and other organ meats, wheat germ, dried lentils, chicken, eggs, cheeses, peanuts, English walnuts, plums, prunes, cranberries, coffee.

Eat Spinach, Not Meat
High-alkaline foods, such as spinach and beet greens, tend to "recirculate" nicotine in the body, maintaining high levels of the addictive stuff; thus, such foods tend to lessen the need for nicotine intake, says David Daughton, Ph.D., a nicotine researcher at the University of Nebraska Medical Center. Other foods that make the urine more acid, like meat, tend to flush away nicotine, increasing cravings for cigarettes. Thus a diet rich in alkaline foods and low in acid foods may help you cut down on cigarettes gradually. If you quit "cold turkey", it probably doesn't make any difference, he says.

In one test by Dr. Daughton, smokers given sodium bicarbonate to make their bodies more alkaline had a much easier time quitting, and after five weeks nearly all had kicked the habit. Only one subject was smoking even two cigarettes a day. All others, who did not get the alkaline substance, were still smoking.

Also, Stanley Schachter, Ph.D. professor of psychology at Columbia University, showed that people with high body acidity smoked more than did people with alkaline body chemistry. "In the acid condition, there is an increase of roughly 17 per cent in smoking [roughly seven or so cigarettes more per day] for a two-pack-per-day smoker," he said.

Don't Mix Cokes with Nicotine Gum

If you are using nicotine gum to suppress your cravings for cigarettes, acid foods can block the effectiveness of the gum, causing you to smoke more cigarettes to get your nicotine fix. Don't eat highly acidic foods and beverages for at least fifteen minutes before using the gum. That especially means colas, coffee, fruit juices and beer. So advise experts at the National Institute on Drug Abuse. They found that men who rinsed their mouths with coffee or cola before chewing the gum absorbed virtually none of the gum's nicotine. This defeats the gum's purpose of weaning smokers off cigarettes by giving them small nicotine doses; smokers are then forced to smoke more to get their normal dose of nicotine.

VAGINITIS

If you have ever heard that yoghurt fights yeast infections, believe it. It's an old folktale, but it really works, says Dr. Eileen Hilton, an infectious disease specialist at Long Island Jewish Medical Center in New York. Eating 8oz (225g) of yoghurt a day can keep such infections away.

In her study, she asked one group of women with recurring vaginitis – also known as candidal, or "yeast," infections – to eat 8oz (225g) of plain yoghurt every day for six months. Another group ate none. The yoghurt eaters had a threefold lower incidence of vaginitis than the non-yoghurt eaters. Women who ordinarily had three vaginitis flare-ups in a six-month period had only one or none when on the yoghurt regimen.

Important: The yoghurt must contain live active acidophilus bacterial cultures, as did the yogurt used in the study. It is these L. *acidophilus* bacteria that Dr. Hilton identifies as the active infection fighters in yoghurt. Yoghurts are not required to contain acidophilus cultures, although some manufacturers do add them. Check the label to be sure. You can make your own yoghurt using acidophilus cultures sold in many health food stores. The cultures must also be live to have any therapeutic effects. Heating the yoghurt kills the cultures, leaving the yogurt pharmacologically inactive against vaginitis.

HOW TO USE THE DRUGS IN FOODS TO STAY HEALTHY

Here are some of the many ways foods can behave as common medicines. In all cases, the specific pharmacological activity of foods noted here has been reported by scientific studies. A major source of such studies is the NAPRALERT (Natural Products Alert) database at the University of Illinois at Chicago, which contains more than 100,000 scientific journal articles on the pharmacological activity of plants. A computer search of that database by pharmacological activity (antibiotic activity and so forth) revealed the vast majority of foods on the following lists. Other foods were included because their activity was cited in the large database of medical and scientific publications at the National Library of Medicine, or by scientists at academic institutions and government bodies, such as the National Cancer Institute and the U.S. Department of Agriculture.

These compilations can guide you to foods with potential pharma–cological activity. However, it is often unclear from the present data how potent a certain food-effect may be, how much you would have to eat to get an effect and that effect's significance in the body. In some cases, the food's active chemicals have been identified, as well as the mechanism through which it works. In other cases, even though foods and their constituents exhibit specific pharmacological activity, the precise mechanisms remain mysterious.

ANTIBIOTICS

You may recall that, according to rumour, our first major antibiotic, penicillin, was derived from mouldy bread. That's probably myth, but commercial penicillin used today is derived from a strain picked up on a mouldy cantaloupe melon. With the commercial success of penicillin in the 1940s, scientists scrambled to find other natural bacteria killers to convert into drugs. One of the most promising candidates was garlic. Actually, in 1858 Louis Pasteur had noted that bacteria died when exposed to garlic. In 1944, Chester J. Cavallito isolated a potent antibiotic in garlic, the odoriferous allicin. But allicin was so short-lived and elusive that it could not be made into a drug. It has to be administered in its native packaging – as a raw garlic clove.

Garlic is one of nature's strongest, most complex, broad-spectrum antibacterial agents. Tests show that garlic kills or cripples at least 72 infectious bacteria that spread diarrhoea, dysentery, botulism, tuberculosis and encephalitis, among other diseases. Onion, too, is an exceptionally strong antibiotic and antiseptic and was used to treat infections in wounded Russian troops during World War II. Honey and wine were used on ancient Greek and Roman battlefields to clean and heal wounds. Food compounds destroy bacteria by several mechanisms, mainly by disrupting the bacteria's synthesis of protein, folic acid and transpeptidase so they cannot multiply. Blueberries and cranberries not only can inhibit bacteria, but also block their attachment to human cells.

FOODS WITH ANTIBACTERIAL ACTIVITY
Apple, banana, basil, beetroot, blueberry, cabbage, carrot, cashew, celery, chilli pepper, chives, coconut, coffee, cranberry, cumin, dill, garlic, ginger, honey, horseradish, liquorice, lime, black mustard seed, nori (seaweed), nutmeg, olive, papaya, plum, purslane, onion, sage, sugar, tea, watermelon, wine, yoghurt.

SOME FOOD COMPOUNDS WITH ANTIBACTERIAL ACTIVITY
Allicin (garlic), Lactobacillus (yoghurt), Eugenol (clove), Anthocyanates (red wine).

ANTICANCER AGENTS

Cancer is a slow progression that starts with the "initiation" of a single cell by cancer-causing substances. Foods and food compounds can interfere with this cancer process at about ten stages of development, according to John D. Potter, M.D., of the University of Minnesota. Food compounds can prevent would-be cancer agents from being "activated". They can block the mutation of a cell's DNA (genetic material). They can stimulate enzymes in the body that flush cancer-causing chemicals out of the body. They can prevent cancer-causing oncogenes from being switched on. They can combat bacteria related to stomach cancer. They can manipulate hormones and neutralize toxic agents that promote cancer. They can reduce the ability of cancerous cells to proliferate and form tumours. They can even help prevent cancer cells from spreading to establish new cancers. Anticancer compounds are heavily concentrated in fruits and vegetables.

MAJOR FOODS WITH ANTICANCER ACTIVITY

Garlic, cabbage, liquorice, soya beans, ginger, umbelliferous vegetables (carrots, celery, parsnips), onions, tea, turmeric, citrus fruits (orange, grapefruit, lemon), whole wheat, flax, brown rice, solanaceous vegetables (tomato, aubergines, peppers), cruciferous vegetables (broccoli, cauliflower, Brussels sprouts), oats, mints, oregano, cucumber, rosemary, sage, potato, thyme, chives, cantaloupe melon, basil, tarragon, barley, berries, seafood, olive oil.

SOME FOOD CHEMICALS WITH ANTICANCER ACTIVITY

Allylic sulphides (garlic, onions, chives), carotenoids (green leafy vegetables, carrots, sweet potatoes), catechins (tea, berries), coumarins (carrots, parsley, citrus fruits), ellagic acid (grapes, strawberries, raspberries, walnuts), indoles (cabbage, broccoli, cauliflower, kale, Brussels sprouts), isothiocyanates (mustard, horseradish, radishes, other cruciferous vegetables), lignans (soya beans, flaxseed), limoinoids (citrus fruits), protease inhibitors (soya beans, legumes, nuts, grains, seeds), sulphoraphane (broccoli, green onions, kale, red cabbage, Brussels sprouts, ginger, cauliflower, red-leaf lettuce).

VITAMINS, TOO, CAN FOIL CANCER

Vitamins are potent anticancer agents. Vitamin C, one of the best studied, has myriad tricks against cancer. For example, it can block the transformation of amines and nitrite into nitrosamines, deadly carcinogens that can cause every type of cancer known. It can neutralize free radical cancer-causing agents in cell membranes, halting the first step in cancer. It can also help regulate immunity, and prevent oncogenes and viruses from transforming healthy cells into cancerous cells. It can suppress the growth and virulence of tumours in animals; for example, in mice dosed with vitamin C, it took one-third longer for spontaneous cancers to appear. In other tests, cancers in vitamin C-treated animals were smaller, less invasive and less apt to spread.

"Vitamin C has multiple complex effects on a variety of biologic activities, perhaps more widespread than those of any other nutrient," concluded a 1990 American National Cancer Institute report on vitamin C and cancer.

ANTICOAGULANTS

Aspirin, one of our great "blood-thinning" or anticoagulant drugs, came from the bark of a willow tree. It was not until the 1970s, with the discovery of hormone-like substances called prostaglandins, that scientists began to understand how aspirin works. They now know the drug has anti-platelet-aggregation powers. It discourages platelets, our smallest blood components, from clumping together or aggregating; thus, they are less sticky and less able to build clots that can clog arteries. That's one reason doctors think low doses of aspirin help ward off heart attacks and strokes. Only one-tenth of an aspirin – a mere 30mg – inhibits platelet clumping. Aspirin works by blocking action of a prostaglandin-like substance called thromboxane which otherwise would stimulate platelets to stick together.

With this discovery, it was not a big leap to suggest that other plants and foods could also work through the prostaglandin system to dampen blood platelets' enthusiasm to congregate. Like aspirin, some food compounds are antagonists to thromboxane; others, such as garlic and onions, contain several anti-platelet-clumping compounds that work in different biochemical ways.

FOODS WITH ANTICOAGULANT (ANTI-PLATELET-AGGREGATION) ACTIVITY
Cinnamon, cumin, fish oil, garlic, ginger, grape, melon (green and yellow), mushroom (black "tree-ear" or moer), onion, tea, watermelon, wine (red).

SOME FOOD CHEMICALS WITH ANTICOAGULANT (ANTI-PLATELET-AGGRE-GATION) ACTIVITY
Adenosine (garlic, onion, black "tree-ear" mushrooms), ajoene (garlic), catechins (tea), omega-3 fatty acids (fatty deep-water fish), resveratrol (grape skins, red wine).

ANTIDEPRESSANTS

Most commonly, foods seem to manipulate mood by affecting serotonin, one of the brain's most interesting neurotransmitters. Eating foods that deplete serotonin in the nervous system can put people in a down mood, depressed and anxious. Foods that lead to normal amounts of serotonin in the brain heighten mood, somewhat the same way drugs do. Serotonin-active drugs are often used to treat depression.

Peptides in the gut, released when you eat, can also act directly on both the brain and the vagus nerve that sends messages to the brain. Although not everyone agrees on exactly why it happens, it is widely accepted that carbohydrates can act as mood elevators, particularly to relieve certain types of depression, such as the blues that come with premenstrual syndrome and the down moods of seasonal affective disorder (SAD). More recently it's been established that other food components, such as folic acid, can profoundly affect mood, presumably by regulating serotonin levels through complex interplays of brain chemistry.

FOODS WITH ANTIDEPRESSANT ACTIVITY
Caffeine, ginger, honey, sugar.

ANTIDEPRESSANT CHEMICALS IN FOODS
Carbohydrates (sugar, pasta, bread, cereal, biscuits, cake), caffeine (coffee, tea, chocolate), folic acid (green leafy vegetables and legumes), selenium (seafood, grains, nuts).

ANTIDIARRHOEAL AGENTS

Some foods effectively fight diarrhoea because they contain tannins and other compounds that are astringents; thus, they drain water out of the gut, solidifying faeces, and also help restrict the intestinal tract's contractions (motility) that push contents along. Such astringent agents account for dried blueberries' effectiveness as a treatment for diarrhoea. (Note: Only dried blueberries have high concentrations of astringent agents; fresh blueberries do not.) Certain other foods seem to work by fighting bacteria in the intestines and by exerting a soothing effect.

FOODS WITH ANTIDIARRHOEAL ACTIVITY
Blueberries (dried), cinnamon, fenugreek seeds, garlic, ginger, liquorice, nutmeg, rice, tea, turmeric.

ANTIHYPERTENSIVES

Many pharmaceutical blood pressure medications work in roundabout indirect ways, says William J. Elliott, assistant professor of medicine and pharmacology at the University of Chicago, and have "troubling side effects, such as fainting, drowsiness or impotence". By contrast, he finds that food, at least in animal studies, can lower blood pressure in a much more direct, simple fashion just by dilating blood vessels. That's what celery does, he says. He discovered that a celery compound called phthalide relaxes smooth muscles of the blood vessel lining, widening the vessel and thereby lowering blood pressure. Further, Dr. Elliott found, the compound accomplishes this by blocking the action of an enzyme that makes catecholamines, which are stress hormones. These hormones make blood vessels constrict, raising blood pressure. Thus, celery seems to lower blood pressure by suppressing production of the stress hormones that would raise blood pressure.

Interestingly, garlic and onion may lower blood pressure in similar fashion. Both possess adenosine, also a smooth-muscle relaxant.

FOODS WITH BLOOD-PRESSURE-LOWERING ACTIVITY
 Celery, fenugreek, fish oil, garlic, grapefruit, olive oil, onion, garlic.

ANTIOXIDANTS

Nothing protects your health and extends life more than a steady supply of antioxidants to your cells. Food antioxidants are a huge extended family of chemical warriors that directly oppose oxygen-charged molecules hell-bent on damaging cells. Antioxidants are a major police force of the body, thought to help deflect virtually all chronic diseases, including heart disease, cancer, bronchitis, cataracts, Parkinson's disease. and the ageing process itself A deficiency of these antioxidants can leave you extremely vulnerable, especially if you are exposed to hazards like cigarette smoke, industrial chemicals, air pollutants.

Vitamins and minerals can double as antioxidants. So can enzymes and myriad exotic compounds that have various biochemical duties. Antioxidants are heavily concentrated in plant foods; they are also found in seafood, and occasionally in animal foods.

FOODS WITH HIGH CONCENTRATIONS OF ANTIOXIDANTS AND STRONG ANTIOXIDANT ACTIVITY

Avocado, asparagus, basil, berries, Brazil nut, broccoli, Brussels sprouts, cabbage, carrot, chilli pepper, clove, collard greens, cumin, fish, garlic (exceptionally strong), ginger, kale, lettuces (dark green), liquorice, marjoram, nutmeg, oat, onion (exceptionally strong), orange, peanut, pepper, peppermint, pumpkin, sage, sesame seed, spearmint, spinach, sweet potato, tomato, watermelon.

GARLIC: ANTIOXIDANT POWERHOUSE

Garlic is a champion carrier of antioxidants, possessing at least 15 different antioxidant chemicals. "This antioxidant activity may be garlic's primary underlying mechanism against disease." – Dr. David Kritchevsky, Wistar Institute, Philadelphia

---

SOME MAJOR ANTIOXIDANTS IN FOODS

Beta Carotene: An orange pigment, linked to preventing heart attacks, irregular heartbeats, strokes and cancer, especially lung cancer, beta carotene boosts immune functioning and extinguishes singlet oxygen-type free radicals. Cancer victims (notably with cancers of the lung. stomach, oesophagus, small intestine, cervix and uterus) often have low blood levels of beta carotene, reflecting low beta carotene in their diets. According to one study, beta carotene levels in the blood of lung cancer victims was one-third lower than that in healthy individuals. Similarly, a recent British study found men with the most beta carotene in their blood only 60 per cent as likely to develop cancer, especially lung cancer, as those with the lowest blood beta carotene.

Major Food Sources of Beta Carotene. Dark orange and dark green leafy vegetables. Sweet potatoes, carrots, dried apricots, collard greens, kale, spinach and pumpkin have the most. Lesser amounts are found in pink grapefruit, mangoes, green lettuces and broccoli. The darker orange or green the fruit or vegetable, the more beta carotene it contains. In green vegetables, chlorophyll covers up and camouflages the underlying orange colour. Actually varying amounts of beta carotene were present in every one of 28 common fruits and vegetables tested by the USDA.

NOTE: *Beta carotene is not destroyed by cooking, according to USDA tests.*

Glutathione. Glutathione is an important anti-cancer agent. Dean P. Jones, Ph.D., associate professor of biochemistry at Emory University School of Medicine, says glutathione can deactivate at least thirty cancer-causing substances! The compound prevents lipid peroxidation and acts as an enzyme to deactivate free radicals. Thus it offers potential protection against heart disease, cataracts and asthma, as well as cancer and other diseases linked to free-radical damage. Glutathione also helps block damage from toxic compounds such as environmental pollutants by detoxifying them in the body. In test-tube experiments, glutathione almost completely stopped replication of the AIDS virus.

Major Food Sources of Glutathione. Avocado, asparagus and watermelon. Per ordinary serving, this trio contains the most glutathione according to an analysis of 98 popular foods by Dr. Jones. Other foods highest in glutathione: fresh grapefruit and oranges, strawberries, fresh peaches. okra, white potatoes, squash, cauliflower, broccoli and raw tomatoes. Some meats, particularly boiled ham, lean chops and veal cutlets, also had moderately high amounts of glutathione.

NOTE: *Only fresh and frozen fruits and vegetables have high concentrations of glutathione. In Dr. Jones's tests, canned and processed foods typically had only one-eighth as much of the potent antioxidant as the fresh and frozen variety. Cooking and mincing or juicing foods also destroys some glutathione.*

Indoles. One of the earliest classes of anticancer food compounds discovered, indoles are highly successful in blocking cancer in animals. They work by detoxifying cancer-causing agents. In humans, indoles are especially likely to help prevent colon and breast cancer, in the latter case by influencing oestrogen metabolism.

Major Food Sources of Indoles. The so-called cruciferous family, which includes broccoli, Brussels sprouts, cabbage, cauliflower, cress, horseradish, kale, kohlrabi, mustard, radish, swede and turnip.

NOTE: *Studies at the University of Manitoba found that boiled cruciferous vegetables lost about half of their indoles in cooking water.*

Lycopene. Increasingly, lycopene has been hailed as an anticancer agent. For example, Johns Hopkins researchers found lycopene severely lacking in the blood of those with pancreatic cancer. They also observed lycopene to be low in those with rectal and bladder cancer. Researchers at the University of Illinois at Chicago have detected low lycopene blood levels in women with a high risk of a precancerous condition called cervical intra-epithelial neoplasia. Some consider lycopene a stronger antioxidant than beta carotene.

Major Food Sources of Lycopene. The most widely eaten highly concentrated source is tomatoes, although watermelon is richer in lycopene on a weight basis. Tomatoes have 3.1g of lycopene per 100g; watermelon has 4.1g. Lycopene is the stuff that gives them their red colour. Small amounts are also present in apricots. Lycopene is not responsible for the colour of red berries.

NOTE: *Lycopene is not destroyed by cooking or canning. Stewed tomatoes have just as much lycopene as raw tomatoes, USDA tests show.*

Quercetin. Quercetin (pronounced KWER-se-tin) is one of the strongest biologically active members of the flavonoid family, concentrated in fruits and vegetables. Quercetin is probably a prime reason for the formidable therapeutic powers of onions. Some onions are so full of quercetin that the compound accounts for up to 10 per cent of their dry weight, according to tests by Terrance Leighton, Ph.D., professor of biochemistry and molecular biology at the University of California at Berkeley.

Quercetin has versatile anti-disease potential. "Quercetin is one of the most potent anticancer agents ever discovered," says Dr. Leighton. It inactivates several cancer-causing agents, preventing damage to cell DNA, and inhibits enzymes that spur tumour growth. Quercetin is also anti-inflammatory, antibacterial, antifungal and antiviral. It works through the immune system to dampen allergic responses (by inhibiting release of histamine from cells), and thus appears to help combat allergies such as hay fever. Indeed, quercetin is chemically similar to cromolyn, an anti-allergic drug that is known to inhibit histamine. This power plus its anti-inflammatory activity may account for onion's reputed therapeutic impact against asthma and allergies.

Quercetin is antithrombotic, helping block formation of blood clots. As an antioxidant, it absorbs oxygen free radicals and helps keep fat from becoming oxidized (lipid peroxidation). Thus, quercetin is reported to thwart artery damage from oxygen free radicals and oxidized LDL cholesterol, helping keep arteries clean and open.

Major Sources of Quercetin. Yellow and red onions (not white onions) shallots, red grapes (not white grapes), broccoli and Italian yellow squash. Oddly, garlic, onion's close cousin, does not contain quercetin.

NOTE: *Quercetin is not destroyed by cooking or freezing.*

Ubiquinol-10 (Co-enzyme Q10). This little-known food constituent is one of the best antioxidants to help detoxify bad LDL cholesterol. It is found in high concentrations in LDL particles, and appears to be the most efficient of the antioxidants, even more so than vitamin E, in keeping LDL cholesterol safe from dangerous oxidation, says Harvard's Balz Frei. Ubiquinol-10 also helps regenerate vitamin E, so they work together. Ubiquinol-10 may be one more reason certain fatty fish help ward off heart disease.

Major Sources of Ubiquinol-10. Sardines, mackerel, peanuts, pistachio nuts, soya beans, walnuts, sesame seeds, some meats.

Vitamin C. A versatile and powerful antioxidant, vitamin C seems to protect against asthma, bronchitis, cataracts, heart arrhythmias, angina (chest pain), male infertility and birth defects transmitted by men, and cancer of all types. It has also stopped the growth of the AIDS virus in test tubes. Vitamin C's antioxidant ability, many experts think, helps keep LDL cholesterol from becoming oxidized, making it a major deterrent to clogged arteries and cardiovascular disease. Vitamin C and vitamin E work together to revitalize and replenish each other.

Major Sources of Vitamin C. Red and green sweet peppers, broccoli, Brussels sprouts, cauliflower, strawberries, spinach, citrus fruits, cabbage.

NOTE: *Cooking (boiling, steaming, blanching) destroys about half of a vegetable's vitamin C. However, it does not matter how much water you use; broccoli cooked in 5 tablespoons of water loses just as much vitamin C as that cooked in 1½ pints (850ml) of water, tests show. Best bet: microwaving, which destroyed from zero to about 15 per cent of broccoli's vitamin C.*

Vitamin E (Tocopherol). Because of its antioxidant activity, vitamin E is heralded as a leading protector of the heart and arteries. People with higher blood levels of vitamin E are less likely to have arrhythmia and angina as well as heart attacks. Vitamin E, unlike vitamin C and beta carotene, is fat soluble and thus can help protect fat molecules against disease-fostering oxidative damage. For example, vitamin E is a mighty enemy of oxygen free radical chain reactions that can rip through cells, oxidizing their membranes. The presence of vitamin E can stop this catastrophic chain reaction. "Vitamin E is like a little fire extinguisher in a cell's membrane," says Joe McCord, an antioxidant expert at the University of Colorado.

Vitamin E is present in LDL cholesterol, which means it can help keep the LDL cholesterol fat molecules from becoming oxidized or toxic and thus able to launch events that end up in clogged and injured arteries.

Major Sources of Vitamin E. Vegetable oils, almonds, soya beans, sunflower seeds.

ANTI-INFLAMMATORY AGENTS

Before the last couple of decades and the discovery of hormone-like substances called prostaglandins and leukotrienes, it was impossible to comprehend how foods such as fish oil could possibly influence inflammatory diseases like arthritis and asthma. It is now known that prostaglandins and leukotrienes are manufactured by enzymatic breakdown of a fatty acid called arachidonic acid. What you eat determines how much of the arachidonic acid is present and what type of prostaglandins and leukotrienes; cell messengers that regulate the immune and inflammation process, are created.

If you eat a lot of meat and omega-6 type vegetable oils, you are likely to create more arachidonic acid that sets off chain reactions, resulting in specific leukotrienes that trigger inflammation. On the other hand, certain foods, such as fish oil, can manipulate the prostaglandin system to block the cascade of events that ends in troops of leukotrienes being dispatched to destroy tissue and produce inflammation. A food like ginger can intervene in at least three stages to block the complex biochemical inflammatory process.

On the other hand, capsaicin, the stuff that gives chilli peppers their fire, works through a different mechanism, according to researchers who have tested a new class of anti-inflammatory drugs derived from capsaicin.

FOODS THAT HAVE ANTI-INFLAMMATORY ACTIVITY
Apple, blackcurrant, fish oil (omega-3 fatty acids), garlic, ginger, onion, pineapple, sage.

FOOD CHEMICALS WITH ANTI-INFLAMMATORY ACTIVITY
Capsaicin (hot chilli peppers), omega-3 fatty acids (fatty fish such as mackerel, sardines and salmon), quercetin (onion).

ANTITHROMBOTIC AGENTS

Certain foods can lower fibrinogen in the blood, the stuff that forms the basis of blood clots. Additionally, food can stimulate the fibrino–lytic system which dissolves blood clots. High levels of fibrinogen and low fibrinolytic activity are found in those more likely to have atherosclerosis and heart attacks.

FOODS THAT DISCOURAGE BLOOD CLOTTING
Chilli pepper, fish oil, garlic, ginger, grape juice, onion, wakame (brown seaweed), wine (red).

ANTIULCERANTS

Some fascinating discoveries by British and Indian researchers have documented how food and food constituents strengthen the stomach's resistance to noxious ulcer-producing juices. For example, British investigators detected a 20 per cent thicker stomach lining in animals fed powder made from plantains, the banana-like fruit. Indian researchers photographed the rejuvenation of ulcerated cells in guinea pigs. The healing was due to increased mucins, substances that shield the stomach lining from damage, produced by drinking cabbage juice. Thus, one way foods can fight ulcers is by strengthening the stomach lining so it is not so easily eaten away by attacks from acids. Certain foods accomplish this by stimulating the proliferation of cells in the stomach lining and triggering the rapid release of mucus which covers the cells with a protective coating, sealing them off from acid harm.

Further, antibacterial foods such as yoghurt, tea, cabbage and liquorice may be more appropriate medicine against ulcers and gastritis, an inflammation of the stomach lining, than previously imagined. That's because physicians have discovered that a microbe known as H. pylori appears to be a cause of the two maladies in many cases. Ulcer treatment now often includes antibiotics. Antibacterial foods might also help cure the ulcer.

FOODS WITH ANTI-ULCER ACTIVITY
Bananas and plantains, cabbage and other cruciferous vegetables (broccoli, cauliflower, Brussels sprouts, kale and turnips), fenugreek seeds, fig, ginger, liquorice, tea.

ANTIVIRAL AGENTS

What you feed a virus that has made a home in your body can help determine whether it is switched on or off, starves or flourishes, and thus does or does not cause disease. In fascinating studies of women infected with a virus that can lead to cervical cancer, Charles Butterworth, M.D., at the University of Alabama, discovered that the virus was squelched if it was in the presence of adequate supplies of folic acid, a B vitamin in green leafy vegetables and legumes. Dr. Butterworth explains that when folic acid is lacking, chromosomes are more likely to break at "fragile" points. This allows the virus to slip into the healthy cells' genetic material, promoting initial changes that precede cancer. Those with low levels of folic acid in their red blood cells were five times more likely to develop such precancerous cell changes than those with higher folic acid levels.

The herpes virus is another case in point. Richard S. Griffith, M.D., professor emeritus of medicine at Indiana University Medical School, firmly believes diet determines whether this virus grows and causes trouble or remains dormant and harmless. It has been shown in lab studies, he says, that the amino acid arginine makes the herpes virus grow, and that the amino acid lysine stops its growth. He theorizes that lysine wraps itself around the cell, forming a barrier that the virus cannot penetrate.

Yoghurt has antiviral activity, for one reason, because it spurs activity of natural killer cells that are particularly vicious in attacking viruses.

FOODS WITH ANTIVIRAL ACTIVITY
Apples, apple juice, barley, blackcurrants, blueberries, chives, coffee, collards, cranberries, ginger, garlic, gooseberries, grapes, grapefruit

juice, lemon juice, mushrooms (notably shiitake), orange juice, peaches, pineapple juice, plums, plum juice, raspberries, sage, seaweed, spearmint, strawberries, tea, wine (red).

FOOD CHEMICALS WITH ANTIVIRAL ACTIVITY
Glutathione (asparagus, avocado, watermelon, broccoli, oranges), lentinan (shiitake mushrooms), quercetin (red and yellow onions, red grapes, broccoli, yellow summer squash), protease inhibitors (beans, corn, nuts, seeds).

CARMINATIVES

Herbs and spices have long been used in ancient medicine as carminatives, agents that help expel gas, relieving flatulence. The main pharmacological agent is thought to be oils in the plants that relax smooth muscles, letting gas escape. In some cases the gas erupts upward through a relaxed sphincter muscle between the oesophagus and the stomach. Then it is called a burp or a belch. Carminatives also have an antispasmodic, muscle-relaxing effect in the intestine.

FOODS WITH ANTI-GAS (CARMINATIVE) ACTIVITY
Anise, basil, chamomile, dill, fennel seeds, garlic, peppermint, sage.

CHOLESTEROL MODIFIERS

Food can lower bad-type LDL cholesterol, raise good-type HDL cholesterol and help prevent the oxidation of LDL cholesterol that makes it more destructive to arteries. Modern drugs mimic nature. Several years ago, scientists at the U.S. Department of Agriculture's lab at the University of Wisconsin in Madison discovered that food substances called tocotrienols suppress an enzyme that hampers the liver's manufacture of cholesterol. Cells needing cholesterol then suck it out of the bloodstream, and cholesterol blood levels go down. Other foods create different chemicals that seem also to turn down internal cholesterol production. Further, that is precisely how the potent cholesterol-reducing drug Mevacor (lovastatin) also works.

On the other hand, some foods, such as oats, are thought to deplete supplies of bile acids in the intestinal tract that otherwise would be turned into cholesterol.

Along new and more exciting lines, food antioxidants may help keep bad-type LDL cholesterol from becoming oxidized and toxic to arteries. Here are three possible ways food antioxidants may work, according to Harvard's Dr. Balz Frei. First, they may block formation of the bad guys, the reactive oxygen or "free radicals" that turn LDL toxic. The antioxidants could do this by attacking enzymes, in particular one called lipoxygenase, that create the LDL-altering agents. Second, antioxidants could trap the dangerous oxidants in the blood or artery wall where they are made. It is thought that one baddie, known as superoxide, is generated by cells in the arterial wall. Vitamin C, says Dr. Frei, might "soak it up".

Third, eating antioxidants could bolster the defences of LDL molecules so they can better resist destructive oxidation. As Dr. Frei notes, molecules of LDL cholesterol contain, in addition to fats and proteins, natural antioxidants such as vitamin E and beta carotene. Eating more of these antioxidant nutrients might further fortify the LDL molecules to fight off the oxidizing attackers that corrupt and render the LDL cholesterol so dangerous to arteries.

FOODS THAT CAN LOWER BAD LDL CHOLESTEROL
Almond, apple, avocado, barley, dried beans, carrot, garlic, grapefruit pulp, oats, olive oil, rice bran, shiitake mushrooms, soya beans, walnuts.

FOODS THAT MAY KEEP LDL CHOLESTEROL FROM BECOMING TOXIC
Foods high in vitamin C, foods high in beta carotene, foods high in vitamin E, foods high in co-enzyme Q-10, foods high in monounsaturated fat (olive oil, avocado, almond), red wine.

DIURETICS

Technically, plants do not function as diuretics the same way prescription drugs do, says Purdue University plant expert, Dr. Varro Tyler. Pharmaceutical diuretics increase the excretion of water and salt. Plant diuretics should more accurately be called "aquaretics," says Dr. Tyler, because they stimulate only a loss of water, not sodium. Some do this by irritating the cellular filters (glomeruli) of the kidney. Thus, they do not have the same potency as pharmaceutical diuretics, but their irritating mechanism could be detrimental if you have kidney disease. A fairly potent food "aquaretic" is parsley, says Dr. Tyler. He says you will get an effect by drinking parsley tea. Put a couple of heaping teaspoons of dried parsley in a cup of boiling water. He also rates theophylline (in tea) as a better diuretic than caffeine. Both lose their activity quickly when you become accustomed to them, he says.

FOODS WITH DIURETIC ACTIVITY
Anise, celery, coffee, coriander, cumin, aubergine, chicory, garlic, juniper berries, lemon, liquorice, nutmeg, onion, parsley, peppermint, tea.

DECONGESTANTS

It's been known for centuries that hot, spicy, pungent foods can help clear the lungs and breathing passages. They do so by thinning mucus and encouraging it to move along. Just notice what happens when you eat a hot food; your eyes tear up, your nose begins to run. The same thing happens in your lungs. It is thought that hot foods trigger nerve endings in the oesophagus and stomach, causing the watery reactions.

FOODS THAT HAVE MUCOKINETIC (MUCUS-CLEARING) ACTIVITY
Chilli pepper, curry spices, garlic, horseradish, mustard, onion, black pepper, thyme.

HORMONES

Numerous plants contain phytoestrogens that are similar in molecular structure to that of human oestrogen but have a weaker and different effect. Thus plant oestrogens, being less potent, are slower to generate benefits; they appear safer, however, lacking synthetic oestrogen's potential for producing adverse side effects. Additionally, some food, notably vegetables of the cabbage family, increase the rate at which your body burns up and disposes of oestrogen circulating in the body. Legumes, especially soya beans, have particularly strong oestrogenic activity, and are now the commercial source for compounds used to make birth control pills.

FOODS WITH OESTROGENIC ACTIVITY
Anise, apple, broccoli, Brussels sprouts, cabbage, carrot, cauliflower, coffee, corn, cumin, flax seed, garlic, liquorice, oats, pineapple, peanut, potato, rice, sesame seed, soya beans.

IMMUNE STIMULANTS

A primary indicator of health is how well your immune system marshals defences to fight off enemies such as viruses and tumour cells. The possibilities are evident in yoghurt. Eating yoghurt stimulates at least two vital components of immunity – natural killer cells and gamma interferon. 1lb 450g a day with live active cultures raised interferon levels fivefold in human trials. Yoghurt also strengthened the activity of natural killer cells (NK) that attack viruses and tumour cells. Joseph Scimeca, Ph.D., nutrition researcher at Kraft General Foods, Inc., explains that natural killer cells circulating in the body detect tumour cells, then seek out and destroy them just as Pac-Man gobbles up prey in the video game. Natural killer cells are one of the best defences against tumour cells and viruses, he says. Remarkably, even yoghurt that has been heated to kill 95 per cent of the bacterial cultures still activates natural killer cells, Dr. Scimeca discovered.

FOODS THAT STIMULATE IMMUNITY
Garlic, shiitake mushrooms, yoghurt.

FOOD CHEMICALS THAT STIMULATE IMMUNITY
Beta carotene (carrots, spinach, kale, pumpkin, sweet potatoes), vitamin C (peppers, oranges, broccoli, spinach), vitamin E (nuts, oils), zinc (shellfish, grains).

PAINKILLERS

New discoveries about two common food compounds illustrate how food can block the perception of pain. One is caffeine, recently discovered to be a mild painkiller independently of its common use in combination with other analgesic drugs. The other is capsaicin, the fiery chemical in hot chilli peppers, which is now being widely tested as a potential painkiller.

Caffeine seems to work as a painkiller by masquerading as a chemical called adenosine, thus interrupting the transmission of pain signals to the brain. The body pumps out adenosine as a sign of distress. For example, explains Dr. Luiz Belardinelli, professor of medicine at the University of Florida Medical School, let's say you are running and you feel a stab of pain in your chest. It's adenosine telling you to slow down. "The pain is a sign something is wrong," he says. However, if you drink enough caffeine it overrides that pain signal. Like a gang of thugs, molecules of caffeine push adenosine off cells' receptor sites, and take their place, disconnecting the pain signals. The receptor sites accept caffeine because it chemically resembles adenosine, although it does not have the same biochemical function. This is fine if drinking caffeine cures your headache, but may not be good if your heart's pain signals are blocked by caffeine. Dr. Belardinelli fears that caffeine is such a good painkiller it may keep people from noticing heart distress, and thus may contribute to silent myocardial ischemia, in which a person has a heart attack without experiencing painful symptoms.

For years people have put hot pepper extract on their gums to cure toothache. Now it is known that capsaicin (the hot stuff) in peppers is a local anesthetic and a promising new painkiller. Capsaicin squelches pain by draining nerve cells of something called substance P which relays pain sensations to the central nervous system. Thus, capsaicin helps block the perception of pain. Recently, the hot pepper essence has been injected or made into medications to help combat cluster headaches, diabetic neuropathy, chronic itching, rheumatoid arthritis and neuralgia.

FOODS WITH ANALGESIC (PAINKILLING) ACTIVITY
Coffee (caffeine), chilli peppers (capsaicin), clove, garlic, ginger, liquorice, onion, peppermint, sugar.

SALICYLATES

Aspirin in your food? Absolutely. Certain foods, mainly fruits, have aspirin-like activity. The proof is that when people who are sensitive to aspirin eat such foods, they have reactions similar to those caused by taking aspirin. Therefore, allergists warn aspirin-sensitive people to shun foods heavily laced with salicylates, the stuff aspirin is made of.

On the other hand, scientists are intrigued by the prospect that salicylates in food may offer some of the same protection as taking aspirin. New research suggests that regular low doses of aspirin (half an aspirin a day or perhaps less) help prevent heart attacks, strokes, even colon cancer. Perhaps continual low doses of food salicylates also stop some of our health headaches. The presence of this natural drug might be one more reason certain plant foods guard against cardiovascular disease and cancer, say experts. Salicylates have anticoagulant, anti-inflammatory and analgesic effects. They also may affect prostaglandins in ways that retard the grow of tumours.

FOODS EXTREMELY HIGH IN NATURAL ASPIRIN (SALICYLATES)
Blueberries, cherries, dried currants, curry powder, dried dates, gherkins (small pickles), liquorice, paprika, prunes, raspberries.

FOODS MODERATELY HIGH IN SALICYLATES
Almonds, apples (notably Granny Smith), oranges, peppers (sweet and hot), persimmons, pineapples, tea.

NOTE: *Generally, fruits contain considerable amounts of salicylates; vegetables do not. (Canning and heating do not appear to affect salicylate concentrations.)*

SURPRISE! THERE'S VALIUM IN YOUR FOOD

So you think the tranquillizer Valium is a twentieth-century invention? Wrong. Nature holds the patent. Apparently, humans and animals have been eating the drug in food for eons. German scientists came upon this eerie and astonishing fact when they examined the brain tissue of people who died before 1940. Valium did not come on the market until the 1960s. Yet, indisputably, the pre-Valium-age brains contained traces of natural benzodiazepines – mood-altering chemicals of which Valium is the prime example. Somehow it got there a good number of years before Hoffmann-La Roche began production.

Additionally, the scientists – Dr. Ulrich Klotz and Elizabeth Unseld, at the Fischer-Bosch Institute of Clinical Pharmacology in Stuttgart – detected the tranquillizers in the brains of wild and domesticated animals, including dogs, cats, deer, cows and chickens, as well as in eggs, cow's milk and the blood of people who had never taken the drug.

How did it get there? The most reasonable explanation is that the chemicals must be present in plants eaten for food; trace amounts then were "trapped" in the brain. So the scientists screened foods for benzodiazepines. They found them in potatoes, brown lentils, yellow soya beans, rice, corn, mushrooms and cherries, albeit in minuscule amounts. Why did Mother Nature lace food with tiny doses of tranquillizers? Dr. Klotz speculates that food-borne tranquillizers might serve as brain messengers, neurotransmitters or neuromodulators but any pharmacological effect, if it exists, must be very subtle. According to Dr. Klotz's calculations, you would have to eat at least 220lb (100 kg) of potatoes at one sitting to get the effect of a normal dose of 5–10mg of Valium. Frankly, he says, at this point, nobody knows if there is "a biological role" for the natural tranquillizers. Nature's purpose for putting them there is still a scientific mystery

SEDATIVES AND TRANQUILLIZERS

If Mother Nature was thoughtful enough to lace our food with the tranquillizer Valium, albeit in infinitesimal amounts, and to put a mild sedative, quercetin, in onions, who knows how many other undiscovered brain-calming agents may also be present in food? It's possible that some natural sedatives work like morphine by attaching to opiate receptors in the brain. Others probably stimulate the activity and/or levels of neurotransmitters, such as serotonin, that calms the brain. Honey, sugar and other carbohydrates are thought by some to affect serotonin, inducing tranquillity and sleep in most people. Sugar or glucose may also work directly on the neurons in the brain's hypothalamus. Additionally, some foods contain peptides or release peptides in the gut that can send messages from the intestinal tract directly to the nervous system and brain.

FOODS WITH CALMING AND SEDATIVE PROPERTIES
Anise, celery seed, clove, cumin, fennel, garlic, ginger, honey, lime peel, marjoram, onion, orange peel, parsley, sage, spearmint, sugar, tea (decaffeinated).

Additionally, any foods high in carbohydrates – sugar and starches – have sedative effects on most people.

DISEASE-FIGHTING POWERS IN SIXTY COMMON FOODS

Since foods are exceedingly complex packages of chemicals, they do not deliver a single biological punch, as do specially formulated pharmaceutical drugs designed to accomplish a specific purpose. Instead, food stimulates diverse biological activity. Here are the varied pharmacological powers that have been attributed to common foods, according to the latest evidence.

Apple. Reduces cholesterol, contains anti-cancer agents. Has mild antibacterial, antiviral, anti-inflammatory, oestrogenic activity. High in fibre, helps avoid constipation, suppresses appetite. Juice can cause diarrhoea in children.

Asparagus. A super source of glutathione, an antioxidant with strong anticancer activity.

Aubergine. Aubergine substances called glycoalkaloids, made into a topical cream medication, have been used to treat skin cancers such as basal cell carcinoma, according to Australian researchers. Also, eating aubergine may lower blood cholesterol and help counteract some detrimental blood effects of fatty foods. Aubergine also has anti–bacterial and diuretic properties.

Avocado. Benefits arteries. Lowers cholesterol, dilates blood vessels. Its main fat, monounsaturated oleic acid (also concentrated in olive oil), acts as an antioxidant to block artery-destroying toxicity of bad-type LDL cholesterol. One of the richest sources of glutathione, a powerful antioxidant, shown to block thirty different carcinogens and to block proliferation of the AIDS virus in test tube experiments. Also a vasodilator.

Banana and Plantain. Soothes the stomach. Good for dyspepsia (upset stomach.) Strengthens the stomach lining against acid and ulcers. Has antibiotic activity.

Barley. Long known as a "heart medicine" in the Middle East. Reduces cholesterol. Has antiviral and anticancer activity. Contains potent antioxidants, including tocotrienols.

Beans (*legumes, including navy, black, kidney, pinto beans and lentils*). Potent medicine in lowering cholesterol. 3oz (85g) of cooked beans daily reduces cholesterol an average 10 per cent. Regulates blood sugar levels. An excellent food for diabetics. Linked to lower rates of certain cancers. Very high in fibre. A leading producer of intestinal gas in most people.

Blueberry. Acts as an unusual type antibiotic by blocking attachment of bacteria that cause urinary tract infections. Contains chemicals that curb diarrhoea. Also antiviral activity and high in natural aspirin.

Broccoli. A spectacular and unique package of versatile disease-fighters. Abundant in numerous strong, well-known antioxidants, including quercetin, glutathione, beta carotene, indoles, vitamin C, lutein, glucarate, sulphoraphane. Extremely high anticancer activity, particularly against lung, colon and breast cancers. Like other cruciferous vegetables, it speeds up removal of oestrogen from the body, helping suppress breast cancer. Rich in cholesterol-reducing fibre. Has antiviral, anti-ulcer activity. A super source of chromium that helps regulate insulin and blood sugar. Note: cooking and processing destroys some of the antioxidants and anti-oestrogenic agents, such as indoles and glutathione. Most protective when eaten raw or lightly cooked, as in stir frying and microwaving.

Brussels Sprouts. As one of the cruciferous family, possesses some of the same powers as broccoli and cabbage. Definitely anti-cancer, oestrogenic and packed with various antioxidants and indoles.

Cabbage (*including bok choy*). Revered in ancient Rome as a cancer cure. Contains numerous anticancer and antioxidant compounds. Speeds up oestrogen metabolism, is thought to help block breast cancer and suppress growth of polyps, a prelude to colon cancer. In studies, eating cabbage more than once a week cut men's colon cancer odds 66 per cent. As little as two daily tablespoons of cooked cabbage protected against stomach cancer. Contains anti-ulcer compounds; cabbage juice helps heal ulcers in humans. Has antibacterial and antiviral powers. Can cause flatulence in some. Sauerkraut (high in tyramine) can help trigger migraine headaches. Note: Some antioxidant, anticancer and oestrogenic activity of compounds (indoles, in particular) are destroyed by cooking. Raw cabbage, as in cole slaw, appears to have stronger overall pharmacological activity.

Carrot. A super food source of beta carotene, a powerful anticancer, artery-protecting, immune-boosting, infection-fighting antioxidant with wide protective powers. A carrot a day slashed stroke rates in women by 68 per cent. One medium carrot's worth of beta carotene cuts lung cancer risk in half, even among formerly heavy smokers. High doses of beta carotene, as found in carrots, substantially reduces odds of degenerative eye diseases – cataracts and macular degeneration – as well as chest pain (angina). Carrots' high soluble fibre depresses blood cholesterol, promotes regularity. Note: Cooking does not destroy beta carotene; in fact, light cooking can make it easier for the body to absorb.

Cauliflower. A member of the famous cruciferous family, it contains many of the same cancer-fighting, hormone-regulating compounds as its cousins, broccoli and cabbage. Specifically thought to help ward off breast and colon cancers. Note: Heavy cooking destroys some pharmacological activity. Eat raw, lightly cooked or microwaved.

Celery. A traditional Vietnamese remedy for high blood pressure. Celery compounds reduce blood pressure in animals. Comparable human dose: two to four stalks a day. Has a mild diuretic effect. Contains eight different families of anticancer compounds, such as phthalides and polyacetylenes, that detoxify carcinogens, especially cigarette smoke. Eating celery before or after vigorous exercise can induce mild to serious allergic reactions in some.

Chilli Pepper. Revs up the blood-clot-dissolving system, opens up sinuses and air passages, breaks up mucus in the lungs, acts as an expectorant or decongestant, helps prevent bronchitis, emphysema and stomach ulcers. Most of chilli pepper's pharmacological activity is credited to capsaicin (from the Latin "to bite"), the compound that makes the pepper taste hot. Capsaicin is also a potent painkiller, alleviating headaches when inhaled, and joint pain when injected. Hot paprika made from hot chilli peppers is high in natural aspirin. Antibacterial, antioxidant activity. Putting hot chilli sauce on food also speeds up metabolism, burning off calories. Contrary to popular belief, chilli peppers do not harm the stomach lining or promote ulcers.

Chocolate. Contains chemicals thought to affect neurotransmitters in the brain. Added to milk, chocolate helps counteract lactose intolerance. Chocolate does not seem to raise cholesterol or cause or aggravate acne. Dark chocolate is very high in copper, which may help ward off cardiovascular disease. Triggers headaches in some. Aggravates heartburn. Implicated in cystic breast disease.

Cinnamon. A strong stimulator of insulin activity, thus potentially helpful for those with Type II diabetes. Mild anticoagulant activity.

Clove. Long used to kill the pain of toothache and as an anti-inflammatory against rheumatic diseases. Has anticoagulant effects, (anti-platelet aggregation), and its main ingredient, eugenol, is anti-inflammatory.

Coffee. Most, but not all, of coffee's pharmacological impact comes from its high concentration of caffeine, a psychoactive drug of great power. Caffeine, depending on an individual's biological makeup and peculiar sensitivity, can be a mood elevator and mental energizer. Improves mental performance. One cup of morning coffee gives the brain a "jump start". Caffeine is an emergency remedy for asthma. Also, regular coffee drinkers have less asthma and wheezing. Dilates bronchial passages. Mildly addictive. Triggers headaches, anxiety and panic attacks in some. In excess may cause psychiatric disturbances. Definitely promotes insomnia. Coffee stimulates stomach acid secretion (both caffeinated and decaf). Can aggravate heartburn. Promotes bowel movements in many, causes diarrhoea in others.

"Extensive research on caffeine . . . has found no significant health hazard from normal caffeine consumption." – Professor Peter B. Dews, Ph.D., Harvard Medical School

---

No solid evidence links coffee or caffeine to cancers. Caffeine may promote fibrocystic breast disease in some women. There's scant evidence of cardiovascular danger from moderate caffeine and coffee – under four to six cups a day. Coffee brewed by drip method appears to have little or no detrimental impact on blood cholesterol.

WHERE YOU GET CAFFEINE

	Milligrams (average)
Coffee – 5fl oz (140ml) (a cup not a mug)	
Brewed	
drip	115
percolated	80
decaffeinated	3
Instant	
regular	65
decaffeinated	2
Tea 5fl oz (140ml)	
Infused – bags or leaves	60
Instant – 1 tsp, instant powder	30
Soft drinks	
Cola (regular and diet)	46
Mountain Dew	54
Chocolate	
cocoa beverage – 5fl oz (140ml)	4
milk chocolate – 1oz (30g)	6
plain chocolate – 1oz (30g)	20

Collard Greens. Full of diverse anticancer, antioxidant compounds, including lutein, vitamin C, beta carotene. In animals blocks the spread of breast cancer. Like other green leafy vegetables, associated with low rates of all cancers. High in oxalates, not recommended for those with kidney stones.

Corn. Anticancer and antiviral activity, possibly induced by corn's content of protease inhibitors. Has oestrogen-boosting capabilities. A very common cause of food intolerance linked to symptoms of rheumatoid arthritis, irritable bowel syndrome, headaches and migraine-related epilepsy in children.

Cranberry. Strong antibiotic properties with unusual abilities to prevent infectious bacteria from sticking to cells lining the bladder and urinary tract. Thus, it helps prevent recurring urinary tract (bladder) infections. Also has antiviral activity.

Date. High in natural aspirin. Has laxative effect. Dried fruits, including dates, are linked to lower rates of certain cancers, especially pancreatic cancer. Contains compounds that may cause headaches in susceptible individuals.

Fenugreek Seeds. A spice common in the Middle East and available in many supermarkets. Has antidiabetic powers. Helps control surges of blood sugar and insulin. Also antidiarrhoeal, anti-ulcer, antidiabetic, anticancer, tends to lower blood pressure, helps prevent intestinal gas. Note: Fenugreek was the main ingredient, besides alcohol, in Lydia E. Pinkham's Vegetable Compound, a remedy for "female complaints" that came on the American market in 1875.

Fig. Long used in folklore to fight cancer. Both extract of figs and the fig compound benzaldehyde have helped shrink tumours in humans, according to Japanese tests. Also laxative, anti-ulcer, antibacterial and antiparasitic powers. Triggers headaches in some people.

Fish and Fish Oil. An exceedingly remarkable therapeutic and preventive food. Intervenes in heart disease, preventing heart attack deaths (two servings a week); 1oz (30g) a day has been shown to cut risk of heart attacks 50 per cent. Oil in fish can relieve symptoms of rheumatoid arthritis, osteoarthritis, asthma, psoriasis, high blood pressure, Raynaud's disease, migraine headaches, ulcerative colitis, possibly multiple sclerosis. May help ward off strokes. A known anti-inflammatory agent and anticoagulant. Raises good type HDL cholesterol. Slashes triglycerides dramatically. May help guard against development of glucose intolerance and Type II diabetes. Some fish are high in antioxidants, such as selenium and co-enzyme Q-10. Exhibits anticancer activity especially in blocking development of colon cancer and spread of breast cancer. Note: Fish highest in omega-3 fatty acids appear most protective: These include sardines, mackerel, herring, salmon, tuna. Sardines are high in oxalates, and may promote kidney stone formation in susceptible individuals.

Garlic. An all-around wonder drug, used to treat an array of ills since the dawn of civilization. A proven broad-spectrum antibiotic that combats bacteria, intestinal parasites and viruses. In high doses it has cured encephalitis. Lowers blood pressure and blood cholesterol, discourages dangerous blood clotting. Two or three cloves a day cut the odds of subsequent heart attacks in half in heart patients.

Contains multiple anticancer compounds and antioxidants and tops the American National Cancer Institute's list as a potential cancer-preventive food. Lessens chances of stomach cancer in particular. A good cold medication. Acts as a decongestant, expectorant, antispasmodic, anti-inflammatory agent. Boosts immune responses. Helps relieve gas, has antidiarrhoeal, oestrogenic and diuretic activity. Appears to lift mood and has a mild calming effect. High doses of raw garlic (more than three cloves a day) have caused gas, bloating, diarrhoea and fever in some. Note: To fight bacteria, raw garlic is better. However, cooking does not diminish garlic's blood-thinning and other cardioprotective capabilities, and, in fact, may enhance them by releasing antithrombotic ajoene. Sauteeing garlic in oil also boosts its potency as a decongestant. Nor are anticancer properties lost by cooking, say experts. For example, U.S. cancer–authority Dr. Herbert Pierson favours cooked garlic over raw garlic.

Ginger. Used for centuries in Asia to treat nausea, vomiting, headache, chest congestion, cholera, colds, diarrhoea, stomach ache, rheumatism, and nervous diseases. Ginger is a proven anti-nausea, anti-motion sickness remedy that matches or passes drugs such as Dramamine. Helps thwart and prevent migraine headaches and osteoarthritis. Relieves symptoms of rheumatoid arthritis. Acts as an antithrombotic and anti-inflammatory agent in humans; is an antibiotic in test tubes (kills salmonella and staph bacteria), and an anti-ulcer agent in animals. Also, has antidepressant, antidiarrhoeal and strong antioxidant activity. Ranks very high in anticancer activity.

Grape. A rich storehouse of antioxidant, anticancer compounds. Red grapes (but not white or green grapes), are high in antioxidant quercetin. Grape skins contain resveratrol, shown to inhibit blood-platelet clumping (and consequently, blood clot formation) and boost good-type HDL cholesterol. Red grapes are antibacterial and antiviral in test tubes. Grapeseed oil also raises good-type HDL cholesterol.

Grapefruit. The pulp contains a unique pectin (in membranes and juice sacs – not in juice) that lowers blood cholesterol and reverses atherosclerosis (clogged arteries) in animals. Has anticancer activity, and appears particularly protective against stomach and pancreatic cancer. The juice is antiviral. High in various antioxidants, especially disease-fighting vitamin C. May aggravate heartburn.

Honey. Strong antibiotic properties. Has sleep-inducing sedative and tranquillizing properties. Caution: Do not feed honey to infants under age one; there is a danger of potentially deadly botulism.

Kale. An amazingly rich source of various antioxidant, anticancer chemicals of various types. Has more beta carotene than spinach and twice as much lutein, the most of any vegetable tested. Kale is also a member of the cruciferous family, endowing it with anticancer indoles that help regulate oestrogen and fight off colon cancer. It ranks very high as a potential cancer preventive and all-around disease-fighting vegetable.

Kiwi Fruit. Commonly prescribed in Chinese traditional medicine to treat stomach and breast cancer. High in vitamin C which has multiple antidisease activity.

Liquorice. A potent, multi-faceted medicine. Strong anticancer powers, possibly because of a high concentration of glycyrrhizin. Mice drinking glycyrrhizin dissolved in water have fewer skin cancers. Also kills bacteria, fights ulcers and diarrhoea. May act as a diuretic. Eating too much liquorice can be dangerous, as it raises blood pressure. Also it is not advised for pregnant women. Note: Only real liquorice has these powers. Liquorice sweets may be fake, made with anise instead of real liquorice. Check the label. Real liquorice says "liquorice mass". Imitation liquorice is labeled "artificial liquorice" or "anise".

Melon (*green and yellow, such as cantaloupe and honeydew*). Has anticoagulant (blood-thinning) activity. Orange melons contain antioxidant beta carotene.

Milk. Cancer-fighting powers, possibly against colon, lung, stomach and cervical cancers, especially in low-fat milk. One study detected less cancer among low-fat milk drinkers than nonmilk drinkers. May help prevent high blood pressure. Skimmed milk may lower blood cholesterol. Milk fat promotes cancer and heart disease.

Milk is also an unappreciated terror in triggering "allergic" reactions that induce joint pain and symptoms of rheumatoid arthritis, asthma, irritable bowel syndrome, and diarrhoea. In children and infants milk is suspected to cause or contribute to colic, respiratory problems, sleeplessness, itchy rashes, migraines, epileptic seizures, ear infections and even diabetes. Contrary to popular belief, milk stimulates production of stomach acid and retards healing of ulcers.

Mushroom (*Asian, including shiitake*). Long esteemed in Asia as a longevity tonic, heart medicine and cancer remedy. Current tests show Asian mushrooms, such as shiitake, help prevent and/or treat cancer, viral diseases, such as influenza and polio, high blood cholesterol, sticky blood platelets and high blood pressure. Eaten daily, shiitake, fresh (3oz (85g)) or dried (⅓oz (10g)) cut cholesterol by 7 and 12 per cent respectively. A shiitake compound, lentinan, is a broad-spectrum antiviral agent that potentiates immune functioning. Used to treat leukemia in China and breast cancer in Japan. Shiitake extract (sulphated B-glucans) has been declared by Japanese scientists more effective as an AIDS drug than the common drug AZT. Eating black mo-er ("tree ear") mushroom "thins the blood". Note: No therapeutic effects are known for the common button mushroom. Some claim this species has cancer-causing potential (hydrazides) unless cooked.

Mustard (*including horseradish*). Recognized for centuries as a decongestant and expectorant. Helps break up mucus in air passages. A good remedy for congestion caused by colds and sinus problems. Also antibacterial. Revs up metabolism, burning off extra calories. In one British test about three-fifths of a teaspoon of ordinary yellow mustard increased metabolic rate about 25 per cent, burning 45 more calories in three hours.

Nuts. Anticancer and heart-protective properties. A key food among Seventh-Day Adventists, known for their low rates of heart disease. Walnuts and almonds help reduce cholesterol, contain high concentrations of antioxidant oleic acid and monounsaturated fat, similar to that in olive oil, known to protect arteries from damage. Nuts generally are high in antioxidant vitamin E, shown to protect against chest pain and artery damage. Brazil nuts are extremely rich in selenium, an antioxidant linked to lower rates of heart disease and cancer. Walnuts contain ellagic acid, an antioxidant and cancer-fighter, and are also high in omega-3 type oil. Nuts, including peanuts, are good regulators of insulin and blood sugar, preventing steep rises, making them good foods for those with glucose intolerance and diabetes. Peanuts also are oestrogenic. Nuts have been found lacking in the diets of those who later develop Parkinson's disease. Peanuts are a prime cause of acute allergic reactions in susceptible individuals.

Oats. A couple of bowls of oat bran or three bowls of oatmeal a day can depress cholesterol 10 per cent or more, depending on individual responses. Oats help stabilize blood sugar, have oestrogenic and antioxidant activity. They also contain psychoactive compounds that may combat nicotine cravings and have antidepressant powers. High doses can cause gas, abdominal bloating and pain in some. Oats, like other cereals, can trigger food intolerances in susceptible persons, causing chronic bowel distress.

Olive oil. An artery protector that lowers bad LDL cholesterol without lowering good HDL cholesterol. Helps keep bad cholesterol from being converted to a toxic or "oxidized" form. Thus, helps protect arteries from plaque. Reduces blood pressure, helps regulate blood sugar. Has potent antioxidant activity. May help ward off cancer.

Onion (including chives, shallots, spring onions, leeks). One of civilizations oldest medicines, reputed in ancient Mesopotamia to cure virtually everything. An exceptionally strong antioxidant. Full of numerous anticancer agents. Blocks cancer dramatically in animals. The onion is the richest dietary source of quercetin, a potent antioxidant (in shallots, yellow and red onions only – not white onions). Specifically linked to inhibiting human stomach cancer. Thins the blood, lowers cholesterol, raises good-type HDL cholesterol (preferred dose: half a raw onion a day), wards off blood clots, fights asthma, chronic bronchitis, hay fever, diabetes, atherosclerosis and infections. Anti-inflammatory, antibiotic, antiviral, thought to have diverse anticancer powers. Quercetin is also a sedative. Onions aggravate heartburn, may promote gas.

Orange. A complete package of every class of natural cancer inhibitor known – carotenoids, terpenes and flavonoids. Also rich in antioxidant vitamin C and beta carotene. Specifically tied to lower rates of pancreatic cancer. Orange juice protected mice sperm from radiation damage. Because of its high vitamin C, oranges may help ward off asthma attacks, bronchitis, breast cancer, stomach cancer, athero–sclerosis, gum disease, and boost fertility and healthy sperm in some men. Oranges and orange juice may aggravate heartburn.

Parsley. Anticancer because of its high concentrations of antioxidants, such as monoterpenes, phthalides, polyacetylenes. Can help detoxify carcinogens and neutralize certain carcinogens in tobacco smoke. Also, has diuretic activity.

Parsnip. Excellent anticancer potential. Contains six types of anticancer agents.

Pineapple. Suppresses inflammation. Both the fruit and a main constituent, an antibacterial enzyme called bromelain, are anti-inflammatory. Pineapple aids digestion, helps dissolve blood clots and is good for preventing osteoporosis and bone fractures because of its very high manganese content. It is also antibacterial and antiviral and mildly oestrogenic.

Plum. Antibacterial. Antiviral. Works as a laxative.

Potato (white). Contains anticancer protease inhibitors. High in potassium, thus may help prevent high blood pressure and strokes. Some oestrogenic activity.

Prune. A well-known laxative. High in fibre, sorbitol and natural aspirin.

Pumpkin. Extremely high in beta carotene, the antioxidant reputed to help ward off numerous health problems, including heart attacks, cancer, cataracts.

Raspberry. Antiviral, anticancer activity. High in natural aspirin.

Rice. Antidiarrhoeal, anticancer activity. Like other seeds, contains anticancer protease inhibitors. Of all grains and cereals, it is the least likely to provoke intestinal gas or adverse reactions (intolerances), causing bowel distress such as spastic colon. Rice bran is excellent against constipation, lowers cholesterol and tends to block development of kidney stones.

Rhubarb. Extremely high in oxalates which help promote formation of kidney stones in susceptible individuals. Little or no laxative effect.

Seaweed and Kelp (brown or Laminaria type seaweed). Antibacterial and antiviral activity in brown Laminaria type seaweed known as kelp. It kills herpes virus, for example. Kelp may also lower blood pressure and cholesterol. Wakame boosts immune functioning. Nori kills bacteria and seems to help heal ulcers. A chemical from wakame seaweed is a clot-buster, in one test twice as powerful as the common drug heparin. Most types of seaweed have anticancer activity. Seaweed is very high in iodine and might aggravate acne flare-ups.

Soya bean. Packed with pharmacological activity. Rich in hormones, it boosts oestrogen levels in postmenopausal women. Has anticancer activity and is thought to be especially antagonistic to breast cancer, possibly one reason rates of breast and prostate cancers are low among the Japanese. Soya beans are the richest source of potent protease inhibitors which are anticancer, antiviral agents. In many human tests, soya beans lower blood cholesterol substantially. In animals, soya beans seem to deter and help dissolve kidney stones.

Spinach. Tops the list, along with other green leafy vegetables, as a food most eaten by people who don't get cancer. A super source of antioxidants and cancer antagonists, containing about four times more beta carotene and three times more lutein than broccoli, for example. Rich in fibre that helps lower blood cholesterol. Extremely high in oxalate, thus, not recommended for people with kidney stones. Note: Some of its antioxidants are destroyed by cooking. Eat raw or lightly cooked.

Strawberry. Antiviral, anticancer activity. Often eaten by people less likely to develop all types of cancer.

Sugar. A sedative, sleep inducer, painkiller, tranquillizer, antidepressant. Very antibacterial. Helps heal wounds when applied externally. Like other carbohydrates, sugar helps induce cavities. Also may be related to Crohn's disease. Triggers rises in blood sugar and stimulates insulin production.

Sweet Pepper. Super-rich in antioxidant vitamin C. Therefore, a great food for fighting off colds, asthma, bronchitis, respiratory infections, cataracts, macular degeneration, angina, atherosclerosis and cancer.

Sweet Potato (*also popularly called yams*). A blockbuster source of the antioxidant beta carotene, linked to preventing heart disease, cataracts, strokes and numerous cancers. 4½oz (130g) of mashed sweet potatoes contains about 14mg of beta carotene, or about 23,000 international units (IUs), according to Department of Agriculture figures.

Tea (*including black, oolong and green tea, not herbal teas*). Amazing and diverse pharmacological activity, mainly due to catechins. Tea acts as an anticoagulant, artery protector, antibiotic, anti-ulcer agent, cavity-fighter, antidiarrhoeal agent, antiviral agent, diuretic (caffeine), analgesic (caffeine), mild sedative (decaffeinated). In animals tea and tea compounds are potent blockers of various cancers. Tea drinkers appear to have less atherosclerosis (damaged, clogged arteries) and fewer strokes. Excessive tea drinking because of its caffeine could aggravate anxiety, insomnia and symptoms of PMS. Tea may also promote kidney stones because of its high oxalate content.

Note: Green tea, popular in Asian countries, is highest in catechins, followed by oolong and ordinary black tea. Thus, green tea is considered most potent. One human study, however, found no difference in benefits to arteries from green or black tea. Black tea is the type you find anywhere sold as loose tea or in tea bags. Green tea is less available, but may be found in Asian markets, specialty food stores and some supermarkets. It's also served in Asian restaurants.

Tomato. A major source of lycopene, an awesome antioxidant and anticancer agent that intervenes in devastating chain reactions of oxygen free radical molecules. Tomatoes are linked in particular to lower rates of pancreatic cancer and cervical cancer.

Turmeric. Truly one of the marvellous medicinal spices of the world. Its main active ingredient is curcumin which gives turmeric its intense cadmium yellow colour. Curcumin, studies show, is an anti-inflammatory agent on a par with cortisone, and has reduced inflammation in animals and symptoms of rheumatoid arthritis in humans. In other tests, it lowered cholesterol, hindered platelet aggregation (blood clotting), protected the liver from toxins, boosted stomach defences against acid, lowered blood sugar in diabetics, and was a powerful antagonist of numerous cancer-causing agents. It is known to have varied anticancer activity.

Watermelon. High amounts of lycopene and glutathione, antioxidant and anticancer compounds. Also mild antibacterial, anticoagulant activity.

Wheat. High-fibre whole wheat, and particularly wheat bran, rank as the world's greatest preventives of constipation. The bran is potently anti-cancer. Remarkably, in humans, wheat bran can suppress polyps that can develop into colon cancer. In women wheat bran appears to antagonize breast cancer by diminishing supplies of oestrogen. It is also antiparasitic. On the negative side, wheat ranks exceedingly high as a trigger of food intolerances and allergies, resulting in symptoms of rheumatoid arthritis, irritable bowel syndrome and neurological illnesses.

Wine. In moderation – a glass or two a day – benefits cardiovascular system. Both red and white wine boost heart-protecting HDL cholesterol. Red wine, in particular, seems to help ward off heart disease, blood clots and strokes because grape skins contain blood-thinning agents. (Grape skins are used in making red wine, but not white wine.) Boosts oestrogen levels, which may accentuate wine's HDL-raising effects. Kills bacteria, inhibits viruses. May also discourage gallstones. Red wine is a trigger of migraine headaches in some individuals. In excess, wine, because of its alcohol, can cause heart, liver and brain damage.

Yoghurt. An ancient wonder food, strongly antibacterial and anticancer. 8oz (225g) or so of yoghurt a day boosts immune functioning by stimulating production of gamma interferon. Also spurs activity of natural killer cells that attack viruses and tumours. A daily 8oz (225g) of yoghurt reduced colds and other upper respiratory infections in humans. Helps prevent and cure diarrhoea. A daily cup of yoghurt with acidophilus cultures prevents vaginitis (yeast infections) in women. Helps fight bone problems, such as osteoporosis, because of high available calcium content. Acidophilus yoghurt cultures neutralize cancer-causing agents in the intestinal tract. Plain old yoghurt with L. bulgaricus and S. thermophilus cultures, both live and dead, blocked lung cancers in animals. Yoghurt with live cultures is safe for people with lactose intolerance.

"Yoghurt is just about a panacea for women. It boosts immunity, delivers lots of available calcium and helps prevent vaginitis." – Georges Halpern, M.D., University of California at Davis.

APPENDIX
Foods with the Most Pharmacological Vitamins, Minerals and Oils

FOODS HIGH IN BETA CAROTENE

(milligrams per 3½oz/100g)

Apricots dried	17.6 (about 28 halves)
Peaches, dried	9.2 (about 7 halves)
Sweet Potatoes, cooked	8.8
Carrots	7.9 (about 1¼ medium carrots)
Collard greens	5.4
Kale	4.7
Spinach, raw	4.1
Apricot, raw	3.5 (about 3 medium)
Pumpkin	3.1
Cantaloupe	3.0 (about ⅒ melon)
Beet greens	2.2
Squash, winter	2.4
Cos lettuce	1.9 (equal of 10 leaves)
Grapefruit, pink	1.3 (about ½ grapefruit)
Mango	1.3 (about ½ mango)
Green lettuces	1.2 (about 10 leaves)
Broccoli, cooked	0.7
Brussels sprouts	0.5 (about 5 sprouts)

FOODS HIGH IN CALCIUM

(milligrams per serving)

Ricotta chesse: 4oz (115g)	337
Parmesan cheese: 1oz (30g)	336
Milk: 8fl oz (225ml)	300
Calcium-fortified orange juice: 8fl oz (225ml)	300
Mackerel with bones: canned 3oz (85g)	263
Yoghurt, no fat: 4oz (115g)	225
Salmon with bones, canned: 3oz (85g)	191
Collards, frozen, cooked: 3oz (85g)	179

Dried figs: 5 figs   135
Sardines, with bones: 1oz (30g)   130
Tofu, firm: 4oz (115g)   118
Turnip greens, fresh, cooked: 3oz (85g)   99
Kale, cooked: 3oz (85g)   90
Broccoli, fresh, cooked: 3oz (85g)   89
Okra, frozen, cooked: 3oz (85g)   88
Baked Beans: 6oz (170g)   80
Soya beans, cooked: 3oz (85g)   65
Chickpeas, cooked: 3oz (85g)   60
White beans, cooked: 3oz (85g)   45
Pinto beans, cooked: 3oz (85g)   40

Note: All dairy foods are high in calcium. All cheeses average about 200mg of calcium per 1oz (30g), although some are higher, for example, Parmesan and Romano.

FOODS HIGH IN FOLIC ACID

	(micrograms per serving)
Chicken livers, simmered: 3oz (85g)	539
Bulgur, cooked: 6oz (170g)	158
Okra, frozen, cooked: 3oz (85g)	134
Orange juice, fresh or canned: 8fl oz (225ml)	136
Spinach, fresh, cooked: 3oz (85g)	130
White beans, cooked: 3oz (85g)	120
Red kidney beans, cooked: 3oz (85g)	114
Orange juice, frozen, diluted: 8fl oz (225ml)	109
Soya beans, cooked: 3oz (85g)	100
Wheat germ: 1oz (30g)	100
Asparagus, fresh, cooked: 3oz (85g)	88
Turnip greens, fresh, cooked: 3oz (85g)	85
Avocado, Florida: ½ fruit	81
Brussels sprouts, frozen, cooked: 3oz (85g)	79
Lima beans, dry, cooked: 3oz (85g)	78
Chickpeas, cooked: 3oz (85g)	70
Sunflower seeds: 1oz (30g)	65
Orange segments: 4oz (115g)	54
Broccoli, fresh, cooked: 3oz (85g)	53
Mustard greens, fresh, cooked: 3oz (85g)	51

Beetroot, fresh, cooked: 3oz (85g)   45
Raspberries, frozen: 2½oz (75g)   33

Note: Many cereals also typically have 100 micrograms of folic acid per serving. Check cereal labels for content.

FOODS HIGH IN POTASSIUM

	(milligrams per serving)
Blackstrap: 3oz (85g)	2,400
Potato, baked: 1 medium	844
Cantaloupe: ½ fruit	825
Avocado, Florida: ½ fruit	742
Beet greens, cooked: 3oz (85g)	654
Peaches, dried: 5 halves	645
Prunes, dried: 10 halves	626
Tomato juice: 8fl oz (225ml)	536
Yoghurt, low-fat: 8oz (225g)	530
Snapper: 3½ (100g)	522
Lima beans, dried, cooked: 3oz (85g)	517
Salmon: 3½oz (100g)	490
Soya beans, cooked: 3oz (85g)	486
Swiss chard, cooked: 3oz (85g)	483
Apricots, dried: 10 halves	482
Orange juice, fresh: 8 floz (225 ml)	472
Pumpkin seeds: 2oz (55g)	458
Sweet potato, cooked: 3½oz (100g)	455
Banana: 1 fruit	451
Acorn squash: 3oz (85g)	446
Almonds: 2oz (85g)	426
Spinach, cooked: 3oz (85g)	419
Herring: 3½oz (100g)	419
Milk, skimmed: 8 floz (225 ml)	418
Mackerel: 3½oz (100g)	406
Peanuts: 2oz (55g)	400

FOODS HIGH IN SELENIUM

	(micrograms 3½oz/100g)
Brazil nuts	2,960
Puffed wheat	123
Tuna, light, canned in water	80
canned in oil	76
Tuna, white, canned in water	65
canned in oil	60
Sunflower seeds, roasted	78
Oysters, cooked	72
Chicken liver, cooked	72
Wheat flour, whole grain	71
Clams, canned	49

Note: Organ meats are generally high in selenium as are whole grains. Most fruits and vegetables are generally low in selenium; the highest is garlic with 14 micrograms per 3½oz (100g).

FOODS HIGH IN ZINC

	(milligrams per serving)
Oysters, smoked: 3oz (85g)	103
Oysters, raw, without shell: 3oz (85g)	63
Crabmeat, steamed: 2 medium	4
Crabmeat, cooked: 3oz (85g)	6
Pot roast, braised: 3oz (85g)	7
Calf's liver, cooked: 3oz (85g)	7
Turkey, dark meat, roasted: 3½oz (100g)	5
Pumpkin and squash seeds: 1oz (30g)	3

Note: Meat and poultry are generally high in zinc. Many cereals have about 4 milligrams of zinc per serving. Check the label.

FOODS HIGH IN VITAMIN C

	(milligrams per serving)
Guava: 1 fruit	165

Red sweet pepper: 1 pepper	141
Cantaloupe: ½ fruit	113
Pimientos, canned: 4oz (115g)	107
Sweet green pepper: 1 pepper	95
Papaya: ½ fruit	94
Strawberries, raw: 5oz (140g)	84
Brussels sprouts: 6 sprouts	78
Grapefruit juice: from 1 fruit	75
Kiwi fruit: 1 fruit	74
Orange: 1 fruit	70
Tomatoes, cooked: 8oz (225g)	45
Orange juice, in carton or from concentrate: 4 floz (115 ml)	52
Broccoli: 3oz (85g) cooked	49
Tomato juice: 8fl oz (225 ml)	45
Grapefruit: ½ fruit	42
Broccoli: 3oz (85g) raw	41
Cauliflower, raw: 3oz (85g)	36
Peas, green, raw: 3oz (85g)	31
Kale, cooked: 3oz (85g)	27

FOODS HIGH IN VITAMIN D

	*International Units (IU) per 3½oz (100g)
Eel	4,700
Pilchard	1,500
Sardines, fresh	1,500
Herring, fresh	1,000
Salmon, red	800
Salmon, pink	500
Mackerel	500
Salmon, chinook	300
Herring, canned	225
Salmon, chum	200
Tuna	200
Milk (nonfat, low-fat, whole): 8fl oz (225ml)	100

*Multiply by 0.025 for mg

FOODS HIGH IN VITAMIN E

Vitamin E is fat-soluble and thus is concentrated in vegetable oils, nuts and seeds. Legumes and brans are also fairly high. Vitamin E is almost nonexistent in animal foods. Although fruits and vegetables are fairly low in vitamin E, they still provide about 11 per cent of Vitamin E in Western diets. About 64 per cent comes from oils, margarines and shortenings, and about 7 per cent comes from grains.

(milligrams per 3½oz/ 100g)

Nuts and Seeds

Sunflower seeds	52
Walnuts	22
Almonds	21
Filberts (hazelnuts)	21
Cashews	11
Peanuts, roasted	11
Brazil nuts	7
Pecans	2

Brans and Legumes

Wheat germ	28
Soya beans, dried	20
Rice bran	15
Lima beans, dried	8
Wheat bran	8

Oils

Wheat germ	250
Soya bean	92
Corn	82
Sunflower	63
Safflower	38
Sesame	28
Peanut (groundnut)	24

TYPES OF FATTY ACIDS IN OILS

Oil	Saturated	(percentages) Monounsaturated	Omega-6	Omega-3
Flax	9	18	16	57
Rapeseed	6	62	22	10
Soya	15	24	54	7
Walnut	16	28	51	5
Olive (extra virgin)	14	77	8	1
Groundnut	18	49	33	0
Corn	13	25	61	1
Safflower	10	13	77	0
Sesame	13	46	41	0
Sunflower, regular	11	20	69	0

Note: It's easy to see that corn, safflower and sunflower seed oils have the most omega-6 fatty acids and the least omega-3, making them more hazardous in general. Flax and rapeseed oils have the best ratios of omega-3 to omega-6. Olive oil is highest in heart-protecting monounsaturated fat.

OMEGA-3 FATTY ACIDS IN SEAFOOD

Fresh or Frozen	(milligrams per 3½oz/100g)
Roe, finfish, mixed species	2,345
Mackerel, Atlantic	2,299
Herring, Pacific	1,658
Herring, Atlantic	1,571
Mackerel, Pacific and jack	1,441
Sablefish	1,395
Salmon, chinook (king)	1,355
Mackerel, Spanish	1,341
Whitefish, mixed spices	1,258
Tuna, bluefin	1,173
Salmon, sockeye (red)	1,172
Salmon, pink	1,005
Turbot, Greenland	919
Shark, mixed species	843
Salmon, coho (silver)	814
Bluefish	771

Bass, striped	754
Smelt, rainbow	693
Oysters, Pacific	688
Swordfish	639
Salmon, chum	627
Wolfish	623
Bass, freshwater, mixed species	595
Seabass, mixed species	595
Trout, rainbow	568
Pompano, Florida	568
Squid, mixed species	488
Shrimp, mixed species	480
Mussels, blue	441
Oysters, Eastern	439
Tilefish	430
Pollock, Atlantic	421
Catfish, channel	373
Lobster, spiny, mixed species	373
Pollock, Alaska (walleye)	372
Crab, snow (queen)	372
Halibut, Atlantic and Pacific	363
Carp	352
Rockfish, Pacific, mixed species	345
Mullet	325
Crab, blue	320
Snapper, mixed species	311
Crab, Dungeness	307
Ocean perch, Atlantic	291
Tuna, skipjack	256
Grouper	256
Whiting, mixed species	224
Tuna, yellowfin	218
Cod, Pacific	215
Scallops, mixed species	198
Haddock	185
Cod, Atlantic	184
Crawfish	173
Eel, mixed species	147
Octopus	157
Clams	142

Canned Fish	(milligrams per 3½oz/100g)
Anchovies, canned in olive oil (drained)	2,055
Herring, Atlantic, pickled	1,389
Salmon, pink (including liquid and bones)	1,651
Sardines, Pacific in tomato sauce (drained, without bones)	1,604
Salmon, sockeye (drained with bones)	1,156
Sardines, Atlantic in soya bean oil (drained with bones)	982
Tuna (albacore), white in water (drained)	706
Tuna, light, in soya bean oil (drained)	128
Tuna, light in water (drained)	111

Source: U.S. Department of Agriculture

REFERENCES

More than ten thousand scientific studies were consulted for this book; thus, it is impossible to list them all. However, here are some of the most important and interesting published scientific sources that are available in medical libraries. Only the first author of each study is given. The book also contains much unpublished information obtained through interviews with researchers and news reports in scientific publications.

ARTICLES

Arthritis

Belch, J.: Fish oil and rheumatoid arthritis: Does a herring a day keep rheumatologists away? *Annals of the Rheumatic Diseases* 1990; 49:71–72.

Darlington, L G.: Dietary therapy for arthritis. *Nutrition and Rheumatic Diseases* 1991; 17(2):273–85.

Golding D. N.: Is there an allergic synovitis? *Journal of the Royal Society of Medicine* 1990; 83:312–14.

Kjeldsen-Krah, J.: Controlled trial of fasting and one-year vegetarian diet in rheumatoid arthritis. *Lancet* 1991; 338(8772): 899–902.

Kremer, J. M.: Clinical studies of omega-3 fatty acid supplementation in patients who have rheumatoid arthritis. *Rheumatic Disease Clinics of North America* 1991; 17(2):391–402.

Panush, R. S.: Diet therapy for rheumatoid arthritis. *Arthritis and Rheumatism* 1983; 26(4):462–70.

Panush, R S.: Food induced ("Allergic") arthritis: clinical and serologic studies. *The Journal of Rheumatology* 1990; 17:291–94.

Panush, R S.: Food induced ("allergic") arthritis: inflammatory synovitis in rabbits. *The Journal of Rheumatology* 1990; 17:285–90.

Panush, R. S.: Food-induced (allergic) arthritis: inflammatory arthritis exacerbated by milk. *Arthritis and Rheumatism* 1986; 29(2): 220–25.

Parke, A. L: Rheumatoid arthritis and food: a case study. *British Medical Journal* (clinical research) 1981; 282(6281):2027–29.

Ratner, D.: Does milk intolerance affect seronegative arthritis in lactase-deficient women? *Israel Journal of Medical Sciences* 1985; 21:532–34.

Srivastava, K. C., et al., Ginger (Zingiber officinale) and rheumatic disorders. *Medical Hypotheses* 1989; 29:25–28.

Williams, R: Rheumatoid arthritis and food: a case study. *British Medical Journal* 1981; 283:563.

Asthma and Bronchitis

Dorsch, W.: Antiasthmatic effects of onions. *International Archives of Allergy and Applied Immunology* 1989; 88:228–30.

Dorsch, W.: New Antiasthmatic drugs from traditional medicine? *International Archives of Allergy and Applied Immunology* 1991; 94:262–65.

Dry, J.: Effect of a fish oil diet on asthma: results of a 1-year double-blind study. *International Archives of Allergy and Applied Immunology* 1991; 95(2–2):156–57.

Lee, T. H.: Effects of dietary fish oil lipids on allergic and inflammatory diseases. *Allergy Proceedings* 1991;12(5):299–303.

Rodriquez, J.: Allergy to cow's milk with onset in adult life. *Annals of Allergy* 1989; 62(3): 185a–b.

Schwartz, J.: Caffeine intake and asthma symptoms. *Annals of Epidemiology* 1992; 2(5):627–35.

Schwartz, J.: Dietary factors and their relation to respiratory symptoms. *American Journal of Epidemiology* 1990;132(1):67–76.

Wilson, N.: Objective test for food sensitivity in asthmatic children: increased bronchial reactivity after cola drinks. *British Medical Journal* 1982; 284:1226–28.

Ziment, I.: History of the treatment of chronic bronchitis. *Respiration* 1991; 58(1):37–42).

Ziment, I.: Five thousand years of attacking asthma: an overview. *Respiratory Care* 1986; 31(2):117–136.

Blood Cholesterol

Anderson, J. W.: Serum lipid response of hypercholesterolemic men to single and divided doses of canned beans. *American Journal of Clinical Nutrition* 1990: 51(6):1013–19.

Barrie, N. D.: Effects of garlic oil on platelet aggregation, serum lipids and blood pressure in humans. *Journal of Orthomolecular Medicine*, 1987; 2(1):15–21.

Colquhoun, D. M.: Comparison of the effects on lipoproteins and apolipo-proteins of a diet high in monounsaturated fatty adds, enriched with avocado and a high–carbohydrate diet. *American Journal of Clinical Nutrition* 1992; 56:671–77.

Davidson, M. H.: The hypocholesterolemic effects of B-glucan in oatmeal and oat bran. *Journal of the American Medical Association* 1991: 285(14):1833–39.

Gadkari, J. V. The effect of ingestion of raw garlic on serum cholesterol level, clotting time and fibrinolytic activity in normal subjects. *Journal of Postgraduate Medicine* 1991; 37(3):128–31.

Herrmann, W.: The influence of dietary supplementation with omega-3 fatty acids on serum lipids, apolipoproteins, coagulation and fibrinolytic parameters. *Zeitschrift Fur Klinische Medizin* 1991: 46(19):1363–69.

Ripsin, C. M.: Oat products and lipid lowering: a meta-analysis. *Journal of the American Medical Association* 1992; 267(24):3317–27.

Robertson, J.: The effect of raw carrot on serum lipids and colon function. *American Journal of Clinical Nutrition* 1979; 32:1889–92.

Sendl, A.: Inhibition of cholesterol synthesis in vitro by extracts and isolated compounds prepared from garlic and wild garlic. *Atherosclerosis* 1992; 94(1):79–85.

Steinberg, Daniel: Antioxidants in the prevention of human atherosclerosis. *Circulation* 1992; 85(6):2338–44.

Blood Clots

Ernst, E.: Plasma fibrinogen – an independent cardiovascular risk factor. *Journal of Internal Medicine* 1990; 227:365:72.

Lou, F. Q.: A study on tea-pigment in prevention of atherosclerosis. *Chinese Medical Journal* 1989; 102(8):579–83.

Gadkari, Jayashree.: Effect of ingestion of raw garlic on serum cholesterol level, clotting time and fibrinolytic activity in normal subjects. *Journal of Postgraduate Medicine* 1991; 37(3):128–31.

Houwelingen, R.: Effect of a moderate fish intake on blood pressure, bleeding time, hematalogy and clinical chemistry in healthy males. *American Journal of Clinical Nutrition* 1987; 46:424–36.

Kiesewetter, H.: Effects of garlic on blood fluidity and fibrinolytic activity: a randomised placebo-controlled, double-blind study. *British Journal of Clinical Practice* 1990; 44(suppl. 69)(8): 24–29.

Lipinska, I.: Lipids, lipoproteins, fibrinogen and fibrinolytic activity in angio-graphically assessed coronary heart disease. *Artery* 1987; 15(1):44–60.

Makheja, A.: Antiplatelet constituents of garlic and onions. *Agents Actions* 1990; 29(3–4): 360–63.

Marckmann, P.: Effects of total fat content and fatty acid composition in diet on factor VII coagulant activity and blood lipids. *Atherosclerosis* 1990; 80(3):227–33.

Mehrabian, M.: Dietary regulation of fibrinolytic factors. *Atherosclerosis* 1990; 84:25–32.

Seigneur, M.: Effect of the consumption of alcohol, white wine, and red wine on platelet function and serum lipids. *Journal of Applied Cardiology* 1990; 5:215–22.

Siemann, E. H.: Concentration of the phytoalexin resveratrol in wine. *American Journal of Enol Vitic* 1992; 43(1):49–52.

Visudhiphan, S.: The relationship between high fibrinolytic activity and daily capsicum ingestion in Thais. *American Journal of Clinical Nutrition* 1982; 35: 1452–58.

Young, W.: Tea and atherosclerosis. *Nature* 1967; 216:1015–16.

Blood Pressure

Alderman, M. H.: Moderate sodium restriction. Do the benefits justify the hazards? *American Journal of Hypertension* 1990; 3:499–504.

Auer, W.: Hypertension and hyperlipidaemia: garlic helps in mild cases. *British Journal of Clinical Practice Supplement* 1990; 44(8):3–6.

Beilin, L. J.: Alcohol and hypertension. *Clinical and Experimental Hypertension Theory and Practice* 1992; A14(1&2):119–38.

Bulpitt, C J.: Vitamin C and blood pressure. *Journal of Hypertension* 1990; 12:1071–75.

Harvard Health Letter: *A special report: high blood pressure*, 1990. Harvard Medical School, Health Publications Group.

Knapp, H.R. Omega-3 fatty acids, endogenous prostaglandins; and blood pressure regulation in humans. *Nutrition Reviews* 1989; 47(10):301–13.

Krishna, G.G.: Increased blood pressure during potassium depletion in normotensive men. *New England Journal of Medicine* 1989; 329(18):1177–82.

Law, M. R.: By how much does dietary salt reduction lower blood pressure? *British Medical Journal* 1991; 302:819–924.

Margretts, B. M.: Vegetarian diet in mild hypertension: a randomised controlled trial. *British Medical Journal* 1986; 293:1468–71.

Martin, J. B.: Mortality patterns among hypertensives by reported level of caffeine consumption. *Preventive Medicine* 1988; 17(3):310–20.

Patki, P. S.: Efficacy of potassium and magnesium in essential hypertension: a double-blind, placebo controlled, crossover study. *British Medical Journal* 1990; 301(6751):521–23.

Sacks, F. M.: Dietary fats and blood pressure: a critical review of the evidence. *Nutrition Reviews* 1989; 47(10):291–300.

Tobian, L: Salt and hypertension. Lessons from animal models that relate to human hypertension. *Hypertension* 1991;17(suppl. 1):152–58.

Brain and Behaviour

Bachorowski, J.: Sucrose and delinquency: behavioral assessment. *Pediatrics* 1990; 86(2):24–53.

Gans, D. A.: Sucrose and delinquency: oral sucrose tolerance test and nutritional assessment. *Pediatrics*; 86(2):254–61.

Greenwood, C: Influence of dietary fat on brain membrane phospholipid fatty acid composition and neuronal function in mature rats. *Nutrition* 1989; 5(4):278–81.

Harper, A. E.: Claims of antisocial behavior from consumption of sugar: an assessment. *Food Technology*, Jan. 1986:142–49.

Spring, B.: Psychobiological effects of carbohydrates. *Journal of Clinical Psychiatry* 1989; 50:(suppl. 5):27–33.

Spring, B.: Carbohydrates, tryptophan, and behavior: a methodological review. *Psychological Bulletin* 1987; 102(2):234–56.

Cancer, General

Block, G.: Fruit, vegetables, and cancer prevention: a review of the epidemiological evidence. *Nutrition and Cancer* 1992; 18:1–29.

Caragay, A. B.: Cancer-preventive foods and ingredients. *Food Technology* 1992; 46:65–68.

Henson, D.E.: Ascorbic acid: biologic functions and relation to cancer. *Journal of the National Cancer Institute* 1991; 83(8):547–50.

Lau, Benjamin H. S.: Garlic compounds modulate macrophage and T-lymphocyte functions. *Molecular Biotherapy* 1991; 3:103–7.

Lubin, F.: Consumption of methylxanthine-containing beverages and the risk of breast cancer. *Cancer Letter* 1990; 53(2–3):81–90.

Messina, M.: The role of soy products in reducing risk of cancer. *Journal of the National Cancer Institute* 1991, 83(8):541–46.

Mettlin C. J.: Patterns of milk consumption and risk of cancer. *Nutrition and Cancer* 1990; 13(1–2):89–99.

Schwartz, J. L.: Beta carotene and/or vitamin E as modulators of alkylating agents in SCC-25 human squamous carcinoma cells. *Cancer Chemotherapy and Pharmacology* 1992; 29(3):207–13.

Steinmetz K. A.: Vegetables, fruit and cancer. I. Epidemiology. *Cancer Causes Control* 1991; 2(5):325–57.

Steinmetz, K. A.: Vegetables, fruit, and cancer. II. Mechanisms. *Cancer Causes Control* 1991; 2(6):427–42.

Wattenberg, L. W.: Inhibition of carcinogenesis by minor anutrient constituents of the diet. *Proceedings of the Nutrition Society* 1990; 49(2):173–83.

Zhang, Yuesheng: A major inducer of anticarcinogenic protective enzymes from broccoli: isolation and elucidation of structure. *Proceedings of the National Academy of Sciences* 1992 89:2399–2403.

Cancer, Breast

Adlecreutz, H.: Diet and breast cancer. *Acta Oncologica* 1992; 31(2):175–81.

Barnes, S.: Soybeans inhibit mammary tumors in models of breast cancer. *Progress in Clinical and Biological Research* 1990; 347:239–53.

Bresnick, E: Reduction in mammary tumorigenesis in the rat by cabbage and cabbage residue. *Carcinogenesis* 1990;11(7):1159–63.

Holm, L. E.: Treatment failure and dietary habits in women with breast cancer. *Journal of the National Cancer Institute* 1993; 85(1):32–36.

Howe, G. E.: Dietary factors and risk of breast cancer combined analysis of 12 case-control studies. *Journal of the National Cancer Institute* 1990; 82(7):561–69.

Karmali, R. A.: Omega-3 fatty acids and cancer. *Journal of Internal Medicine* 1989; 225 (suppl. 1):197–200.

Kushi, L. H.: Dietary fat and postmenopausal breast cancer. *Journal of the National Cancer Institute* 1992; 84(14):1092–99.

Lee, H. P.: Dietary effects on breast-cancer risk in Singapore. *Lancet* 1991; 337:1197–200.

Michnovicz, J. J.: Induction of estradiol metabolism by dietary indole-3 carbinol in humans. *Journal of the National Cancer Institute* 1990; 82(11):947–49.

Rose, D. P.: Effect of dietary fat on human breast cancer growth and lung metastasis in nude mice. *Journal of the National Cancer Institute* 1991; 83(20):1491–95.

Rose, D. P.: High-fiber diet reduces serum estrogen concentrations in pre-menopausal women. *American Journal of Clinical Nutrition* 1991; 54(3):520–25.

Cancer, Colon

Alberts, D. S.: Effects of dietary wheat bran fiber on rectal epithelial cell proliferation in patients with resection for colorectal cancers. *Journal of the National Cancer Institute* 1990; 82:1280–85.

Anti, M.: Effect of omega-3 fatty acids on rectal mucosal cell proliferation in subjects at risk for colon cancer. *Gastroenterology* 1992; 103:883–91.

DeCosse, J. J.: Effect of wheat fiber and vitamins C and E on rectal polyps in patients with familial adenomatous polyposis. *Journal of the National Cancer Institute* 1989; 81(17):1290–97.

Freudenheim, J. L.: Lifetime alcohol intake and risk of rectal cancer in western New York. *Nutrition and Cancer* 1990; 13:101–9.

Howe, G. R: Dietary intake of fiber and decreased risk of cancers of the colon and rectum: evidence from the combined analysis of 13 case-control studies. *Journal of the National Cancer Institute* 1992; 84(24):1887–96.

Nicholas, C. M.: Intervention studies in adenoma patients. *World Journal of Surgery* 1991; 15:29–34.

Willett, W. C.: Relation of meat, fat, and fiber intake to the risk of colon cancer in a prospective study among women. *New England Journal of Medicine* 1990; 323:1664–72.

Cancer, Lung

Goodman, M. T.: Dietary factors in lung cancer prognosis. *European Journal of Cancer* 1992: 28(2/3):495–501.

Harris R W.: A case-control study of dietary carotene in men with lung cancer and in men with other epithelial cancers. *Nutrition and Cancer* 1991; 15(1):63–68.

Knekt, P.: Dietary antioxidants and the risk of lung cancer. *American Journal of Epidemiology* 1991; 134:471–79.

Ziegler, R. G.: Carotenoid intake, vegetables, and the risk of lung cancer among white men in New Jersey. *American Journal of Epidemiology* 1986; 123:1080–93.

Ziegler, R. G.: Does beta-carotene explain why reduced cancer risk is associated with vegetable and fruit intake? *Cancer Research* 1992; 52(suppl.7):2060s–66s.

Colic

Campbell, J. P.: Dietary treatment of infant colic: a double blind study. *Journal of the Royal College of General Practitioners* 1989; 39(318):11–14.

Clyne, P. S.: Human breast milk contains bovine IgG. Relationship to infant colic? *Pediatrics* 1991; 87:439–44.

Jakobsson, I.: Food antigens in human milk. *European Journal of Clinical Nutrition* 1991; 45(suppl. 1): 29–33.

Leung, A.: Infantile colic. *American Family Physician* 1987; 36(3):153–56.

Constipation and Diverticular Disease

Brown, S. R.: Effect of coffee on distal colon function. *Gut* 1990; 31:450–53.

Edwards, C. A.: Fibre and constipation. *British Journal of Clinical Practice* 1988; 42(1):26–32.

Jain, N. K.: Sorbitol intolerance in adults. *The American Journal of Gastroenterology* 1985; 80(9):678–81.

Miller, D. L: Small-bowel obstruction from bran cereal. *Journal of the American Medical Association* 1990; 263(6):813–14.

Painter, N. S.: Unprocessed bran in treatment of diverticular disease of the colon. *British Medical Journal* 1972; 2:137–40.

Tomlin, J.: Comparison of the effects on colonic function caused by feeding rice bran and wheat bran. *European Journal of Clinical Nutrition* 1988; 42:857–61.

Diabetes

Bailey, C. J.: Traditional plant medicines as treatments for diabetes. *Diabetes Care* 1989; 12(8):553–64.

Close, E.J.: Diabetic diets and nutritional recommendations: what happens in real life? *Diabetic Medicine* 1992; 9(2):181–88.

Dahlquist, G. G.: Dietary factors and the risk of developing insulin dependent diabetes in childhood. *British Medical Journal* 1990; 300:1302–6.

Feskens, E. J. M.: Inverse association between fish intake and risk of glucose intolerance in normoglycemic elderly men and women. *Diabetes Care* 1991; 14(11):935–41.

Holbrook, T. L: A prospective population-based study of alcohol use and non-insulin dependent diabetes mellitus. *American Journal of Epidemiology* 1990; 132(5):902–9.

Jenkins, D. J. A.: Lente carbohydrate: a newer approach to the dietary management of diabetes. *Diabetes Care* 1982; 5:634.

Karjalainen, J.: A bovine albumin peptide as a possible trigger of insulin-dependent diabetes mellitus. *New England Journal of Medicine* 1992; 327(5):302–7.

Mahdi, G. S.: Role of chromium in barley in modulating the symptoms of diabetes. *Annals of Nutrition and Metabolism* 1991; 35:65–70.

Marshall, J. A.: High-fat, low-carbohydrate diet and the etiology of noninsulin dependent diabetes mellitus: the San Luis Valley Diabetes Study. *American Journal of Epidemiology* 1991; 134(6):590–603 .

Sharma, R. D.: Effect of fenugreek seeds on blood glucose and serum lipids in type I diabetes. *European Journal of Clinical Nutrition* 1990; 44(4):301–6.

Virtanen, S. M.: Feeding in infancy and the risk of type I diabetes mellitus in Finnish children. *Diabetic Medicine* 1992; 9(9):815–19.

Wolever, T. M. S.: Beneficial effect of a low glycaemic index diet in type-2 diabetes. *Diabetic Medicine* 1992; 9:451–58.

Diarrhoea

Brown, K. H.: Dietary management of acute childhood diarrhea: optimal timing of feeding and appropriate use of milks and mixed diets *Journal of Pediatrics* 1991; 118:92S–98S.

Casteel, H. B.: Oral rehydration therapy. *Pediatric Clin North Am* 1990; 37(2):295–311.

Hirschhorn, N.: Progress in oral rehydration therapy. *Scientific American* 1991; 264(5):50–56.

Hyams, J. S.: Carbohydrate malabsorption following fruit juice ingestion in young children. *Pediatrics* 1988; 82(1):64–68.

Jain, N. K.: Sorbitol intolerance in adults. *American Journal of Gostroenterology* 1985; 80(9):678–81.

Kneepkens, C. M.: Apple juice, fructose, and chronic nonspecific diarrhoea. *European Journal of Pediatrics* 1989; 148(6):571–73.

Kotz, C. M.: In vitro antibacterial effect of yogurt on Escherichia coli. *Digestive Diseases and Sciences* 1990; 35(5):630–37.

Lewis, P.: Starvation ketosis after rehydration with diet soda. *Pediatrics* 1991; 88(4):806–7.

Lifshitz, F.: Role of juice carbohydrate malabsorption in chronic nonspecific diarrhea in children. *Journal of Pediatrics* 1992; 120(5):825–29.

Saibil, F.: Diarrhea due to fiber overload. *New England Journal of Medicine* 1989; 320(9):599.

Wolfe, M. S.: Acute diarrhea associated with travel. *American Journal of Medicine* 1990; 88(suppl. 6A): 34S–37S.

Gallstones

Liddle R A.: Gallstone formation during weight-reduction dieting. *Archives of Internal Medicine* 1989; 149(8):1750–53.

Maclure, K. M.: Dietary predictors of symptom-associated gallstones in middle-aged women. *American Journal of Clinical Nutrition* 1990; 52(5):916–22.

Mogadam, M.: Gallbladder dynamics in response to various meals: is dietary fat restriction necessary in the management of gallstones? *American Journal of Gastroenterology* 1984; 79(10):745–47.

Pixley, F.: Dietary factors in the aetiology of gallstones: a case control study. *Gut* 1988, 29(11):1511–15.

Sichieri, R.: A prospective study of hospitalization with gallstone disease among women: role of dietary factors, fasting period, and dieting. *American Journal of Public Health* 1991; 81(7):880–84.

Gas

Bond, J. H.: Relation of food ingestion to intestinal gas production and gas related symptoms. *Journal of Environmental Pathology, Toxicology and Oncology* 1985; 5:157–64.

Jha, K.: Flatulence production abilities of different Indian foods and effect of certain spices on flatulence. *Indian Journal of Pathology and Microbiology* 1980; 23:279–88.

Levitt, M. D.: Studies of a flatulent patient. *New England Journal of Medicine* 1976; 295(5):260–62.

Olson, A. C.: Nutrient composition of and digestive response to whole and extracted dry beans. *Journal of Agriculture and Food Chemistry* 1982; 30:26–32.

Headache

Egger, J.: Is migraine food allergy? A double-blind controlled trial of oligoantigenic diet treatment. *Lancet* 1983; 2:865–69.

Egger, J.: Oligoantigenic diet treatment in children with epilepsy and migraine. *Journal of Pediatrics* 1989: 114:51–58.

Griffiths, R. R.: Low-dose caffeine physical dependence in humans. *Journal of Pharmacology and Experimental Therapeutics* 1990; 255(3):1123–32.

Henderson, W. R.: Hot dog headache: Individual susceptibility to nitrite. *Lancet* 1972; 2:1162–63.

Koehler, S. M.: The effect of aspartame on migraine headache. *Headache* 1988; 28(1):10–14.

Lipton, R B.: Aspartame as a dietary trigger of headache. *Headache* 1989: 29(2):90–92.

Littlewood, J.: Red wine as a cause of migraine. *Lancet* 1988; 1(8585):558–59.

McCabe, B. J.: Dietary tyramine and other pressor amines in MAOI regimens: a review. *Journal of the American Dietetic Association* 1986(8):1059–64.

Mustafa, T.: Ginger (zingiber officinale) in migraine headache. *Journal of Ethnopharmacology* 1990; 29(3):267–73.

Radnitz, C. L: Food-triggered migraine: a critical review. *Annals of Behavioral Medicine* 1990; 12(2):51–65.

Saper, J. R.: Daily chronic headache. *Neurol Clin* 1990; 8(4):891–901.

Scopp, A. L.: MSG and hydrolyzed vegetable protein induced headache: review and case studies. *Headache* 1991; 31(2):107–10.

Shulman, K. I.: Dietary restriction, tyramine, and the use of monoaine oxidase inhibitors. *Journal of Clinical Psychopharmacology* 1989: 9:397–402.

Smith, R.: Caffeine withdrawal headache. *Journal of Clinical Pharmacy and Therapeutics* 1987; 12:53–57.

Heart Disease

Bairati, I.: Double blind, randomized, controlled trial of fish oil supplements in prevention of recurrence of stenosis after coronary angioplasty. *Circulation* 1992; 85:950–56.

Burr, M. L: Effects of changes in fat, fish, and fibre intakes on death and myocardial reinfarction: diet and reinfarction trial (Dart). *Lancet*, Sept. 1989:757–61.

Ettinger, P. O.: Arrhythmias and "the holiday heart": alcohol associated cardiac rhythm disorders. *American Heart Journal* 1978; 95:555–62.

Fraser, G. E.: A possible protective effect of nut consumption on risk of coronary heart disease. *Archives of Internal Medicine* 1992; 152:1416–23.

Gey, K. F.: Inverse correlation between plasma vitamin E and mortality from ischemic heart disease in cross cultural epidemiology. *American Journal of Clinical Nutrition* 1991; 53(Suppl. 1): 326S–34S.

Gramenzi, A.: Association between certain foods and risk of acute myocardial infarction in women. *British Medical Journal* 1990; 300(6727):771–73.

Grobbee, D. E.: Coffee, caffeine and cardiovascular disease in men. *New England Journal of Medicine* 1990; 323(15):1026–32.

Hojnacki J. L.: Effect of drinking pattern on plasma lipoproteins and body weight.*Atherosclerosis* 1991; 88(1):49–59.

Leaf, A.: Cardiovascular effects of omega-3 fatty acids. *New England Journal of Medicine* 1988; 318:549–57.

Milner, M. R.: Usefulness of fish oil supplements in preventing clinical evidence of restenosis after percutaneous transluminal coronary angioplasty. *American Journal of Cardiology* 1989; 64(5):294–99.

Myers, M. G.: Coffee and coronary heart disease. *Archives of Internal Medicine* 1992; 152:1767–72.

Myers, M. G.: Caffeine and cardiac arrhythmias. *Annals of Internal Medicine* 1991; 114:147–50.

Orlando, J.: Effect of ethanol on angina pectoris. *Annals of Internal Medicine* 1976; 84:652–55.

Riemersma, R A.: Risk of angina pectoris and plasma concentrations of vitamins A, C, and E and carotene. *Lancet* 1991; 337(8732):1–5.

Sacks, F.: More on chewing the fat. *New England Journal of Medicine* 1991; 325(24):1740–41.

Simopoulos, A. P.: Omega-3 fatty acids in growth and development and in health and disease. *Nutrition Today*, May/June 1988:12–18.

Singh, R. B.: Randomized controlled trial of cardioprotective diet in patients with recent acute myocardial infarction: results of one year follow up. *British Medical Journal* 1992; 304:1015–19.

Stampfer, M. J.: A prospective study of moderate alcohol consumption and the risk of coronary disease and stroke in women. *New England Journal of Medicine*; 319(5):267–73.

Steinberg, D.: Alcohol and atherosclerosis. *Annals of Internal Medicine* 1991; 114:967–76.

Verlangieri, Anthony: Effects of d-a-tocopherol supplementation on experimentally induced primate atherosclerosis. *Journal of American College of Nutrition*, 1992; 11(2):130–37.

Wilson, P. W. F.: Is coffee consumption a contributor to cardiovascular disease? *Archives of Internal Medicine* 1989; 149:1169–72.

Heartburn

Allen, M. L: The effect of raw onions on acid reflux and reflux symptoms. *American Journal of Gastroenterology* 1990; 85(4): 377–80.

Becker, D. J.: A comparison of high and low fat meals on postprandial esophageal acid exposure. *American Journal of Gastroenterology* 1989: 84(7):782–85.

Kitchin, L. I.: Rationale and efficacy of conservative therapy for gastroesophageal reflux disease. *Archives of Internal Medicine* 1991; 151:448–54.

Murphy, D. W.: Chocolate and heartburn: evidence of increased esophageal acid exposure after chocolate ingestion. *American Journal of Gastroenterology* 1988; 83(6):633–36.

Price, S. F.: Food sensitivity in reflux esophagitis. *Gastroenterology* 1978; 75:240–43.

Vitale, G. C.: The effect of alcohol on nocturnal gastroesophageal reflux. *Journal of the American Medical Association* 1987; 258:2077–79.

Immunity, Infections and Colds

Desencios, J. C.: The protective effect of alcohol on the occurrence of epidemic oyster-borne hepatitis A. *Epidemiology* 1992; 3(4):371–74.

Halpern, G. M.: Influence of long-term yoghurt consumption in young adults. *International Journal of Immunotherapy* 1991; VII(4):205–10.

Lau, B. H. S.: Garlic compounds modulate macrophage and T-lymphocyte functions. *Molecular Biotherapy* 1991; 3:103–7.

Malter, M.: Natural killer cells, vitamins, and other blood components of vegetarian and omnivorous men. *Nutrition and Cancer* 1989; 12(3):271–78.

Saketkhoo, K.: Effects of drinking hot water, cold water, and chicken soup on nasal mucus velocity and nasal airflow resistance. *Chest* 1978; 74:408–10.

Kidney Stones

Curhan, G.: A prospective study of dietary calcium and other nutrients and the risk of symptomatic kidney stones. *New England Journal of Medicine* 1993; 328:833–38.

Ebisuno, S.: Results of long-term rice bran treatment on stone recurrence in hypercalciuric patients. *British Journal of Urology* 1991; 67(3):237–40.

Gleeson, M. J.: Effect of unprocessed wheat bran on calciuria and oxaluria in patients with urolithiasis. *Urology* 1990; 35(3):231–34.

Goldfarb, S.: Dietary factors in the pathogenesis and prophylaxis of calcium nephrolithiasis. *Kidney International* 1988; 34:544–55.

Goldfarb, S.: The role of diet in the pathogenesis and therapy of nephrolithiasis. *Endocrinology and Metabolism Clinics of North America* 1990; 19(4):805–20.

Hughes, J.: Diet and calcium stones. *Canadian Medical Association Journal* 1992; 146(2):137–43.

Iguchi, M.: Clinical effects of prophylactic dietary treatment on renal stones. *Journal of Urology* 1990; 144(2 Pt. 1):229–32.

Schwille, P. O.: Environmental factors in the pathophysiology of recurrent idiopathic calcium urolithiasis (RCU) with emphasis on nutrition. *Urological*

Research 1992; 20:72–83.

Shuster, J.: Soft drink consumption and urinary stone recurrence: a randomized prevention trial. *Journal of Clinical Epidemiology* 1992; 45:911–16.

Trinchieri, A.: The influence of diet on urinary risk factors for stones in healthy subjects and idiopathic renal calcium stone formers. *British Journal of Urology* 1991; 67:230–36.

Wasserstein, A. G.: Case-control study of risk factors for idiopathic calcium nephrolithiasis. *Mineral and Electrolyte Metabolism* 1987; 13:85–95.

Mood, Anxiety and Depression

Benton, D.: The impact of selenium supplementation on mood. *Biological Psychiatry* 1991; 29:1092–98.

Bruce, M. S.: The anxiogenic effects of caffeine. *Postgraduate Med Journal* 1990, 66 (suppl. 2):S18–24.

Carney, M. W. P.: Vitamin deficiency and mental symptoms. *British Journal of Psychiatry* 1990; 156:878–82.

Cowen, R.: Receptor Encounters. *Science News* 1989; 136:248–52.

Griffiths, R. R.: Low dose caffeine discrimination in humans. *Journal of Pharmacology and Experimental Therapeutics* 1990; 252(3):970–8.

Ratliff-Crain, J.: Cardiovascular reactivity, mood, and task performance in deprived and nondeprived coffee drinkers. *Health Psychology* 1989; 8(4):427–47.

Roy-Byrne, P. P.: Exogenous factors in panic disorder: clinical and research implications. *Journal of Clinical Psychiatry* 1988; 49:56–61.

Wurtman, R. J.: Carbohydrates and depression. *Scientific American*, Jan. 1989: 68–75.

Young, S. M.: Some effects of dietary components (amino acids, carbohydrate, folic acid) on brain serotonin synthesis, mood, and behavior. *Canadian Journal of Physiology and Pharmacology* 1991; 69:893–903.

Young, S. M.: Folic acid and psychopathology. *Progress in Neuropsychopharmacology and Biological Psychiatry* 1989; 13:841–63.

Osteoporosis

Heaney, R. P.: Calcium in the prevention and treatment of osteoporosis. *Journal of Internal Medicine* 1992; 231:169–80.

Johnston, C. C. Jr.: Calcium supplementation and increases in bone mineral density in children. *New England Journal of Medicine* 1992; 327(2):119–20.

Nielsen, F. H.: Boron – an overlooked element of potential nutritional importance. *Nutrition Today*, January/February 1988: 4–7.

Spastic colon (IBS)

Bianchi, P.G.: Lactose intolerance in adults with chronic unspecified abdominal complaints. *Hepatogastroenterology* 1983; 30(6):254–57.

Friedman, G.: Diet and the irritable bowel syndrome. *Gastroenterology Clinics of North America* 1991; 20(2):313–24.

Fritznelis, G.: Role of fructose-sorbitol malabsorption in the irritable bowel syndrome. *Gastroenterology* 1990; 99:1016–20.

Hunter, J. O.: Irritable bowel syndrome. *Proceedings of the Nutrition Society* 1985; 44:141–43.

Hunter, J. O.: Food allergy – or enterometabolic disorder? *Lancet*, Aug. 24, 1991: 495–96.

Jones, V. A.: Food intolerance: a major factor in the pathogenesis of irritable bowel syndrome. *Lancet*, Nov. 20,1982: 1115–17.

Nanda, R: Food intolerance and the irritable bowel syndrome. *Gut* 1989; 30:1099–1104.

Sex, Fertility and Menstrual Problems

Bowen, D. J.: Variations in food preference and consumption across the menstrual cycle. *Physiology & Behavior* 1990; 47:287–91.

Dawson, E. B.: Relationship between ascorbic acid and male fertility. *World Review of Nutrition and Dietetics* 1990; 62:1–26.

Fraga, C. G.: Ascorbic acid protects against endogenous oxidative DNA damage in human sperm. *Proceedings of the National Academy of Sciences* 1991; 88:11003–6.

McCallum, K. A.: Hot flushes are induced by thermogenic stimuli. *British Journal of Urology* 1989; 64:507–10.

Meikle, A. W.: Effects of a fat-containing meal on sex hormones in men. *Metabolism* 1990; 39(7):943–46.

Van Thiel, D. H.: The phytoestrogens present in de-ethanolized bourbon are biologically active: a preliminary study in a postmenopausal woman. *Alcoholism, Clinical and Experimental Research* 1991; 15(5):822–23.

Wilcox, G.: Oestrogenic effects of plant foods in postmenopausal women. *British Medical Journal* 1990; 301:905–6.

Wurtman, J. J.: Effect of nutrient intake on premenstrual depression. *American Journal of Obstetrics and Gynecology* 1989; 161:1228–34.

Stroke

Acheson, R. M.: Does consumption of fruit and vegetables protect against stroke? *Lancet*, 1983:1191–93.

Hillborn, M.: Alcohol abuse and brain infarction. *Annals of Medicine* 1990; 22(5):347–52.

Khaw, K.: Dietary potassium and stroke associated mortality. *New England Journal of Medicine* 1987; 216:235–40.

Sato, Y.: Possible contribution of green tea drinking habits to the prevention of stroke. *Tohoku Journal of Experimental Medicine* 1989; 157(4):337–43.

Ulcers

Cheney, G.: Anti-peptic ulcer dietary factor. *Journal of the American Dietetic Association* 1950; 26:668–72.

Elta, G. H.: Comparison of coffee intake and coffee-induced symptoms in patients with duodenal ulcer, nonulcer dyspepsia, and normal controls. *American Journal of Gastroenterology* 1990; 85(10):1339–42.

Graham, D. Y.: Spicy food and the stomach. *Journal of the American Medical Association* 1988; 260(23):3473–75.

Holzer, P.: Intragastric capsaicin protects against aspirin-induced lesion formation and bleeding in the rat gastric mucosa. *Gastroenterology* 1989; 96:1425–33.

Ippoliti, A. F.: The effect of various forms of milk on gastric-acid secretion. *Annals of Internal Medicine* 1976; 84:286–89.

Kaess, H.: Food intolerance in duodenal ulcer patients, non-ulcer dyspeptic patients and healthy subjects. *Klinische Wochenschrift* 1988; 66:208–11.

Kumar, N.: Effect of milk on patients with duodenal ulcers. *British Medical Journal*; 1986; 293:666.

Marotta, R. B.: Diet and nutrition in ulcer disease. *Medical Clinics of North America* 1991; 75(4):967–79.

McArthur, K.: Relative stimulatory effects of commonly ingested beverages on gastric acid secretion in humans. *Gastroenterology* 1982; 83:199–203.

Morgan, A. G.: Comparison between cimetidine and caved-s in the treatment of gastric ulceration, and subsequent maintenance therapy. *Gut* 1982; 23:545–51.

Pearson, R C.: Preference for hot drinks is associated with peptic disease. *Gut* 1989; 30:1201–5.

Sarin, S. K.: Diet and duodenal ulcer. *Journal of the Association of Physicians of India*

1985; 33(2):164–67.

Rydning, A.: Dietary Fiber and peptic ulcer. *Scandinavian Journal of Gastroenterology* 1986; 21:1–5.

Singer, M. V.: Action of beer and its ingredients on gastric acid secretion and release of gastrin in humans. *Gastroenterology* 1991; 101:935–42.

Sok Wan Han: Protective effect of diallyl disulfide against ethanol-induced gastric mucosal damage in rats. *Bulletin of Clinical Research CMC* 1990; 18(2):223–36.

Vazquez-Olivencia, W.: The effect of red and black pepper on orocecal transit time. *Journal of the American College of Nutrition*, 1992; 11(2):228–31.

BOOKS

Burkitt, Denis, M.D. *Eat Right — To Stay Healthy and Enjoy Life More.* New York: Arco Publishing, 1979.

Carper, Jean. *The Food Pharmacy.* New York: Bantam Books, 1988.

Graedon, Joe, and Teresa Graedon. *Graedon's Best Medicine,* New York: Bantam Books, 1991.

Grossman, Richard. *The Other Medicines.* New York: Doubleday, 1985.

Heimlich, Jane. *What Your Doctor Won't Tell You.* New York: HarperPerennial, 1990.

Hoffman, Ronald L., M.D. *Seven Weeks to a Settled Stomach.* New York: Simon and Schuster, 1990.

Hoffman, Ronald L., M.D. *Tired All the Time: How to Regain Your Lost Energy,* New York: Poseidon Press, 1993.

Kronhausen, Eberhard, Ed. B. and Phyllis Kronhausen, Ed. D., with Harry B. Demopoulos, M.D. *Formula for Life,* New York: Morrow, 1989.

Lands, William E. M. *Fish and Human Health,* Orlando, Fla: Academic Press, 1986.

Murray, Michael, N. D. and Pizzorno,Joseph, N. D. *Encyclopedia of Natural Medicine,* Rocklin, Calif: Prima Publishing. 1991.

Naj, Amal. *Peppers: A Story of Hot Pursuits,* New York: Alfred A. Knopf, 1992.

National Research Council. *Diet and Health,* Washington, D.C.: National Academy Press, 1989.

Perdue, Lewis. *The French Paradox and Beyond,* Sonoma, Calif.: Renaissance Publishing, 1992.

Spiller, Gene A. *The Mediterranean Diets in Health and Disease*, New York: Van Nostrand Reinhold, 1991.

Spiller, Gene A. *The Superpyramid Eating Program*, New York: Random House,

Reader's Digest. *Magic and Medicine of Plants*. Pleasantville, N.Y.: The Reader's Digest Association, Inc., 1986.

Swank, Roy Laver, M.D., and Dugan, Barbara Brewer. *The Multiple Sclerosis Diet Book*, New York: Doubleday, 1987.

Thompson, W. Grant, M.D. *Gut Reactions: Understanding Symptoms of the Digestive Tract*. New York: Plenum Press, 1989.

Tyler, Varro E., Ph.D. *The Honest Herbal*, third edition. Binghamton, N.Y.: Pharmaceutical Products Press, 1993.

Weil, Andrew, M.D. *Natural Health, Natural Medicine*, Boston: Houghton Mifflin Company, 1990.

Wurtman, Judith J., Ph.D. *Managing Your Mind and Mood Through Food*. New York: Rawson Associates, 1986.

INDEX